Inhale And Relax

CLASSIC

PRESCRIPTIONS and INDUCTIONS

for

HYPNOTHERAPY

Compiled and Edited By Dennis L. Franks

AuthorHouse™ LLC
1663 Liberty Drive
Bloomington, IN 47403
www.authorhouse.com
Phone: 1-800-839-8640

Published by AuthorHouse   03/24/2014

ISBN: 978-1-4918-1876-3 (sc)
ISBN: 978-1-4918-1875-6 (e)

Library of Congress Control Number: 2013917517

PREFACE

This compendium contains various inductions (by which a person is induced into a euphoric state) in preparation to receive a prescribed course of action, by way of therapy; as in the treatment or reduction of various stressful conditions. However, inductions may also be applied simply as a means of attaining complete therapeutic relaxation.

Contained herein are an assortment of inductions which will bring a client to a hypnotic state quite rapidly; or slowly, as in a shallow state of dreaminess, or into complete somnambulism, depending upon the prescription to be applied.

156 prescriptions are included, alphabetically listed, in addition to 22 Weight-Loss prescriptions, herein listed randomly. Prescriptions are complete and self-contained although at times it is suggested that they be combined with other equally relevant prescriptions.

Apart from straightforward prescriptions, additional empowering techniques are described such as 'Healing Hands' (thanks to Michael Stellitano of Las Vegas), and the Rapid Eye Movement technique which induces hypnosis immediately and also eliminates fear/anxiety due to its connection with the brain frontal lobe. Common techniques, i.e., numbness, etc., are also described. Of further interest is a Celestial exploration as delineated by the Rosicrucians.

Readership would include a wide array of individuals interested in uplifting the lives of those in need. Hypnosis is commonly practiced in the medical professions as well as public protection, child protective services, public education, armed forces and, of course, private therapy clinics. This book is intended to not only enhance those arenas but to advance their practices further by imparting knowledge that may be beneficial to their careers.

As not all circumstances can be covered in any one volume, the writing of additional prescriptions of specific need will undoubtedly occur. Therefore, guidance is provided for the writing of such prescriptions and/or inductions as needed for specific instances. **INHALE And RELAX,** is also intended to allay that necessity by providing prime examples for your use.

GENERAL CONTENTS

INDUCTION SCRIPT CONTENTS

PRESCRIPTION CONTENTS

PRESCRIPTION CONTENTS

PRESCRIPTION CONTENTS

PRESCRIPTION CONTENTS

SCRIPT NAME

WEIGHT LOSS
PRESCRIPTION CONTENTS

OVERVIEW

Who was it, once said, "I've never *Metaphysical* I didn't like"? Was that a mistranslation from a different lifetime? A Freudian slip, perhaps? Or was it an echo from a wry sense of humor? Fortunately, not all of life need be serious. The essence of this compendium, however, does have two serious sides in that it is relevant to only two major subjects: **INDUCTIONS** and **PRESCRIPTIONS**.

Many books . . volumes, in fact, have been written on various subjects to do with hypnosis; therapeutic analysis or psychoanalysis and psychological applications including, case histories, summations, etc. There are methods, processes, examples and explanations given as documented by major study groups, universities and laboratories from all over the world. All of which confirms one similar and basic truth and that is . . . it works.

None of the above mentioned subjects are going to be dealt with herein for the following reason. Inductions and prescriptions are systematically guarded and treated secretively by their owners. For the student or beginning therapist just starting out, it can be a frustrating world when trying to gain this vital information . . exception being only those adept at creative writing.

Let us begin by opening a few basic questions. i.e., Who are Hypnotherapists? How are they trained and what do they do? In answer to the last question first : a hypnotherapist begins a session by consulting with the client to determine the nature of the problem; then prepares the client to enter an hypnotic state by, first, explaining how hypnosis works and, second, what the client will experience. He/she then tests the client to determine the degree of physical and emotional suggestibility. This is followed by inducing an hypnotic state in the client (Induction). Individualized methods and techniques of hypnosis are here applied. Based on interpretation of testing results coupled with analysis of client's initial problem, the written prescription is introduced once the client is relaxed at the proper depth level of induction. The hypnotherapist may also indulge in training the client for self-hypnosis, should conditions warrant. Professional Hypnotherapists are trained in State approved schools or through the training programs of professional associations. Professional associations also impose continuing education requirements, mandate peer performance testing and sets specific standards for ethical practices. No professional Hypnotherapist is authorized by his/her professional society to practice outside the scope appropriate for his/her level of formal education. In addition, the hypnotherapist is encouraged to provide a disclosure statement to clients regarding the nature of said education and training.

What it means, according to New World Dictionary: Hyp-no-ther-a-py; The treatment of disease (dis-ease) through the use of hypnosis. Hyp-no-sis; A sleep-like condition, psychically induced, usually by another person, in which the subject is in a state of altered consciousness and responds, with certain limitations, to the suggestions of the hypnotist.

The majority of people seeking therapy generally come at a low point in their lives. They may be in pain or anguish, or suffer a high degree of stress. Their issues may be tough to address for both the therapist and the client. Traditional training for the therapist follows a medical model for dealing with this level of distress and pain. The therapist may be a medical expert - or not. Nonetheless, the intent is to diagnose, treat and, hopefully, cure the client. A client's circumstance may range from seriously impaired to quite normal. Regardless of how well a client is functioning, he or she seeks therapy for that part of life which is dysfunctional, wounded or hurting.

Depending upon the reason a client has for making an appointment, a therapist may become a hypnotist or, perhaps, merely an ear for listening. Then again, he or she may become simply an advisor. One segment of the populace attracted to therapy is commonly known as the 'walking-wounded' or the 'worried-well'. These are higher functioning adults who consider themselves 'happy and normal' but want more for themselves, perhaps feeling blocked in some part of their lives. These people won't seek out the aid of a psychotherapist because they don't consider themselves to be psychologically 'ill'. For the most part, however, people will consider a hypnotherapist to help them overcome lesser problems occurring in their daily lives such as, weight loss, acne, job stress or a myriad of other issues. Unbeknownst to them is the coupling factor of a psychological reasoning of cause for their malady. Thus, necessitating a step beyond a case of pimples or upset stomachs, up into the realm of understanding and treatment of the underlying condition.

The true nature and resulting 'cure' are brought about through the client's own subconscious via hypnotherapeutic practices. Following a regime of needed sessions, clients respond with robust improvements over their specific problem as well as in personal growth, insight, confidence, productivity, interpersonal relations and solid enjoyment of their daily life activities. Successful sessions invariably produce return sessions.

PRACTICAL HINTS FOR A SUCCESSFUL HYPNOTIC INDUCTION

While witnessing an induction in process, it often appears that the hypnotherapist is inserting a lot of meaningless 'mumbo-jumbo' words to relax the client without any real intent. Not so! A proper induction follows a definite plan of procedure.

Most clients will be more comfortable with a first induction that is primarily a progressive relaxation script. That is, a slower process designed to support the desired comfort level.

For hypnosis to be successful, two important factors must be kept in mind: first, the client must be comfortable with hypnosis itself and, second, the client must also be comfortable with the hypnotherapist.

The following suggestions have proven helpful in achieving successful hypnotic inductions :

1. Ensure the client is absolutely comfortable. Sitting in an uncomfortable position, needing to go to the bathroom or becoming thirsty becomes distracting, thus, preventing the best outcome from occurring. Considerations include a pleasant and relaxing 'ambiance' of decor and room temperature.

2. It will be helpful to remark, "If you follow these simple suggestions, such as, looking at a spot above your eyes or counting to yourself, you will notice how easy it is to find yourself imagining, thinking and feeling that you are going into a very relaxed state."

3. Using a monotone voice stressing the key words of 'relax', 'heavy' and 'deep', in a repeatable manner will enhance the relaxation process.

4. As the client goes deeper in a session, slow the word pace so your voice pitch won't accelerate, sounding like 'Mickey Mouse'.

5. Never tell the client that he/she is difficult to induce. Future sessions are facilitated by using positive conditioning such as, "You are doing very well considering it is your first time. You will do even better the next time."

ADDITIONAL THOUGHTS TO CONSIDER

Confidence is essential. Most clients can pick up on any insecurities and hesitancies of the therapist. Therefore, the hypnotherapist must approach every induction with full confidence and expectancy of complete success.

Expectations. Before beginning an induction procedure, the hypnotherapist should raise the expectancy level of the client by describing, as simply as possible, what the hypnotherapist is going to do, what the client is suppose to feel and what is expected of the client.

Attention. The hypnotherapist must stress that a successful induction rests, most importantly, on the client's intense attention to the suggestions.

Belief. How the client believes is important for success. All suggestions must be made on the basis of the client's belief system, as well as logic and common sense.

Clarity and simplicity during inductions are mandatory in order to avoid induction failures. Suggestions should be simple, concise and clearly expressed, therefore, understood. Use of the client's own pleasant experiences in supporting positive suggestions will allay the client's fears. Gather this information during the initial interview and screening process.

If a suggestion is not being followed, the hypnotherapist should substitute another one and, at the same time, remind the client that he/she is progressing nicely. It is important to always encourage the client in their pursuit of self improvement. Everyone has their individual pace and readiness from which the hypnotherapist must work in supporting anticipated goals.

Some hypnotherapists become lax, being not overtly concerned about the hypnotic induction procedure. However, the initial induction procedure is an important building block in the foundation of a successful session as well as for an on-going professional relationship.

UNDERSTANDING THE ESSENCE OF A SUGGESTION

Suggestions are at the beginning of the chain that directs our lives. Injected suggestions are constantly at work within us and around us, at all times. Even though we are not consciously aware of them, we systematically program ourselves continually, through the use of suggestions.

Our behavior is controlled, knowingly or unknowingly, positively or negatively, by reinforcement and encouragement. Reinforcement is any action or experience that strengthens a habit. Often it is unconscious and counterproductive. Encouragement is a motivational tool used to manipulate an individual's drive. It may be received on an internal or external basis. We can turn this drive to our advantage through a conscious effort for managing our suggestions, reinforcing our goal-directed habits and encouraging ourselves towards higher improvement. It all begins with basic and honest self-evaluation.

There is no driving force over which one has no control. All problems can be solved by, first, accepting them as real and facing them squarely, then by taking the proper action to eradicate them.

The first step against a bad habit is deconditioning; which erases the old imprint, allowing one to begin a new slate. The next step is reconditioning, which imprints new and better thoughts towards a healthier behavior pattern. Hypnotherapy accomplishes this through means of retraining the conditioned reflexes.

A conditioned reflex (habit) can be redefined (deconditioning - reconditioning) by activation of new signals which are generated through new connections being formed within the brain. This quality, which exists in every person, is produced by repetition and will tend to deteriorate unless regularly reinstated or otherwise, reinforced. This last characteristic can be useful or detrimental, depending upon whether it is a positive or a negative reinforcement. The conditioned reflex is responsible for the development of athletic skills as well. A conscious awareness should be maintained at all times of how personal habit training affects anything and everything we think, feel or do, either mental, physical or spiritual.

SCRIPT WRITING OF PRESCRIPTIONS

As in all things of logic, there are basic steps to follow. Generally, these steps are completed at the discretion of the therapist; i.e., rapport and documentation which are followed by discussion and analysis of the sub-reason for the existence of the client's problem or dilemma.

Preparation is then made for writing and administering the suggestions of instruction which are termed, Hypnotic Prescription. Knowing what to say to the client is the most essential part of the therapy process. The proceedings of hypnosis; the various depth tests and considerations for reawakening are the rudimentary mechanics that must be done with finality. Resolution to a cure, however, is only attained through conversation with the subconscious character of the subject. This is, of course, is not the same thing as speaking face to face on a conscious level.

The Prescription dialogue should be written in an intelligent but nonintellectual manner; i.e., confusing terms or words. One should be brief, honest, direct and orate in a slow, procedural pattern. It is commonplace to know that positive thoughts and actions bring about positive changes and reactions. Positive expressions are encouraging, inspiring and hopeful to the client who is seeking to improve a quality-area of life. It is imperative that the hypnotherapist support the client's effort in their behalf.

When a positive attitude is in harmony with a charged atmosphere, the implosion increases the success ratio of any circumstance, especially when conditioning one for improved potential achievement, personal development or spiritual growth. As positive instructions are given, expectations for positive results will increase.

PRIMARY SCRIPT WRITING RULES

1.   Prescription suggestions must be expressed in a positive manner using every conceivable support for bringing out the positive results desired. An example of a positive expression used in a smoking session is; "You will have more and more will power and self-control over the cravings you once had."

An example of a smoking issue 'negative' expression is; "You will find the idea of smoking as being repulsive . . Cigarettes will taste vile and putrid and they will make you cough . . Your eyes will burn and tear . . Inhaling cigarette fumes will make you become nauseous and vomit." Such negative instructions will have but a temporary and short-lived effect. After a period of days or a few weeks at most, the client will become curious to know if these unpleasant and abnormal reactions still remain.

2.   Refer only to the future (you will) for suggestions in behavior and conduct. In so doing, the client remains passive and receptive to the positive suggestions for the desired (future) changes in the client's life. To mention mistakes or past negative behavioral patterns can invite the possibility of a mental challenge and outright rejection.

3.   The hypnotherapist works on one issue at a time. The subconscious mind is similar to a computer in how it receives and processes information. The most efficient and effective methodology is a one-step, one-issue at a time, process. Clients may soon want to address more than one issue, once they are committed to improving their lifestyles. It is important to help them to understand the power of the mind and how the use of hypnosis is based on a conclusive formula that works and that is, one issue at a time.

A synopsis of the above criteria, simply stated, is as follows :

1. Prescriptions must be expressed in a positive manner.
2. Refer only to future time for behavioral changes.
3. Make each prescription one issue at a time.
4. Make contribution of a new, positive thought or idea which will benefit the client.
5. Assure the client there will be some degree of noticeable improvement. Explain that improvements are progressive and will noticeably increase with each passing day.

The following pages contain prewritten and approved INDUCTIONS and PRESCRIPTIONS which have been successfully used for a number of years. These items are now in the public domain wherein written permission for their use is not required nor shall any be granted. It is assumed that the reader be knowledgeable and qualified in the craft of expertise herein described, therefore, academic license for use is laid entirely upon the reader. The author assumes no responsibility or liability in the case of fraudulent or misrepresented use of the enclosed information. The reader (user) assumes all risk and liability and shall render the author harmless by way of disclosure of said information. It is further assumed that the reader shall peruse said information, as written, towards their benefit as well as that of their clientele. As not every situation can be covered in the folds of one book, encouragement is offered to the reader to write anew, adding to this assorted collection as time and talent will allow and to share such knowledge with others where practical.

Dennis L. Franks
Fellow & CMHT
Hypnologist

This is to follow a regular induction, when client does not respond well.

There are many directions you can follow . . when you allow your subconscious mind to do it for you . . Sometimes your conscious mind can be confused . . and you don't really know what to do . . But that's okay because . . your subconscious mind will still respond . .

It is comparable to a time when I was in my car . . going on a weekend vacation . . I was listening to the radio . . knowing I was driving to another place . . where I could relax . . and let go of all the normal things of everyday life . .

It gave me a feeling of freedom . . to let go and not need to think about anything at all . . It was going to be a time for relaxing . . And I was enjoying the freedom of just being out, driving . .

Moving along easily . . Headed to that place of relaxation . . Listening to the soothing sounds . . And not really paying attention to the things going on around me . . Just looking forward to a wonderful time of complete relaxation . . I continued along at a slow but steady pace . .

Everything was so calm and peaceful that . . I didn't notice a sign when I should have . . I was quite certain I was still headed in the right direction . . I didn't remember turning left . . Nor did I remember turning right . . However, the only thing I knew for sure was that I was here . . even though I had no idea where here was . .

I began wishing I was there . . And I felt good . . knowing I would soon be there . . I certainly wanted to get there . . And be there . .

Better pay attention . . because I wanted to make the right turn at the right time . . There were still several turns that needed to be made . . and I wanted them to be right . .

Again, my mind began wandering . . And I thought . . It's getting near time to be going to sleep . . It sure will feel good to go to sleep for a while . .

Would it be best to go to sleep now . . Or should I go a little farther before going to sleep . . By doing that, I'll be much closer to the place I'm going to . . when I awaken . .

Continuing on . . Listening to the music . . The drowsiness kept increasing . . The feelings of sleepiness kept getting stronger . . It would seem so good to sleep for a while . . and let the eyes . . just relax . . and let the mind . . just relax . . It's a good time to sleep . . And it's a good place to sleep . . It feels so good . . to just lay back in the seat . . and let go . . completely . .

I'd like you to begin now, counting down from 100 . . And keep feeling drowsier with each number . . From 100 . . 99 . . Getting very sleepy now . . 98 Becoming drowsier . . 97 Almost asleep . . 96 Feeling more relaxed and comfortable . . 95 Moving into a deeper, more peaceful state . . 94 Conscious awareness is narrowing down now . . 93 Drowsier . . 92 Sleepier . . Keep counting to yourself . . (Pause a minute.)

Just letting the trance develop . . Don't pay any attention to anything . . It's so nice to know you can let go completely . . And let your subconscious mind work for you . .

IF CLIENT NEEDS FURTHER DEEPENING, CONTINUE COUNTING DOWN – SKIPPING AND REVERSING NUMBERS.

Now . . you will feel all the muscle groups in your body letting go of any tension . . Take a deep breath . . Hold it a moment and now, gently exhale . . You will notice your body wanting to relax . .

I am going to count from one to 20 . . And as I count each number . . you will relax deeper . . and DEEPER . . with each number you hear . . 1-2-3 . . Tension is leaving your body . . 4-5 . . Resting and relaxing, more deeply now . . Deeper and deeper . . 6-7-8 . . Deeply relaxing . . Going deeper and deeper into a restful state . . So peaceful . . Peaceful and relaxing . . Relax . . Gently relax . . 9 . . Deeper now . . Deeply relaxing . . 10-11-12 . . Gently inhale . . Deeply inhale . . and let it out slowly . . With each breath you take . . you will go deeper . . and deeper . . And as you let it out slowly . . you will relax more and more . . Inhale deeply now . . and let it out, slowly . . 13-14-15 . . You will be free of all pain and discomfort . . as you deeply relax . . Gently relax . . 16 . . Hear nothing but the sound of my voice . . Any other sounds will help you to go deeper . . into complete relaxation . . Complete relaxation . . 17 - 18 Deeper and deeper . . Completely relaxed . . So relaxed . . 19 . . and . . finally . . 20 . . Deep . . deep . . deep . . deeply relaxed hypnosis . .

Your mind is very relaxed now . . and open to receive the helpful and beneficial suggestions I am about to give you . . You may use those suggestions that apply now . . And you may reject those that do not apply . . Or keep them for another time, if they apply then . . Let us begin . .

I want you to use your imagination now . . In your mind . . I want you to see yourself driving . . toward the beach . . It is a beautiful day . . The sun is shining . . and you can hear soft, soothing sounds in the background . .

The sun will soon be setting and you are getting closer and closer . . to the beach . . You will arrive at the beach . . just in time to see the sun . . setting, on the horizon . .

You have arrived . . And you walk onto the beach . . Sitting down on the sand, you watch the bright orange sun as it slowly sinks from the sky, towards the far horizon . . Notice the colors as they begin to change . . from orange to crimson red . .

And as it continues . . descending . . it changes more still . . becoming a deep, dark red-orange color . . As the sun gets nearer to the water . . you notice that it appears to be two suns . . One, still in the sky, and one, on the water . .

You are continuing to feel more calm and peaceful . . And you notice that the sun seems to be disappearing . . right into the water . . The colors are changing dramatically now . . from a deep red to purple, with streaks of flashing yellow . . and finally . . to a deep, darkening blue . . And you are continuing to feel more relaxed . . At peace with the world . .

Everything around you keeps becoming more calm and more still . . The air smells fresh . . and the water is so peaceful and smooth . . The sounds of distant sea birds seem to travel on for ever . .

You are not even noticing . . as you keep feeling more comfortable and tranquil . . that you are feeling more safe and secure . . Your whole body is responding to the comfort of complete relaxation . .

You are realizing, too, that . . this calmness and peacefulness . . are available to you, at all times . . Every time you look at water . . your mind responds to that signal . . and causes you to become even more calm and relaxed . . And you feel very peaceful and at ease . . Every time you look at water . . your nerves become more relaxed and steady . .

I am also giving you another signal . . that you can use to experience immediate relaxation . . at any time . . All you need to do . . is to bring your thumb and one finger together . . And that will cause you to become calm and relaxed . . Do that now . . You will experience a wonderful feeling of peace and tranquility . . just by touching your thumb and finger together . .

Continue relaxing . . just as you are . . In a moment, I will talk to you again . . And I will give you new suggestions that will be helpful . .

ADDRESS PRESCRIPTION, i.e., SELF-CONFIDENCE, SELF-ACCEPTANCE, PAIN RELEASE OR OTHER POSITIVE SUGGESTION.

Now . . close your eyes and relax . . I want to take you to a restful . . quiet place deep in the forest . . where you will find peace and relaxing comfort . . in a totally relaxing world of your own . .

You're going to take a short journey up a mountain trail . . where tall trees are nestled high up . . in the rain clouds. The clouds bump and mesh together . . swirling in shades of pink and soft azure blue . . Occasional drops of rain settle softly . . on your face . . You smile because . . the rain drops make you feel excited and . . happy inside . .

Climbing up the steep mountainside is slow . . and difficult . . It's time now to let go . . Let yourself be free to slowly drift up . . up . . to the tops of the trees . . High above the trees to where . . you are free to sail on the wind . . Look away and you will see the far mountain ranges . . covered in white snow caps, many miles away . . You can see them clearly in the distance . . but you are not going there . . Perhaps another time . . Let yourself slowly drift through the branches of the elm trees . . and the oak trees . . tall and majestic . . You are settling down into the top of a mighty tree with heavy . . spreading branches . . Where birds flutter past in darting flashes . . Chipmunks and squirrels . . find food to store for the winter . . And there, far below you, a gurgling brook trickles . . with singing waters, winding its way through the tall forest grasses . . far, far below . .

You are drifting now . . Sailing on the winds like the leaves . . Drifting slowly, up to the left . . then down to the right . . back and forth, as you slowly, gently sail down . . down . . deeper towards the green grasses of the forest, far below . . Slowly you circle through the huge branches of the trees, drifting in circles . . Swaying to the right . . Sailing up with the wind . . then to the left . . circling . . circling . . The winds carry you gently in a downward motion . . Down . . Down . . until at last your feet touch the soft, lush, green grass that covers the earth . . Here is where you will find peace . . tranquility . . and complete relaxation . . Here, you are as one with all that God . . has created for you . . Here, there are no sounds besides my voice . . and the noise of rushing waters in the distant brook . . Gently it is flowing through the forest . . Any other sounds you may hear will only support you . . in your relaxed and comfortable place . . Your mind and body are open to complete trust . .

Trust in the power of your mind to benefit you on your journey . . Your mind is very relaxed now and . . open to receive the suggestions I am about to give you . . I want you to consider the implications of these suggestions . . And consider what values you might apply after receiving them . . So, let us begin . .

Begin appropriate Prescription or . .

EMERGE

Now, I'm going to count from 1 to 5 . . and on the count of five you will open your eyes to an alert, waking state, feeling clear of mind, relaxed and feeling wonderful, for you are a wonderful person . .

1. You WILL remember everything you have experienced, with clear understanding . .

2. You are connected to your inner strength supporting your best interest.

3. What I have told you is true and is happening right now . . You will benefit greatly from this experience . .

4. Beginning to be more aware of your body as it fully awakens and wants to stir . .

5. Let your feet and hands move freely now . . Stir and stretch as you open your eyes, feeling clear, rested and good about yourself . .

We are participating in an interactive experience . . I am asking you to participate . . by using your vivid imagination in a very active way . . in order to achieve the results you desire . .

Now close your eyes and relax . . In just a moment . . you will imagine all the muscle groups in your body, letting go of any tension . .

Take a deep breath now . . Hold it a moment . . Now, gently, exhale . . and you will notice your body wanting to relax . . Take another gentle and deep breath . . Hold it a moment . . Now, gently, exhale . . and you will feel your body beginning to relax . . Each time you breathe, from here on in . . imagine a golden glow of energy, flowing down from the top of your head . . and flowing into your lungs . . Flowing with the oxygen, throughout your body and spreading relaxation . . Your breath is filling your entire body with a golden glow of relaxation that is penetrating every particle of your being . . and radiating out of your pores . . So very relaxing . . You even notice your body giving off this golden glow of light all around you . . And as you breathe, more deeply now . . you feel this glow continuing to relax you . . more and more . .

Feeling this golden glow of relaxation . . Notice that the muscle groups around your face are relaxing . . Notice how your scalp is relaxing . . your forehead, your eyebrows, your eyelids . . It is so easy and enjoyable to relax . . your cheeks, your nose . . and your mouth . . Especially your mouth . . Notice how the muscles of your mouth and lips are gently relaxing . . Make sure your teeth are not clinched together . . Continue to notice how your body is becoming more and more relaxed . . as your chin and jaws fall into a natural relaxed position . .

And now your neck relaxes . . the front part of your neck . . the back part of your neck . . right on throughout your shoulders . . The golden glow of relaxation moves you into deeper . . and deeper . . sensations . . It feels so good to allow the tension in your neck and

shoulders to just . . let go . . and relax . . completely . . Relax . .
You can feel the tensions completely melting away . .

And allow your arms to relax now . . Your upper arms, your elbows,
your forearms . . Relax your wrists and your hands . . Notice how the
fingers respond to the relaxation . . as it moves throughout your body
in natural acceptance of what is good . . Just imagine your arms
becoming heavy now . . in their relaxation . . Loose and limp . . Loose
. . Limp . . Like a wet washcloth . .

And allow yourself to breath comfortably . . and naturally . . Notice
how deep and regular your breathing is . . as you become more and
more relaxed . . Notice how your breathing has become deeper and
more regular than when we started a little while ago . . Feel your
breathing . . Feel the rhythm of your breathing . . Notice the
contraction and expansion of your diaphragm . . and your chest . .
Allow the chest muscles to relax . . completely . . right down
through to your stomach muscles . . Just relax . . Let go of any
tension that might be in that area . . Just let go and relax . .

Allow your back muscles to relax . . Those large muscle groups in
the upper part of your back . . The golden glow of energy flows right
down your spinal column and into your lower back muscles . . Just
let go . . Let go completely . . Just relax . . Let the golden glow of
energy immerse . . through all of your back muscles . . and your spinal
column . .

Allow all of those smaller groups of muscles in the lower part of
your back to relax as well . . Your hips relax . . Your thighs . .
And especially your legs . . They really need this relaxation, don't
they . . They need this golden glow of energy . . to flow through
them . . as well as your knees . . your calves . . your ankles . .
down to your feet . . and even your toes . . Just allow those muscle
groups to relax completely . . as you begin to drift now . . into deep
. . deep . . relaxation . . Letting your mind and body become one
with the universe . .

Feeling good . . Feeling so good now . . Feeling wonderfully relaxed . .
and feeling no discomfort anywhere . .

Any sounds or noises you may hear, besides my voice or background
music, will only support your comfort zone . . You accept and allow your

body and mind . . to be peaceful and open to trust . . You trust in the power of your mind . . and the power of God . . to benefit you . . Relaxing you . . And you are trusting in the power of God to heal you . .

Many people sitting there, as you are, report certain feelings in their body . . Some report a numbness in their arms or legs . . Some people report a tingling sensation . . such as pins and needles . . Or as moving energy . . Usually in their hands, feet or arms . . And some people report both a numbness and a tingling sensation . . Sometimes alternately . . Some people experience a lightness in their body . . And others experience a heaviness . . If you experience a lightness . . you might feel buoyant . . as though you are floating above your chair . . If you feel a heaviness . . you may feel like you are sinking down into the chair . .

And some people, when they relax . . find they have a need to swallow . . Usually because their mouths get a little dry . . If you have a need to swallow . . it is perfectly okay to do so . . Many people also find that when they let go and totally relax . . their eyes respond by flickering or fluttering . . ever so slightly . . This is an excellent sign of letting go . .

And some people report experiencing some form of sensory distortion or detachment . . from their body . . This, too, is a good sign of letting go and relaxing . .

What is important is that these signs . . all indicate your readiness and willingness . . to allow yourself to go into a deeper hypnosis . . Going into hypnosis is gradual . . yet comfortable . . In a moment, I am going to count . . from one to twenty . . On each count, you can allow yourself to drift into a deeper hypnosis . . at your own pace . .

But before I do that, just imagine a custom-built cloud snuggling up underneath your body . . in the shape of a big easy chair . . It is a very soft and comfortable cloud . . Your personal cloud . .

Your cloud is rising up now . . lifting you high up into the other clouds . . to a very special and beautiful place . . A place that you create . . in any way that makes you feel happy and peaceful . . A place where you feel good . . safe . . secure . . happy . . A place where you feel good and look good . . Just allow this special and personal cloud-chair to snuggle up to your body and . . take you to this very special place of yours . . Your place of beauty . . peace . . safety . . and where you feel totally and completely relaxed . . And very calm . . Now, just allow yourself to relax and enjoy your special place . . (Pause)

And as I begin to count . . you will go deeper and deeper into hypnosis . . with each number you hear . .

1 . . Deeper and deeper now . . 2 All the way down, DEEP . . 3 - 4 Very relaxed . . Tired and drowsy . . 5 - 6 Just letting go now . . 7 - 8 Deeper and deeper . . 9 - 10 Tired and letting go now . . 11 - 12 All the way down . . DEEP now . . 13 - 14 Deeper and deeper . . 15 - 16 Letting go now . . 17 - 18 Deeper and deeper . . Completely relaxed . . RELAXED . . 19 and finally . . 20 DEEP . . DEEP . . DEEP . . Relaxing peace and comfort . .

Your mind is now very relaxed . . and open to receive the helpful and beneficial suggestions I am about to give you . . You may use those suggestions that apply now . . and you may reject those that do not apply . . Or you may accept those that apply for use . . at a later time . . Let us begin . .

BEGIN APPROPRIATE SCRIPT AT THIS POINT. (Complete the script with the following reminder) If there were any suggestions that I gave you today that are not in your best interest, they now disappear out of your subconscious mind . . Your self-protective mechanisms are always in place, allowing you to choose whatever will benefit your improvement . .

EMERGE

I am going to count from 1 to 5 and on the count of 5 you will open your eyes to an alert waking state . . feeling clear of mind . . relaxed . . and wonderful . . I will begin . .

1 - You will remember everything you have experienced today with understanding and clarity . .

2 - You are now connected to your inner strength and higher power . . supporting your best interest . . You will carry that inner strength with you throughout your day . .

3 - Everything I have told you is true and is already happening . . And you are already successful in manifesting the positive suggestions that I have given you, into your daily life and consciousness . .

4 - You are beginning to be more aware of your body as it fully awakens and wants to stir . .

5 - Let your feet and hands move . . Stir and stretch as you open your eyes, feeling clear, rested and wonderful.

Close your eyes and begin inhaling deeply . . deeply . . And exhale slowly . . You will experience a peaceful relaxation coming over your whole body . . each time you exhale . . Do that five or six times . . Continuing to feel more at ease . . more calm . . more safe and secure . .

Now, as you sit there with your eyes closed, you can continue listening, easily and effortlessly . . to my voice . . In fact, you won't need to make any effort to listen to what I say because . . whether you are consciously listening to me or not . . your subconscious mind is totally aware of everything I say to you . .

I am going to give you some suggestions that will help occupy the thoughts of your conscious mind . . while I speak directly to the subconscious level of your mind . .

I want you to use your imagination now . . Imagine that you are lying outside in a hammock on a beautiful, warm summer night . . and you are looking up into the evening sky . . You may see a cloudy sky . . or you may see a clear, deep blue sky . . with stars twinkling . . It is so enjoyable that it really doesn't matter what kind of a sky you see . . whatever comes into your mind is fine . .

Now, imagine that you are watching a huge flying saucer, up above you . . and you want to keep watching that flying saucer . . For a moment, it appears to be standing still in the sky . . just above you . . But you will notice, as it begins to move up . . higher and higher into the sky . .

As it continues to move up higher and higher . . it may begin to revolve slowly . . as it moves farther and farther away from you . . Whatever the flying saucer does . . from this point on . . just allow it to happen . .

Gradually, the flying saucer moves further into the heavens . . And it keeps becoming smaller and smaller . . In a few more minutes, it may disappear behind the clouds . . or perhaps it will blend into the stars . . and disappear that way . .

And as you concentrate on watching the flying object in the sky . . I want you to do something else . . In your mind . . I want you to begin counting down from 100, at about this pace . . 99 . . 98 . . 97 . .

ILLUSTRATE THE COUNT AT ABOUT TWO SECOND INTERVALS.

Begin counting now as you continue watching the flying saucer . . As you are counting backward in your mind and . . watching the flying saucer in the sky . . your conscious mind will concentrate on that . . Releasing your subconscious mind to be free to receive and acknowledge the suggestions and instructions that I give you . . And you will continue moving into a deeper state of hypnosis . .

Continue counting backward now, to yourself . . as you keep watching the flying saucer . . moving in the heavens . . You are relaxing more and more . . going deeper now . . deeper . . deeper . .

NOTE : SOME PEOPLE THINK THEY MUST LISTEN CLOSELY TO WHAT THE HYPNOTHERAPIST IS SAYING. BUT IN AN EFFORT TO LISTEN, THEIR CONSCIOUS LEVEL KEEPS THEM FROM ACHIEVING A DEEP HYPNOTIC STATE. THIS DISTRACTION TECHNIQUE ENABLES THE CLIENT TO REACH A DEEPER HYPNOTIC STATE AND ALSO PERMITS THE SUBCONSCIOUS MIND TO FREELY ACCEPT THE HELPFUL SUGGESTIONS GIVEN BY THE HYPNOTHERAPIST.

(For Clients who tend to Analyze everything the Hypnologist is doing or suggesting.)

Close your eyes now and begin inhaling deeply . . Exhale slowly because every time you inhale . . you bring more oxygen into your lungs . . It passes from your lungs into your heart and your heart pumps it into your circulatory system . . which carries it into every part of your body . . where it is needed . .

As you continue breathing deeply and slowly . . I want to mention how happy I am to have the opportunity to help you understand that I have no power to put you into a hypnotic state . . In reality . . ALL hypnosis is self-hypnosis . . As I am talking to you . . I'm merely giving you guidance . . And as you follow my guidance . . you are actually hypnotizing yourself . . It's really a privilege to have this opportunity to help you learn how to hypnotize yourself, so that you can work out the solution to that problem . .

Sometimes people come to me, expecting me to be able to work out the solution to their problems . . not realizing that I do not know what is causing their problem . . And at the same time, I understand that they, too, do not consciously understand what is causing their problem . . If they knew, they would have already solved the problem and would have no reason to come to see me . . Other people come, thinking they know . . They think they know exactly what is causing their problem and no one can tell them any differently . . They don't seem to understand, when I try to tell them . . the cause of the problem is in the subconscious part of their mind and cannot be known to them, consciously . . And they refuse to accept my guidance when I attempt to show them how their own mind . . can review and examine what has caused the problem . . and to work out the solution . . to help get the problem resolved, permanently . .

So it's nice to be able to work with a person of your intelligence . . who can easily follow my guidance . . and slip into a nice, comfortable state of relaxation . . and listen to the soothing sounds coming from the tape player . . and permit your conscious mind to relax more and more . . as your subconscious mind reviews . . the information from your conscious mind . . and works out the solution to the problem . . in accordance with the suggestions I will give you . .

As I am talking to you . . you can try to be aware of the exact meaning of the words I am saying . . and of all of the changes that are taking place in your mind . . as the problem is being resolved and the pleasant changes are happening . . Or you can merely relax more and . . forget what I am saying . . as you listen to the gentle, soothing sounds . . coming from the tape player . . You will, none the less . . be aware of everything that happens . . even though you may choose to think your own thoughts . . or notice how your feelings and sensations are changing . . pleasantly . . in your left arm . . or perhaps, in your right arm . . as I speak directly to your subconscious mind . .

Every thought . . every sensation in your subconscious mind belongs to you . . They are there for you to use . . or to stop using . . They can be used for your own personal well being . . Or for improving your health . . Or to enable your creative abilities to emerge . . more and more . . Or for improving all of your talents . . skills and abilities . . Or you may choose to simply continue with improving your life, as it is . . without paying very much attention, consciously . . While you are relaxing . . your subconscious mind is letting go . . and IS getting the problem resolved . . in an easy, natural way . .

You may be thinking you have figured out what has been causing the problem . . and not even notice how your subconscious mind is rapidly working out the solution . . Without being aware of it . . your mind may be saying YES . . or it may be saying NO . . Or you may think you are going . . without knowing where you are going . . Or you may feel as though you don't know . . how to let go . . While at the same time . . you subconscious mind IS letting go . . and IS getting the problem resolved . . in an easy natural way . .

Everything you do allows your mind to recognize . . that I can say many different things . . and you do not need to make any effort . . to try to pay close attention to each thing I say . . Because your conscious mind retains only a part of what you hear . . even though your subconscious mind retains everything you hear . . It is also a fact that your mind is continuing to become . . more and more relaxed . . and is becoming much more calm and peaceful . . Knowing that you don't really need to try . . to consciously hear . . or to understand what I am saying . . In fact, there may be times when I am talking to you . . when you may not be consciously aware of my voice at all . . And that is okay because your

subconscious mind is hearing and acknowledging everything I am saying . .
Simply . . relax . . relax . . relax . .

NOTE : IF CLIENT IS WORKING OUT A PROBLEM BY THEM SELF, CONTINUE WITH MUSIC
TAPE AND BRING THEM UP. OTHERWISE, BEGIN TAKING THEM DEEPER AND PROCEED
WITH PRESCRIPTION.

Get yourself in a very comfortable position now and . . close your eyes . . You may begin breathing deeply . . Each time you inhale, hold it for three or four seconds and then`. . exhale slowly . . Notice that each time you inhale, your shoulders lift a little bit . . And each time you exhale . . they go down . . Pay attention to that as you continue inhaling deeply and exhaling slowly . . You can feel that natural relaxation growing and spreading throughout your body . .

You don't even need to try . . Just let it happen and enjoy it . . And remember that you can easily give yourself comfort in this same way, any time you want it or need it . .

You can consciously ignore whatever I am saying to you now because your subconscious mind . . and all inner levels of your mind . . are receiving everything that I say . . You can really enjoy relaxing . . and not even notice that other noises and sounds keep fading away, more and more . .

You can imagine . . if you want to . . that you are doing something you really enjoy . . Perhaps you are sunbathing and swimming at a beautiful lake . . Or, perhaps you are at a rock and roll concert . . listening to your favorite band . . Or you may be taking an easy stroll through a beautiful forest on a warm, summer day . .

MENTION TWO OR THREE OF THE CLIENT'S FAVORITE ACTIVITIES FROM YOUR PRE-INDUCTION CONVERSATION.

You may be already daydreaming that you are doing something you really enjoy . . And while you are doing that . . you know that your mind can be doing something else to help you overcome that problem that is bothering you . . Your inner mind can be reviewing . . examining and exploring . . everything that happened to cause you to begin experiencing that problem . . Your inner mind can assess that information . . privately . . and understand it from a more calm . . relaxed and knowledgeable point of view . . And can work out a pleasant solution to help you overcome that problem . . for now and forever . .

Everyone knows that the more you practice at something . . the more you keep improving . . You are continuing to improve . . in your ability to move into a deeper . . more restful . . more peaceful hypnotic state now . . Yes . . you're improving quite rapidly . .

I'm not sure how fast your mind is working out the solution to your problem . . It's doing it just as rapidly as you are ready to have the problem resolved . . and it is doing it in your own way . .

Your inner mind understands that working out the solution to that problem is for your own benefit . . For your own personal well-being . . and for your own self-improvement . .

I'm not sure exactly how your mind is resolving the problem . . However . . I know that it is being resolved in the most pleasing way for you . . Then you will notice the changes being made in your life . . And you will continue to improve a little more each day . .

When your mind understands all of the causes and affects . . and realizes that the problem is being resolved and essential changes have begun . . your inner mind will cause the index finger on your right hand to lift upward . . toward the ceiling . . and remain there . . until I tell it to go back down . .

CONTINUE WITH SUGGESTIONS FOR BUILDING SELF-CONFIDENCE AND WATCH FOR FINGER TO LIFT. IF FINGER DOES NOT LIFT BY TIME TO CONCLUDE SESSION, GIVE 'THERAPY BETWEEN SESSIONS' SUGGESTIONS BEFORE HAVING CLIENT AWAKEN.

You can close your eyes now . . Begin breathing deeply and slowly . . But before you let go completely and slip into a deep hypnotic state . . just let yourself listen to everything I say to you . . while your eyes are closed . .

It's going to happen automatically . . so you don't need to think about that now . . And you will have no conscious control over what happens . . as you relax . . The muscles in and around your eyes will relax all by themselves . . as you continue breathing deeply . . easily and freely . .

Without thinking about it . . you will soon enter a deep, peaceful, hypnotic trance . . without any effort . . There is nothing important for your conscious mind to do . . There is nothing really important except the activities of your subconscious mind . . And that is just as automatic as dreaming . . You know how easily you can forget dreams . . after you awaken . . But you will not forget what you experience here today . .

You are responding very well, without even noticing it . . You have already altered your rate of breathing . . You are breathing much more easily and freely . . and you are revealing signs that indicate you are beginning to drift into a restful, hypnotic trance . .

You can enjoy relaxing more and more now . . And your subconscious mind will listen to each word I say . . And it becomes less and less important for you to consciously listen to my voice . . Your subconscious mind can hear me, even if I whisper . . And at the same time . . you can hear the soothing sounds from the recorder . .

You are continuing to drift into a more detached state as you examine, privately, in your own mind . . secrets, feelings, sensations and behaviors you didn't know you had . . at the same time . .

Letting go completely now . . Your own mind is solving that problem . . at its own pace . . just as rapidly as it thinks you are ready to accept resolution . . And you are becoming more relaxed and comfortable as you sit there . . with your eyes closed . . Experiencing this deepening comfort, you don't have to move . . or talk . . or let anything bother you . . Your own inner mind . . can respond automatically to everything I say to you . . and you will be pleasantly surprised with your continuous progress . .

You are getting much closer to a deep hypnotic trance now . . And you are beginning to realize that you don't really mind being there . . Being in this peaceful state enables you to experience this rare comfort of complete relaxation . . Being hypnotized is always very enjoyable . . very pleasant . . It is a calming . . peaceful . . soothing and a completely relaxing experience . . Relax . .

It seems natural to include hypnosis in your future . . Every time I hypnotize you, it will keep becoming more enjoyable . . And you will continue experiencing more benefits . . So you will always enjoy having me hypnotize you . . You will always enjoy the sensations of comfort . . of peacefulness . . of calmness . . And all of the other sensations that will come . . automatically, from this wonderful experience . .

Through the years, I have been hypnotized many times . . And it has given me the opportunity to appreciate the tremendous advantages of hypnosis . . And now, you, too, are learning that it is helping you in many different ways . . You will be happy that you decided to do this . . as you continue to progress in your understanding of this experience . .

You are learning something about yourself, aren't you . . You are developing your own understanding of the techniques of therapy . . without knowing you are developing them . . Your comprehension will be a surprise to you . . sooner or later . . A very pleasant surprise . .

Imagine yourself now, in a place you like very much . . near a lake or . . at the ocean . . Perhaps you are floating gently on a sailboat . . on a warm summer day . . with a cool breeze . . just drifting . . You cannot help but relax even more . . here on the water . . drifting . . And you continue becoming even more comfortable . . You are in your own world now . . A world you truly enjoy . .

You are going to find that any time you want to spend a few minutes by yourself . . relaxing . . and feeling very comfortable . . and serene . . you can automatically return to this feeling you are experiencing now . . You can put yourself into this world any time you like . . There may be times when you will want to return to this serene feeling . . And it is yours . . whenever you want it . .

Let go completely now . . as you enjoy this pleasant experience . . Your subconscious mind is receiving everything I tell you . . And you will be pleased with the way you automatically respond to everything I say . . Just relax now and we will continue with . . (prescribed suggestion)

26

RAPID
FINGER – EYE MOVEMENT

THIS IS AN EFFECTIVE AND RAPID INDUCTION TECHNIQUE WHERE THE CLIENT ENTERS HYPNOSIS ALMOST BEFORE HE OR SHE IS AWARE OF IT. THE PROCEDURE INVOLVES EYE FIXATION, DEEP BREATHING AND DIRECT SUGGESTION. IT ALSO EMPLOYS THE ELEMENT OF SURPRISE. DEEPENING IS PRODUCED BY INTERMITTENT MOVEMENT OF THE CLIENT'S HEAD. BEFORE STARTING, HAVE CLIENT REMOVE EYE GLASSES. HOLD YOUR OPEN HAND IN A HORIZONTAL POSITION, ABOUT 12 TO 18 INCHES IN FRONT OF THE CLIENT'S FACE. THERE IS A BRIGHT RED DOT (MADE WITH A FELT TIPPED PEN) ON THE CENTER OF THE END JOINT OF THE EXTENDED INDEX FINGER. THE OTHER FINGERS ARE CLENCHED.

SAY TO THE CLIENT, WHOSE EYES ARE OPEN, "Now watch the red dot and keep looking at the red dot at all times. You are to inhale whenever I raise my finger, and exhale, whenever I lower my finger. Now, keep your eyes on the RED DOT."

START AT THE CLIENT'S EYE LEVEL AT ABOUT 18 INCHES AWAY. RAISE YOUR (RED DOT) FINGER ABOUT 9 INCHES ABOVE EYE LEVEL BUT STAY WITHIN THE CLIENT'S RANGE OF VISION. AT THE SAME TIME, SAY, "INHALE". THEN QUITE RAPIDLY, SAY, "EXHALE". AS YOU LOWER YOUR HAND TO ABOUT 9 INCHES BELOW EYE LEVEL BUT STILL WITHIN CLIENT'S VISUAL RANGE. THEN RAISE YOUR FINGER AGAIN TO ABOVE EYE LEVEL AT A RATE SLIGHTLY FASTER THAN NORMAL INHALATION. TIMING IS IMPORTANT TO CREATE A RESPONSE COMPARABLE TO A SIGH.

REMIND CLIENT TO KEEP LOOKING AT THE DOT. WATCH CLIENT'S EYE TO ENSURE THEY FOLLOW THE MOVEMENT OF THE RED DOT AT THE END OF YOUR FINGER. ALSO PAY CLOSE ATTENTION TO THE CLIENT'S BREATHING. IF CLIENT IS NOT TAKING VERY DEEP BREATHS THEN CONTINUE WITH CYCLES OF INHALATION AND EXHALATION. MOST CLIENTS ARE READY FOR THE NEXT PHASE AFTER 3 OR 4 CYCLES WITH A MAXIMUM OF 6 CYCLES.

THE CLIENT IS NOW BREATHING DEEPLY. AFTER COMPLETING CYCLES, STOP YOUR HAND IN THE UPWARD POSITION. OPEN YOUR HAND, SUDDENLY, AND COVER CLIENT'S EYE WITH THE PALM OF YOUR HAND, SAYING, "SLEEP". HOLD THE CENTER OF YOUR PALM OVER THE CLIENT'S CHAKRA (CENTER OF FOREHEAD JUST ABOVE EYES, ABOUT 10-15 SECONDS WITH OPPOSITE HAND BEHIND CLIENT'S HEAD. NOW, SLOWLY, TURN CLIENT'S HEAD FROM SIDE TO SIDE IN A SOFT, ROLLING MOTION. DO NOT MOVE THE HEAD CONTINUOUSLY. WITH INTERMITTENT MOVEMENT OF THE HEAD, CLIENT WILL QUICKLY UNDERSTAND THAT THEY MUST LET YOU MOVE THE HEAD. THIS WILL ALLOW THE CLIENT TO 'LET GO'.

NEXT SAY, "When I remove my hands, you will go ten times deeper". QUICKLY AND DECISIVELY, REMOVE YOUR HANDS AND SAY, "Ten Times Deeper". OR IF RECLINER IS BEING USED, SAY, "I am going to gently tip the recliner and you will go Ten Times Deeper". YOU MAY ALSO TELL THE CLIENT, "When I turn off the light, you will go Ten Times Deeper".

CLIENT IS QUICKLY INDUCED AND PREPARED TO RECEIVE PRESCRIPTION.

You are about to participate in an interactive experience. I will ask you to participate by using your vivid imagination in a very active way to help achieve the results you desire.

Now, close your eyes and Relax. Just for a moment, imagine all the muscle groups in your body, letting go . . Take a deep breath . . up through your nose . . That's good . . Exhale now . . and take another deep breath . . And again . .

Each time you breath, imagine the oxygen filling your lungs and spreading relaxation throughout your body . . Just feel that relaxation . . as I talk to you . .

Relax all the muscle groups around your face for a moment . . Now, relax your scalp . . your fore head . . your eyebrows . . your eyelids . . and your cheeks . . and your nose . . and your mouth . . Especially those muscle groups around your mouth and lips . . Make sure your teeth are not clinched together . . Now just relax . . Relax your chin and jaw . . Allow all those muscles in your face to just let go . .

And now, your neck relaxes . . The front of your neck and especially . . the back part of your neck . . right down into your shoulders . . Feel your shoulders relaxing completely . . Get rid of all the tension clustered in your shoulders . . It feels so good to do that . .

And allow your arms to relax now . . Your upper arms . . to your elbows . . Your forearms . . Relax your wrists . . your hands . . Even your fingers relax and let go . . Just imagine your arms becoming very heavy . . loose and limp . . Heavy, Loose, Limp . . Like a wet washcloth . . And allow yourself to breath comfortably . . Notice how deep and regular your breathing has become . . Feel your breathing . . Feel the rhythm . . the cadence of your breathing . . Notice the contraction and expansion of your diaphragm . . and your chest . . Allow your chest muscles to relax completely . . right down through to your stomach . . Feel the stomach muscles just relaxing . . Getting rid of any tension that might be in your stomach area or in any of your organs . . Release them all now . .

And now, allow your back muscles to relax . . Those large muscle groups in the upper part of your back . . Right down your spinal column and into your lower back . . Just let go . . Let go completely . .

And allow those smaller muscle groups in the lower part of your back to relax as well . . And your hips and pelvic area relaxes . . Your thighs . . and especially your legs . . They need the relaxation . . Your knees . . your calves . . your ankles and into your feet . . Yes, and even your toes . . Just allow all those muscle groups to relax completely as you begin to drift into a very deep, comfortable state . . Letting yourself go now . . Letting your mind and body become one . . Feeling good . . Feeling oh, so good . .

Many people, sitting there as you are now, report having certain feelings in their body . . Some report a numbness in their arms or legs . . Some people report a tingling sensation, like pins and needles . . usually in their hands or arms . . Some report having both feelings, alternately . . Some people experience a lightness in their body, and others . . more of a heaviness . . You may feel buoyant, as though you are floating above the chair . . Or a heaviness, as though you are sinking into the chair . . with shoulders sagging . .

And some people, when they relax, find they have a need to swallow, because their salivary glands become too dry . . If you have a need to swallow . . it's perfectly okay to do so . . Many people also find, when they let go and relax totally . . their eyeballs relax in the sockets and their eyelids begin to flicker or flutter . . ever so slightly . . This is an excellent sign of Letting go . .

The important implications of these signs is an expression of your willingness and readiness . . to allow yourself to go deeper into hypnosis . . Going into hypnosis is very gradual and . . in a moment . . I am going to take you on a relaxing experience . . to help you go deeper . . Call it a vacation trip . . to a place where you have always wanted to go . .

But before I do that, just imagine a custom-built cloud snuggling up underneath your body . . in the shape of a big easy chair . . It is a very soft and comfortable cloud . . Your personal cloud . .

Your cloud is rising up now . . Lifting you high up into the other clouds . . to a very special and beautiful place . . far across the sea . . You can look down now . . Far below, you can see the blue waters of the ocean . . Far - far below . .

In the distance you can see a high volcanic peak . . rising up out of the waters of the Pacific . . A beautiful island paradise awaits you . .

You are a long way up in the sky . . but descending down now . . Down . . down . . deeper . . deeper . . Towards the volcanic mountain in the distance . . It is getting closer now . . but we must go deeper . . Deeper . . Gliding nearly down to it now . . Still going down . . deeper . . deeper . . deeper . . We are passing the mountain now . . Floating just above the sandy beaches that stretch for miles . . on this lovely tropical island . .

Your private cloud is slowing down . . Coming to a stop now . . just above the many palm trees along the shore line . . It is safe for you to step off the cloud and . . gently float down among the palm tree tops . . Down . . down . . Gently downward . . Deeper and deeper . . Until at last you sink your bare feet . . into the warm, soft sand . . Oh, that feels so good . .

You have arrived on such a glorious day . . Surrounded by tall palms, swaying gently in the soft sea breeze . . that is blowing in off the water . . The water is so blue . . with dolphins following the native surfboard riders . . Here, there is no time . . It is neither past nor future . . It is only now . .

Listen and you hear the softly beating drums and strumming ukuleles coming from canoes floating by, draped with scented passion flowers . .

The Lyre birds and colorful parrots flock nearby . . The smell of passion fruits fill the air with an aroma that calls for you to stay in this beautiful island paradise . . Native girls in grass skirts beckon you with their swaying hips and alluring hands . . This is the place where you have traveled so far to come to . . And you never want to leave . . This truly is . . a paradise on Earth . .

Many miles back up the beach you can see the rising mountain . . far in the distance . . Rising high above the island and the blue waters of the Pacific . . The snow packed glacier on the top of the mountain is a brilliant white color . . It is so beautiful against the pale blue sky with wispy soft clouds surrounding it . .

Now, your attention is drawn to a lone figure . . walking slowly toward you . . Walking up the beach toward you . . Does the person look familiar to you ? . . You wonder . . I want you to walk down the beach now . . Walk towards that person who is coming your way . . You are coming closer together now . . Closer . . The person coming toward you has a very important message to tell you . . And only you . . It may be a friend . . Someone you know . . Or a relative who has passed over . . Perhaps it is a stranger to you . . But the message is important and is meant for you alone to receive . . It may be a man . . or a woman . . or a child . . The figure is coming closer now . . Closer . . Close enough for you to look into their eyes . . Take this time now to communicate . . The information you are to receive will be quite clear . . Accept this message . . And when you are through communicating . . I want you to raise your hand in the air . . I will wait . .   (Pause to wait until the message is received and the hand is raised.)

You have done very well . . The message you have received will be in your subconscious for a very long time . . You will remember everything you have learned . . Everything you have experienced here today . . Later on, after you are awake . . you will recall all of it clearly . .

Let not your heart be troubled . . for the message you have received . . is a blessed event . . Very few people are so fortunate . . that they can speak of such an exciting occurrence . . Indeed, you are fortunate . . You are blessed . .

It is time now to leave this beautiful tropical island . . with its golden sandy beaches and azure blue waters to swim in . . Perhaps one day you will return . . if that is your desire . . It is such a great pleasure . . for me to hypnotize you . . . for I know how much you thoroughly enjoy it . .

(Continue from this point with any Prescription)

EMERGE

Take a few moments now to pay attention to the relaxed feeling all over your body . . Memorize it as carefully as you can . . Store into your memory, the entire feeling of your whole body in complete relaxation . . You enjoy this peaceful feeling . . and you look forward to re-experiencing this wonderful, restful state of mind in the future . . Each time you are hypnotized . . you will go into a deeper level of hypnosis more quickly and more easily . . Continue to relax . .

In a few moments, I will count to five (5) . . and at the count of 5, you will open your eyes . . You will feel wide awake . . and you will feel wonderfully better for this long and relaxing rest . .

You will feel completely relaxed . . both mentally and physically . . You will be more refreshed and more invigorated than you have ever felt before in your life . . You will be totally free from all feelings of stress or anxiety . . You will always find hypnosis to be relaxing . . refreshing . . and invigorating . . An experience you truly enjoy . .

Now, the counting begins . . On the count of 5, your eyes will open . . On the count of 5, you will emerge from this pleasant relaxation, feeling wonderfully refreshed and completely relaxed . . Refreshed, as though you were awakening from a long nap . . Here we go . .

1 - You are coming up now . . You feel the energy and the vigor flowing through your legs . . Flowing up through your body . . Your eyes feel fresh and clear . . From head to foot, you feel refreshed . . Physically refreshed . . Emotionally refreshed . . and Spiritually refreshed . .

2 - Rising up now . . Coming to the surface . .

3 - Feeling wonderful . . wonderful . . For you truly are a wonderful person . .

4 - You are more and more alert . . More and more alert . . You feel vigorous . . energetic . . Relaxed from head to foot . . You are completely refreshed . . rejuvenated . . Your eyes are ready to open . . And you are ready to return to an alert . . wakeful state . .

5 - Open your eyes now, feeling refreshed and alert . .

Before I put you into a deep hypnotic state, I'd like for you to stretch your whole body. Stretch your arms and legs . . Just stretch all over. Then you will be ready to really relax in a deep hypnotic state . . (Pause while client stretches.)

Now you are ready to go into a deep hypnotic state of relaxation. Close your eyes now and begin to inhale deeply, through your nose . . and exhale out through your mouth, very slowly . . That allows your body to take oxygen into your lungs while expelling the nitrogen . . Your body will continue relaxing more each time you breath this way . .

Being in a light state of hypnosis is very pleasant . . But you will probably prefer going into a very deep trance . . where you will automatically experience all the wonderful benefits of complete hypnosis . .

In a moment, I'm going to ask you to open your eyes and pick a spot to look at . . as I am giving you suggestions . . That will help you go into a deep hypnotic state . . I want you to continue breathing deeply . . and slowly . . Even after your eyes are opened . . That will help you to go into a deep hypnotic trance more quickly . .

Now, open your eyes . . and look at any spot you choose . . Any object . . As you look at the spot you choose, your eyes will become heavier . . And they will feel like they want to close . . Don't try to make them close deliberately . . And don't make any effort to keep them from closing . . They are becoming heavier and they will close by themselves . . easily and gently . . As your eyes close, you will experience a pleasant feeling of drowsiness . . as you drift into what seems to be a deep, dreamy state . .

Listen to the soothing sounds of the air conditioner as your conscious mind continues relaxing more and more ... You are not trying to listen to anything in particular . . Only the sound of my voice . . and the words I am saying to you . . If you do not understand the words, that's okay . .

Your subconscious mind is ever alert to every word . . There may be brief moments, at first, when other thoughts come into your mind . . But that will not interfere . . Your subconscious mind will hear each word I say . . And your conscious mind can feel safe and secure as you relax . .

It keeps becoming less important that your eyes are not open . . And becomes less and less important for you to listen to my voice . . Because your subconscious mind will hear everything I say . . and can cause you to respond to everything I tell you . . Your eyelids continue feeling heavier . . Pay no attention if they should flutter a bit . . It is quite normal . .

You are experiencing a pleasant drowsiness coming over your whole body . . That is good . . Other sounds and noises keep fading away . . into the far distance . . as you continue relaxing more and more . . It is a very pleasant feeling for your whole body to keep relaxing . . Your whole body responds to the idea of relaxation . . You continue to feel more calm . . more peaceful . . more at ease . .

As you continue relaxing . . there may be times when it seems like you are going . . into a state of sleep . . And that's okay because your subconscious mind will still hear . . everything I say . . and will enable you to respond to any suggestions . . and instructions I give you . . If I tell you to move, you will be able to move . . If I ask you to speak, you will be able to talk . . You will find it easy to put my suggestions into your own actions . .

There may be times when my voice seems like its a long distance away . . And there may be times when I am talking to you and you will not be consciously aware of my voice . . And that is okay because your subconscious mind hears everything that I say . . And you will be pleased to find that your subconscious mind is receiving what I say and is making it all true . . Your subconscious mind understands that I'm telling you only those things I know you can do . . And you will be able to do everything I tell you . .

You are in the process of making some very important changes . . that will bring you great happiness . . You are making changes that will increase your self awareness . . Changes that are causing the activities of your body to function properly . . so that your physical and mental health . . will continue to improve . .

These are some of the reasons your subconscious mind is receiving everything I tell you . . And you will be quite happy . . with your natural ability . . to achieve everything you desire to achieve . .

It's okay for you to consciously forget what I am saying to you now . . because your subconscious mind will remember . .

Your subconscious mind will easily cause you to respond to everything I tell you . . You can enjoy the comfort of being in a deep hypnotic trance and . . consciously forget whatever I say while you are relaxing . .

You are becoming so completely relaxed that it seems like you are almost asleep . . You're becoming drowsier, just like when you are drifting into a natural sleep . . Becoming drowsier . . sleepier . .

You can really enjoy responding to everything I tell you . . and be pleased . . with the continuous improvements . . in all areas of your life . . Your nerves are becoming more relaxed and steady . . Your muscles are continuing to become more relaxed . .

Being hypnotized is always a very pleasant, very enjoyable, soothing, restful, completely relaxing experience . . You will always enjoy having me hypnotize you . . Every time I hypnotize you . . you continue to enjoy it more . .

Your conscious mind is relaxing completely and your subconscious mind is free . . to limit itself to everything I say . . Your subconscious mind enjoys receiving everything I tell you and . . causes you to put what I say . . into your own actions . .

It is so enjoyable to let go completely . . knowing I am only telling you those things I know you can do . . You find it easy and enjoyable to do everything I tell you . . because your subconscious mind knows it is for your own good . . For your own benefit . . For your own self-improvement . . and for your own personal well being . .

It is natural for your body to be healthy . . It is natural for your body to be slim, trim, firm and strong . . It is normal for all of the processes and activities of your body to function perfectly . .

So, everything I am telling you is already a part of your real nature . . Everything I am telling you is a part of your real personality . . And your subconscious mind . . is receiving everything I am telling you . . and is causing it to be used by you . . to keep improving yourself . . physically . . mentally . . emotionally and spiritually . .

You are breathing more easily and freely now . . Your heart is pumping your blood through the circulatory system, perfectly . . And without any conscious effort . . your muscles and nerves are more relaxed . . and steady . . There is nothing important for your conscious mind to do . .

Everything I am telling you is influencing your thoughts . . your feelings . . and your actions . . in a positive, helpful way . . Even after you awaken from your hypnotic state . . everything I say to you will continue to influence you . . Just as strongly, just as surely and just as powerfully . . as it does while you are hypnotized . . And it will continue becoming more effective each day . . Even when you are wide awake and fully alert . . your subconscious mind will continue reacting to everything I tell you and will cause it to work automatically . . And you will continue to become more successful in all areas of your life . . Your self-confidence and self-acceptance will continue increasing more each day . .

You will use these principles of relaxation, which you are now experiencing, during your daily life . . And will be relaxed . . and calm . . in every situation and circumstance . . in which you find yourself . . Whether you are alone or with others . .

I want you to rest for a moment in silence now and . . let all that I have said, absorb into your subconscious mind . . In a moment or two, we will take a peaceful journey . . to a place you will enjoy . . Just rest now . . I'll be back with you in a short time . . (pause)

I want to take you to a restful . . quiet place, deep in the forest . . where you will find peace and relaxing comfort . . in a totally relaxing world of your own . . You're going to take a short journey up a mountain trail where . . tall trees are nestled high up . . in the rain clouds . . The clouds bump and mesh together . . Swirling in shades of pink and soft azure blue . . Occasional drops of rain settle softly . . onto your face . . But you smile, because the rain drops make you feel excited and . . happy inside . .

Climbing up the steep mountainside is slow . . and sometimes difficult . . But it is time now to let go . . Let yourself be free to slowly drift upward . . Up and up . . to the tops of the trees . . High above the trees now . . where you are free to sail on the wind . . Look away and you will see the far mountain ranges . . covered in white snow caps . . many miles away . . You can see them clearly in the distance, but you are not going there . . Let yourself slowly drift down into the branches of the elm trees . . and the oak trees . . Tall and majestic . . You are settling down slowly into the top of . . the great elm tree with its mighty . . spreading branches . .

Where birds flutter past in darting flashes . . Chipmunks and squirrels . . find safety and food to store for the winter . . And there, far, far below you, a gurgling brook trickles . . with singing waters . . winding through the forest grasses . . far, far below . .

You are drifting now . . Rocking on the winds . . like the leaves . . Drifting slowly, to the left . . Then to the right . . Back and forth, as you slowly, gently, sail down . . down . . deeper . . Deeper now . . toward the green grasses of the forest, far below . . Slowly you circle through the huge branches of the trees . . Drifting in circles . . Swaying to the right . . Sailing up . . up, with the wind . . Then downward . . To the left . . Circling . . Circling . . The winds carry you gently in a downward motion . . Down . . down . . Swirling gently in circles . . Focus on the leaves, swirling beside you as you slowly drift down - downward . . Until, at last, your feet touch the soft, green grasses . . covering the earth . . Here is where you will find peace . . tranquility . . complete relaxation . . Here, you are as one . . with all that God . . has created for you . .

Here, there are no sounds . . besides my voice . . and the noise of rushing waters in the distant brook . . flowing through the forest . . Any other sounds you may hear will only support you . . in your relaxing, comfortable place . . Your mind and body are open to complete trust . . Trust in the power of your mind to benefit you on your journey . . Your mind is very relaxed and . . open to receive the beneficial suggestions . . I will soon give you . . But for now, we will stay here . . in this beautiful valley with its lush, tall grasses . . surrounded by forest creatures who live here . . for here, there is much to experience . . and to learn . . And later on . . to recall . .

Relax here in comfort . . for a while longer . . before we continue . .

(Continue with Prescription)

Settle back comfortably in your chair . . In a moment, I will give you a series of suggestions that will relax each and every portion of your body . . Internalize this deep relaxation . . Just listen effortlessly and your subconscious mind will automatically record and accept the things I say . . Do not try to analyze them . . As you relax, just let things happen, without any thought as to question . . or analysis . .

Focus your attention now, on my voice . . Close your eyes gently, so you can listen effortlessly . . There is nothing you need to look at . . so just let your eyes relax and your eyelids close . .

Now, to begin . . I want you to go inside of yourself . . and just think about peace . . And experience the solitude . . the tranquility . . and the calmness . . Take notice of your breathing . . You are breathing more slowly . . more deeply . . Now, take a deep breath . . and breathe relaxation in . . Hold it . . Now slowly exhale and release all of the tension from your body . . And let your eyes relax still more completely . . That's it . . Now your body is starting to relax . . more and more deeply . . Keep your eyes closed . . and just let your body go . . and relax deeper and deeper . . Deeply relaxed . .

Your body is letting go of all tension . . It is truly relaxing . . Now, take another deep breath . . and hold it until I tell you to exhale . . Now, release that breath . . Slowly exhale . . and let your body go limp and loose . . You are now starting to feel a little drowsy . . Your body feels so very comfortable . . So relaxed . . Now, take another deep breath . . Really deep . . Fill your lungs . . and hold it for a moment of time . . Now, exhale slowly . . That's it . . Release all the air in your body . . And now, you are floating and drifting . . Just float . . Float as if you were riding on a big billowy cloud . . Floating and drifting into deeper relaxation . . You feel so dreamy . . So drowsy . . as you go deeper and deeper into pleasant relaxation . . You are breathing slowly and smoothly . . And with each breath . . you become a little more relaxed . . With each gentle breath . . Floating and drifting into gentle relaxation . .

Your body is relaxing more and more deeply . . Deeper and deeper . . Now, take another deep breath . . and hold it as long as you can . . Now, breathe out slowly . . Feeling your body go limp and relaxed . . You are feeling so pleasantly drowsy and so sleepy . . Notice how very comfortable your body is . .

How the tension is nearly gone from your body . . Just allow yourself to relax completely . . And with every gentle breath . . ripples of soothing relaxation pass throughout your body . . Allowing the muscles of your face to relax . . to let go . . Releasing tension . . Also, relax your neck muscles . . The muscles of your shoulders . . your arms . . hands . . Relax your chest muscles . . and your lungs . . your heart . . down to your stomach . . And relax all of the organs inside of your abdomen . . Your pelvic muscles . . your legs and your feet . . Let them all relax . .

Enjoy this feeling of inner calm and peace . . Internalize this pleasurable feeling . . Going deeper and deeper . . Every muscle . . every nerve . . every fiber of your being . . is now deeply relaxed . . and you are drifting . . floating . . into deeper relaxation . .

You are relaxing still deeper . . Going deeper into pleasant relaxation . . Drifting and floating into dreamy, drowsiness . . Drifting and floating . . And with each and every gentle breath . . you become just a little more relaxed . . Allow this gentle feeling to flow throughout your entire body . . You feel so drowsy . . so peaceful . . as you drift and float with my voice . . You may drift up higher and see a self-image of yourself . . sitting there so peaceful . . so serene . . while you become sleepier and dreamier with every breath you breath out . . And deeper and deeper relaxed with every breath you breathe in . . Deeper . . deeper . . dreamier . . drowsier . . with the gentle rise and fall of your chest . . drifting . . deeper and deeper . . More and more relaxed . .

As you internalize this deep relaxation . . your mind and your body go deeper and deeper . . Just let go . . more and more . . And now, go all the way down . . into that deep, pleasant relaxation . .

You have a feeling of complete inner calmness and peace . . How pleasant it is . . How enjoyable . . Enjoy this wonderful feeling you have created for yourself in your mind . . For every nerve . . every muscle . . and every fiber of your being, is enjoying this restful experience . . This deeply penetrating relaxation . . And with this deep relaxation . . your subconscious mind . . is becoming exquisitely receptive to suggestion . .

You are now so deeply relaxed . . that your subconscious mind is focused . . on every suggestion that I give you . .

As you rest here . . all calm and quiet . . your subconscious mind is awake and listening . . and receptive . . It can easily absorb every suggestion that I give you . . You are resting calmly and quietly . . Nothing will disturb your restful peace . . You need pay no attention to other sounds for they are unimportant . . You will hear my voice clearly . . You will find that you will easily, quickly and willingly follow . . every suggestion that I give you . .

In this deeply relaxed condition . . . your subconscious mind will strengthen the effect of every suggestion that I give you . . All of the suggestions will make the changes we want them to make . .

(CONTINUE AT THIS POINT WITH PROPER THERAPEUTIC SUGGESTIONS)

13. (Induction)　　　SELF CONFIDENCE
Progressive Relaxation

Now . . close your eyes and relax . . In just a moment . . you will feel all the muscle groups in your body letting go of any tension . . Take a deep breath . . Hold it a moment . . Now, gently exhale . . And you will notice your body wanting to relax . .

I am going to count from one to 20 now . . And as I count each number . . you will relax deeper . . and DEEPER . . with each number you hear . . 1-2-3 . . Tension is leaving your body . . 4-5 . . Resting and relaxing more deeply now . . Deeper and deeper . . 6-7 and 8 . . Deeply relaxing . . Going deeper and deeper into a restful state . . So peaceful . . Peaceful and relaxing . . Relax . . Gently relax . . 9 . . Deeper now . . Deeply relaxing . . 10-11-12 . . Gently inhale . . Deeply inhale . . and let it out slowly . . With each breath you take . . you will go deeper . . and deeper . . And as you let it out slowly . . you will relax more and more . . Inhale deeply now . . and let it out, slowly . . 13-14-15 . . You will be free of all pain and discomfort . . as you deeply relax . . Gently relax . . 16 . . Hear nothing but the sound of my voice . . Any other sounds will help you to go deeper . . into complete relaxation . . Complete relaxation . . 17-18 . . Deeper and deeper . . Completely relaxed . . So relaxed . . 19 . . and . . finally . . 20 . . Deep . . deep . . deep . . Deeply relaxed hypnosis . .

Your mind is very relaxed now . . and open to receive the helpful and beneficial suggestions I am about to give you . . You may use those suggestions that apply now . . and you may reject those that do not apply . . Or you may keep them for another time, if they apply then . . Let us begin . .

Congratulations on your commitment to improve your SELF CONFIDENCE. Hypnosis will increase your determination . . your will power . . and your self control . . From this time forward . . you will never again feel lost . . or confused . . about making decisions . . or commitments . . that will impact your life . . Before you leave today you will receive guidelines . . for a strong commitment . . to inject self confidence into your daily life . . Keep in mind that you . . are making this commitment . . for your own benefit . . Consider it to be . . a gift . . to yourself . .

Now, relax deeper . . going into complete relaxation . . drifting and floating into dreamy drowsiness . . and with this complete relaxation, your subconscious mind is becoming exquisitely receptive to suggestion . . You are now so deeply relaxed that your mind is focused on every suggestion that I give you . . As you rest here all calm and quiet . . your subconscious mind is awake and receptive . . It can easily absorb every suggestion that I give you . . You are resting calmly and quietly . . Nothing will disturb your restful peace . . You need pay no attention to other sounds for they are not important . . You can hear my voice clearly . . You will follow every suggestion I give you, easily . . and willingly . . In this relaxed condition, your subconscious mind will strengthen the effect of every suggestion I give you . . All of the suggestions will make the changes in you that you want them to make . . And because of the suggestions . . you will have a better understanding of yourself . . And you'll gain new feelings of confidence in yourself . . In your every word . . your every thought . . your every action . . Your words . . your thoughts . . your actions . . are all correct . .

Your need . . to please others . . while not hurting their feelings . . is important to you . . But knowing that your decisions . . are the right ones . . is much more important . . than . . other people's feelings . . Your actions and deeds . . are also impressive . . to other people . . And once they see your words . . in action . . they will admire you even more . . They will wonder . . at your self assurance . . and your self confidence . . For you are strong . . and persuasive . . You will appreciate yourself . . for who you are . . and for the things you are capable of doing . . Do not have self doubts . . or feelings of insecurity . . Release these feelings from your mind . . now . . The ill-feelings of self doubt are the only things holding you back . . Do not trouble yourself with these feelings . . Release them . . Let them go . . Your home life . . your family . . your friends . . your business . . They are all waiting for you . . Depending on your self-assuring confidence . . to create a better environment for them . . as well as for yourself . .

You have made an absolute commitment . . to create a better life . . for yourself and . . for those you love . . You have made a choice to believe in yourself . . And you are right for having made that choice . .

43

You have the power . . to take complete charge of your life . . without fear of criticism . . from those who do not think as clearly as you do . . You are the leader we have all been seeking . .

Your confidence level is high . . and will benefit every person you meet . . You are determined and committed to succeed . . And you feel very good about the absolute commitment you are making . . You have every reason to feel proud . . You are a wonderful person and . . you and your associations . . can always depend on your . . decision making abilities . .

When the time comes to make a difficult choice . . you will find the answer by . . relaxing . . Then taking a deep . . deep breath . . Slowly letting it out . . Your decision will come to you . . It will be the right one . .

At the times you are re-visited by negative thoughts or impressions . . because of what someone else says or does that upsets you . . you will take a short walk . . Each time your right foot hits the floor or the pavement . . you will say the word, "POSITIVE" . . Either out loud or to yourself . . Repeat the word, 'POSITIVE' . . 'POSITIVE' . . over and over to yourself . . The bad feelings will disappear and your self confidence will be even stronger . .

If there are any suggestions that I gave you today that are not in your best interest, they will now disappear - out from your subconscious mind . . Your self-protective mechanisms are always in place . . allowing you to choose what benefits your improvement . .

AT THIS POINT, PROCEED WITH ADDITIONAL POSITIVE PRESCRIPTION OR EMERGE

Now, I am going to count from 1 to 5 . . and on the count of 5 . . you will open your eyes . . to an alert, waking state . . feeling clear of mind, relaxed and wonderful . . for you are a wonderful and confident person . . I will begin . .

One. You will remember everything you've experienced with complete understanding . .
Two. You are now connected to your inner supporting strength . .
Three. Everything I have told you is true and is already happening.
Four. Beginning to be more aware of your body as it fully awakens.
Five. Let your hands and feet move . . Stir and stretch as you open your eyes, feeling clear, rested and wonderful . .

I feel calm . . I feel relaxed . . I feel in control . . I am relaxed . .
I am in control . . I feel safe . . I feel secure . . I'm letting go . .
As I let go, all my muscle groups begin to relax . . I feel calm . .
I feel relaxed . . I feel in control . . I am letting go completely . .

As my muscle groups relax, a beam of sunlight focuses on my scalp
and spreads relaxation and warmth throughout my body . . It rids me
of all negative thoughts and negative feelings . . leaving me with only
positive thoughts and feelings . . I feel calm . . I feel relaxed . .
I am comfortably in control . .

My mind is now open to receive the helpful and beneficial suggestions I am
about to give myself . .

(Examples)

Item 1.   Practicing Hypnotherapy will benefit me by allowing me to help
other people with what I learn.

Item 2.   By combining Therapy and Hypnosis as a business, many more
people can be reached.

Item 3.   People in situations of stress, indulgence, negative habits or
desiring self improvements will seek the help they need through me.

Item 4.   Hypnotherapy is beneficial to everyone and I will provide my
knowledge and expertise for its greater good.

Item 5.   The power to help many people . . is in my control, for the
benefit of all.

REINFORCEMENT SCRIPT

I feel calm . . I feel relaxed . . I feel in control . . I am relaxed . . I am in control . . I feel safe . . I feel secure . . I'm letting go . . As I let go, all my muscle groups begin to relax . . I feel calm . . I feel relaxed . . I feel in control . .

As my muscle groups relax, a beam of sunlight focuses on my scalp and spreads relaxation and warmth throughout my body . . It rids me of all negative thoughts and negative feelings, leaving me with only positive thoughts and positive feelings . . I feel calm . . I feel relaxed . . I am comfortably in control . .

My mind is now open to receive the helpful and beneficial suggestions I am about to give myself . .

Item 1 . .

Item 2 . .

Item 3 . .

Item 4 . .

Close your eyes and begin inhaling deeply . . deeply . . and exhale slowly . . You will experience a peaceful relaxation coming over your whole body . . each time you exhale . . Do that five or six times . . Continuing to feel more at ease . . more calm . . safe and secure . .

As you continue moving into a deeper . . more peaceful hypnotic state . . your subconscious mind is reviewing many things that are important to you . . Going into your inner mind is comparable to reading a book . . You go to the library wondering, 'What do I want to read? There are so many good books to choose from that you are not sure of just what type of book you want to read . . Possibly, you could start off with a self-improvement' book . . Or maybe you'd like a book in the science fiction area . . Or, say, you're feeling a little romantic so perhaps, you might choose a romance novel . . Or possibly, something in the area of religion would be interesting . .

As you walk through the doors of the library, you are amazed at seeing the many thousands of books . . There are more books than you could read in a lifetime . . And you begin thinking about something you had heard once . . that your subconscious mind is kind of like a library . .

And somewhere else you had read . . that your subconscious mind is comparable to a computer . . It has accumulated and stored knowledge ever since your soul first came into being . . And all of that knowledge is still there . . in your subconscious mind . . It is a part of your own existence and, it truly . . belongs to you . . All of the stored knowledge is there for you . . any time you need it . . It enables you to talk . . just by making a decision to talk . . All you have to do is think the words you want to say and your subconscious mind . . automatically causes your tongue to move to the right positions . . causes your mouth to form in the right configuration . . and causes the right amount of oxygen to pass through your vocal cords so you can make the sounds of the words you want to say . . It is where all of your memories are stored . . to be brought into your conscious mind, when you need them . . It is where your creativity comes from . . and millions of other types of information is stored in your subconscious mind . .

Browsing through this virtual library . . causes your amazement . . as you are now realizing the tremendous amounts of information that . . you actually do possess in your subconscious mind . . It is so much more than your conscious mind has been aware of . . and you understand now, there is so much within you that you have never been consciously aware of . .

You look around the library and you see an escalator . . One side is going down . . and the other side goes up . . You get on the one that goes down . . and as you are moving down . . down to a lower level of the library . . you are wondering, what is in the lowest level . . You have never gone all the way down to the basement . . However, today, you want to go all the way down . . even if it is five or six levels below the main floor . . You are continuing to move downward . . to the first level below the main floor . . And as you are nearing that first level . . you notice thousands of additional books . . And there are beautiful sitting areas . . with soft, fluffy chairs to relax in . . and read . . They look so comfortable . . You begin wondering how long you could sit in one of those big chairs . . before you would fall asleep . .

You decide to continue all the way to the basement before settling down to read . . So you move to the escalator that goes down to the next level . . As you are going down . . you see a sitting area with beautiful looking recliners . . You notice a person sitting there, dozing . . You look more closely and you realize . . the person sitting there is you . .

You are really surprised as you notice your level of comfort . . You seem to be in a dreamlike trance . . You look so comfortable, sitting there . . You have the appearance of being asleep . . yet, in a sense, you seem to be aware . . Perhaps you are just relaxing . . permitting your subconscious mind to review important information . .

The escalator finally reaches that level . . you are tempted to walk over to yourself . . but you appear to be so calm . . so at ease, that you decide to let yourself enjoy the quiet and relaxing comfort . . Other sounds and noises have long since faded away . . without any conscious effort by you . . You are listening only to my voice . . and watching yourself really enjoying this relaxing experience . .

Without any effort by you . . your right hand and arm are beginning to feel very light . . they feel so light . . it seems like your hand wants to float upwards . . toward your face . .

You can be pleasantly surprised to notice it is beginning to lift up toward your face . . while the rest of your body is sinking more deeply . . into the recliner . .

You are still there . . watching yourself . . You find it interesting that your right hand and arm are gradually lifting . . raising up toward your face . . as you stand there watching yourself . . You are realizing that you really do know how to be relaxed and comfortable . .

IF HAND RAISES, TELL IT TO GO BACK DOWN – TO REST IN LAP, AND CONTINUE.

As you look at yourself . . you notice that you have an intense desire to be connected to yourself in a new way . . You begin walking over toward yourself . . and you notice, your body . . that is sitting in the chair, relaxing . . looks to be perfectly developed . . just the way you want your body to be . . It looks healthy . . and strong . .

(MALES) All of the muscles are well developed . . and seem to be perfectly toned . . admirable . .

(FEMALES) Your body looks beautiful with all of the curves in just the right places . . Your legs and thighs are slim and trim . . And your waist is small . . Your abdomen is flat and your breasts are full and firm . . perfectly proportioned for your slim, trim body . .

As you are preparing to move into that body . . you are very much aware that it is just the way you would like it to be . . And you feel confident that you can . . and will . . develop that perfect body . . just as you have envisioned it . .

You have now moved into that body and you breath in deeply as you become even more comfortable . . You are pleased to discover that you are developing . . all of the qualities and characteristics you desire for yourself . . and that you now have great determination . . to develop that perfect . . healthy . . well formed body . .

Suddenly, you realize . . that you were on your way down to the bottom floor of the library . . You get up easily and go back over to the escalator . . and you realize that there is only one more floor to the deepest part of the basement . . You feel yourself going even deeper now . . deeper . . deeper . . Your subconscious mind . . is hearing only my voice . . There may be times when I am talking to you and . . it may seem like my voice is a long distance away . . There may also be times when I am talking to you and . . you won't hear my voice . . consciously . . But that is okay . . Your subconscious mind will hear and interpret everything I say to you . . and cause it to happen in an easy, natural way . .

(Continue with appropriate Prescription)

HAVE THE CHILD CLOSE HIS OR HER EYES AND PRETEND HE IS VISITING WITH A NEW FRIEND. MAYBE THE FRIEND IS A CUDDLY PUPPY OR A KITTEN. OR IT MAY BE A LITTLE TOY RABBIT THAT LIKES BEING CUDDLED.

Now, just keep your eyes closed and pretend that you are enjoying the company of your friend . . You are a very special person and you can really relax and enjoy yourself, feeling calm and peaceful and safe in the company of your new friend . .

While you are having a fun, enjoyable time with your friend, you are listening only to my voice . .

Now, I want you to tell me a little bit about your friend . .
(Pause as client describes his friend.)

Now, ask your friend what name we should use when we talk to him . . Tell me your friends name . .   (Wait for response.)

Okay, that's good . . Now, you can relax even more . . And I want you to ask your friend to help you . . Your friend knows about the problem you've been experiencing, doesn't he . . and your friend, (Name) will be able to tell you how you can get rid of that problem completely . .

Now, as soon as your friend tells you how to get rid of that problem . .   I want you to lift one of your hands up towards the ceiling . . Go ahead and ask him and he will tell you in just a few minutes . . then lift your hand . .
(Pause and wait for response.)

Let yourself continue relaxing . . Bring your friend along now as you begin feeling a peaceful drowsiness all over your body . . Now, you are beginning to see yourself improving . . You are getting rid of that problem . . You are experiencing some pleasant changes right now . . And you will keep improving even more, later on . . after I tell you to open your eyes and come back awake again . .

You are learning more and more from your friend . . You are aware now that your friend really loves you and cares for you . . and is doing everything to help you get rid of that problem completely . . And you will know that you can go back and be with your friend, any time you want to, in the future . . Your friend will always be with you to help you . . Just call his name and he will answer . . Now, I want you to count up to five . . in your mind, and then . . you can open your eyes . . feeling wonderful. Okay ? Begin counting up to five now . .

TO INDUCE THE HYPNOTIC COMA, YOU MUST FIRST GET THE CLIENT INTO A VERY DEEP SOMNAMBULISTIC STATE OF HYPNOSIS. ONCE YOU HAVE INDUCED A VERY DEEP CONDITION, PROCEED AS FOLLOWS :

You are very relaxed and comfortable . . and even in this deep state of relaxation . . you know in your own mind . . that you are capable of reaching . . an even deeper state of relaxation . . than you are in now . .

You know that you can clench your fist . . and make it tighter . . and tighter . . You could clench it so tight that . . it would be impossible to make it any tighter . . That would be the pinnacle of tension in your fist . . Then you could let your fist relax until . . it would be impossible . . to relax it any more . . And that's what we call 'the basement' of relaxation . .

I am going to give you some suggestions and instructions now that will enable your whole body to go down to the very basement of relaxation . . You will become so totally relaxed . . that it would be impossible for you to become any more relaxed . . Every fiber of your body will be completely relaxed . . It will be like a state of euphoria . .

There are three levels of relaxation that are even deeper than the level you are at now . . Let's call them simply . . A, B and C . .

To get down to level A . . you'll have to relax twice as much as you have already . . To get down to level B . . you will relax twice as much as you relax at level A . . And then, when you get down to level C . . you will be much more relaxed than you are at level B . . At level C . . you will be in the very basement . . of relaxation . . Level C is the very deepest, most enjoyable . . most pleasant state of relaxation . . that you can achieve . .

When you reach the basement of relaxation . . there will be signs that will enable me to know . . you have reached the final level . . You don't know what those signs are . . And it isn't anything to concern yourself with . . Every person who has been in the basement of relaxation . . reveals those signs . . And they always enjoy being there . . tremendously . . So, lets get started . .

Imagine yourself getting on an elevator . . and riding down . . down . . to the basement . . You are going, first, to level A . .

Then you'll continue on down to level B . . and from there . . you will travel on down . . deep . . to the basement of relaxation . . Level C . .

You are getting on the elevator now . . The door opens and you get on . . The door closes behind you . . When I count from three down to one . . the elevator will start going down . . By the time you reach level A . . you will be twice as relaxed as you are now . . Tell me when you reach level A, by saying the word, "A", out loud . .

Three . . Two . . One . .   (wait for client to say "A".)

You are doing very well . . reaching a very deep state of relaxation now . . In just a moment . . I will count from three down to one, again . . and you will go down even deeper . . to level B . . You will double your relaxation level again . . when you reach level B . .

It may seem difficult for you to talk . . but again . . I want you to let me know . . When you are relaxed . . twice as much . . as you are now . . you will be at level B . . You will be so relaxed that . . it may be difficult for you to talk . . but I want you to try hard . . and you'll be able to say " B", when you have reached that very deep state of relaxation . .

Three . . Two . . One . .   (wait for client to say "B".)

You have reached a very deep state of relaxation now . . And you can still go even deeper . . The next time I count from three down to one . . you will go down to the very basement of relaxation . . You will continue relaxing . . until your whole, entire body is totally and completely relaxed . . When you know that you are totally relaxed . . you will then be at level C . . So, tell me when you have reached the basement of relaxation . . by saying the word, "C" . .

Three . . Two . . One . .

NOTE : IF CLIENT HAS REACHED HYPNOTIC COMA STATE, HE WILL BE UNABLE TO RESPOND.   IF THE CLIENT SAYS "C", IT INDICATES HE HAS NOT REACHED THE COMA STATE.

AFTER WAITING A FEW MINUTES FOR THE CLIENT TO RESPOND, ASK, "How is your state of relaxation now?"

IF CLIENT IS SOMNAMBULISTIC, HE WILL NOT ANSWER. WITHOUT FURTHER SUGGESTIONS, TEST FOR ANESTHESIA. IN THE COMATOSE STATE.   ANESTHESIA IS AUTOMATIC.   AN EXAMPLE FOLLOWS ;

SUGGEST THE CLIENT LIFT HIS RIGHT LEG. IF CLIENT LIFTS THE LEG, HE IS NOT IN THE COMA STATE.

SUGGEST THE CLIENT OPEN HIS EYES. IN THE COMA STATE, CLIENT WILL NOT OPEN HIS EYES.

NOTE : AFTER THESE TESTS (IF CLIENT IS IN THE COMA STATE) HE IS READY TO RECEIVE YOUR SUGGESTIONS, AS LONG AS YOU GIVE NO SUGGESTION CALLING FOR A VERBAL RESPONSE WHILE CLIENT IS IN THIS STATE OF MIND.

Find a position that is most comfortable for you. In a few moments I will begin to guide you into a deep state of physical and mental relaxation. This session will help you learn the skill of deep relaxation which is so important for Stress Reduction and for your overall health and well being . .

I am going to give you a series of instructions that will relax each and every portion of your body. Now, close your eyes, gently, so you can listen effortlessly . . There is nothing you need to look at . . so . . let your eyes relax as your eyelids close . .

With your eyes closed, you can begin to relax . . although at first, you may be more aware of some things than you were before . . the sounds of the room . . the sound of my voice . . sensations in your hands or feet . . thoughts and images that drift into your mind, automatically . . With your eyes closed, it becomes easier and easier to become more and more aware of a variety of things that would otherwise be overlooked or ignored . . thoughts . . feelings . . sensations . . and the alteration of awareness as your mind begins to experience that gradual . . letting go . .

Just listen effortlessly and your subconscious mind will automatically record and accept the words I say . . Do not try to analyze them . . as you continue to relax . . Just let things happen as they happen . . naturally . . without thought . . without question . . without analyzing . .

Now, take a deep breath through your nose . . Breathe in nice and slow . . filling your lungs all the way . . and, hold it for a moment (pause) . . And now, breathe out slowly through your mouth . . You'll notice your mind and body relaxing as you breathe . . With each breath, you notice yourself feeling deeper and deeper relaxation   . . Your breathing becomes slower but natural in the comfort of relaxation and . . letting go . . Letting go as you become more and more relaxed . . More relaxed with each gentle breath . . It is so easy to do, as you listen to my voice . . Just . . letting go . .

Each time you inhale, you bring more oxygen into your lungs . . And the oxygen passes from your lungs . . into your heart . . Your heart then pumps the oxygen into your circulatory system . . And it is carried   . . into every part of your body . . where it is needed . .

As you exhale . . your muscles, ligaments . . and tendons . . continue relaxing, more and more . .

I have explained a little bit about hypnosis to you . . but I didn't tell you exactly what a hypnotic state is . . The reason I didn't describe a hypnotic state is because . . it is different for each person . . And if I hypnotized you a hundred times . . it would be a little bit different each time . .

You may have been wondering what it would be like to be . . hypnotized . . and even if you had been hypnotized before . . you really don't quite know what it will be like this time . . In fact, you may be in a deep, hypnotic state . . and not even realize it, consciously . . And you can notice a peaceful, relaxing, drowsiness coming over your whole body . . and realize that you are continuing to move . . into a deeper and deeper hypnotic state . .

Each time you exhale, you can continue relaxing more peacefully . . You can feel yourself moving into a deeper, more peaceful, more detached state of relaxation . .

You can listen to the soothing sounds coming from the air conditioner . . and not even notice other sounds and noises . . You notice only the sound of my voice . . while everything else around you fades away into the background . . Nothing will disturb your peaceful rest . .

Notice now, how very comfortable your body is beginning to feel . . Enjoy this pleasant relaxation . . You will experience a sense of inner calm and peace . . A feeling of letting go as you relax . . That's it . . Let go now . . and . . relax . . Mind and body, deeply relaxed . .

And now, breath in all the air that you can, filling up your lungs . . Breathe in through your nose . . and hold it for a moment . . Now, as you slowly exhale, out through your mouth . . all of the air from your body . . you feel yourself relaxing deeper and deeper . . Drifting down into a pleasant, dreamy, drowsy state of mind . . Drifting and drifting . . Drifting and drifting . . Deeper and deeper . . More and more . . relaxed . .

Let all of your muscles become relaxed . . all over your body . . Let go and feel your body going limp . . Now, direct your attention to the top of your head . . and allow a deeper feeling of complete relaxation begin there . . You may see it as a soft, blue glow . . all around and on the top of your head . . And you may follow it as you allow it to go down . . down through your body . . Let the tiny muscles of your scalp relax . . Let the muscles of your forehead relax . . Feel them letting go and relaxing . . Your eyelids are now completely relaxed . . You feel your eyelids sagging down and becoming very heavy . . Now, let a wave of deeper blue relaxation flow into the muscles of your face . . your lips . . and jaw muscles . . feel your jaw relaxing . . and allow your jaw to drop slightly . . Let the relaxation flow down into your neck and shoulders . . and let it flow down your back . . into all the muscles . . Allow relaxation to flow down into your arms . . to your elbows . . to your wrists . . your hands and on down into your fingertips . .

Now, take another deep breath gently in . . and hold it for a moment . . And as you let this breath out . . let there be a feeling of letting go, into deeper relaxation . . Now, breathe normally . .

Feel the rising and falling of your abdomen with each breath . . Let this rising and falling relax your internal organs . . The flowing blue energy will breathe fresh air for relaxation into your chest . . your pelvic area . . your thighs . . knees . . lower legs . . to your ankles . . and to your feet . . All the way down to the tips of your toes . . You may even feel a tingling in your toes . .

Take notice of your breathing . . You are breathing more slowly and regularly . . More and more deeply . . You can feel your body letting go of all tension . . It is truly relaxing and peaceful . .

Now, take another deep breath . . Fill your lungs up . . up . . up . . and hold it for a moment as you feel the energy fill your entire body . . Gently release the breath, feeling relaxed and, letting go of all tension . . Your body is letting go of all tension . . It is truly relaxed and at peace . .

Now, take another deep breath . . filling your lungs with the blue energy of life . . Hold it a moment as you feel the connection with the life force . . Now, let go once more but feel your body go totally limp and loose . . in its relaxing harmony as it enjoys the life force of energy you have brought to it through your breathing . .

You are now beginning to feel a little drowsy . . Your body feels so very comfortable in its relaxed state of being . . So relaxed . . So relaxed . . And you feel yourself floating and drifting . .

Just enjoy the floating sensation . . as if you are on a billowy cloud, made just for you . . Here, you are safe and secure . . Just floating on this wonderful cloud . . Floating and drifting into sensuous relaxation . . You feel so dreamy . . So drowsy . . as you go deeper and deeper into pleasant relaxation . . You are breathing slowly and smoothly . . And with each breath, you become a little more relaxed . . Floating and drifting . . Deeper and deeper . .

Your body is deeply relaxed and the pleasant, heavy, numbness is spreading up through your body . . More and more relaxed . . drowsier . . dreamier . . as you feel your self going down . . down . . Gently down into deeper and deeper relaxation that is wonderful and restful . . Just let go as you follow my voice into a deeper and deeper state of restful, wonderful relaxation . .

With each and every word I speak . . and with each and every gentle breath . . you will feel ripples of soothing energy passing over your body . . Sleepier and dreamier with every breath you breathe in and out . . Your whole body accepts the relaxation of wonderful rest and calmness . . Enjoy this pleasant relaxation . . Let everything go and feel the sense of inner calm and peace . . of relaxing . . Of letting go . . What a marvelous feeling . . It is a marvelous feeling that you have created for yourself . . And you are relaxing more deeply with the enjoyment of your experience . . More and more relaxed . . peaceful . . wonderful feeling . .

As you internalize this deep relaxation . . in your mind and in your body . . you now have a feeling of inner calmness and peace . . How pleasant it is . . How enjoyable . . Enjoy this wonderful feeling . . For every nerve . . every muscle . . every fiber of your being, enjoys this restful peace . . This deep relaxation . . And with this deep relaxation, your subconscious mind is exquisitely receptive to suggestion . .

As you rest now, all is calm and quiet . . Your subconscious mind is awake and listening . . and receptive . . It can easily absorb every suggestion that I give you . . You are resting calmly and quietly . . Nothing will disturb your restful peace . . You need pay no attention to other sounds for they are unimportant . . You hear only the sound of my voice . .

You will find that you can easily, quickly and willingly follow every suggestion that I give you . . In this relaxed condition, your subconscious mind will strengthen the effect of every suggestion . . that I give you . . And all of the suggestions will make the changes we want them to make . .

CONTINUE FROM THIS POINT WITH ESSENTIAL PRESCRIPTION OR EMERGE, AS FOLLOWS:

Take a few moments now to pay attention to the relaxed feeling all over your body . . Memorize it as carefully as you can . . Store into your memory, the entire feeling of your whole body in complete relaxation . . You enjoy this peaceful feeling . . and you look forward to re-experiencing this wonderful, restful state of mind in the future . . Each time you are hypnotized . . you will go into a deeper level of hypnosis more quickly and more easily . .

In a few moments, I will count to five (5) . . And at the count of 5, you will open your eyes . . You will feel wide awake . . and you will feel wonderfully better for this long and relaxing rest . .

You will feel completely relaxed . . both mentally and physically . . You will be more refreshed and more invigorated than you have ever felt before in your life . . You will be totally free from all feelings of stress or anxiety . . You will always find hypnosis to be relaxing . . refreshing . . and invigorating . . An experience you truly enjoy . .

Now, the counting begins . . On the count of 5, your eyes will open . . On the count of 5, you will emerge from this pleasant relaxation, feeling wonderfully refreshed and completely relaxed . . Refreshed, as though you were awakening from a long nap . . Here we go . .

1 - You are coming up now . . You feel the energy and the vigor flowing through your legs . . flowing up through your body . . Your eyes feel fresh and clear . . From head to foot, you are feeling refreshed . . Physically refreshed . . Emotionally refreshed . .

2 - Rising up now . . coming to the surface . .

3 - Feeling wonderful . . wonderful . . For you truly are a wonderful person . .

4 - You are more and more alert . . More and more alert . . You feel vigorous . . energetic . . relaxed from head to foot . . You are completely refreshed . . rejuvenated . . Your eyes are all ready to open . . and you are ready to return to an alert . . wakeful state . .

5 - Open your eyes now, feeling refreshed and alert . .

Close your eyes and begin breathing deeply and slowly . . As you continue breathing deeply and slowly, it allows your entire body to relax, from the top of your head to the bottom of your feet . .

In just a moment, I'm going to ask you to open your eyes and pick out a spot to look at, as you continue to breath deeply and slowly . .

Of course, you are not in a hypnotic state yet . . You want to be more relaxed and comfortable, before going into a deep hypnotic state . .

Notice your hands and arms now . . And if you want to move them to a more comfortable position before we begin . . you can do that now . .

That's good . . And now, you'll be able to relax easier . . Soon you will experience a feeling of drifting off . . Comparable to floating on a cloud . . Just feel yourself floating away . . Floating out beyond space and time . .

You can open your eyes now . . and continue having the experience of floating . . as you gaze at a random spot on the wall . . And you can notice that your eyes keep feeling heavier . . And you will notice a soothing drowsiness coming over your entire body . .

I'll be talking to you . . as you notice your eyes continuing to feel heavier . . They will soon close all by themselves . . And as you continue relaxing . . you may feel yourself drifting . . into a deep hypnotic state . . without even noticing it . .

By permitting your whole mind and body to completely relax . . you will experience many wonderful benefits . . that will become even more effective . . after this session has completed . .

It keeps becoming less and less important for you to consciously listen to my voice . . Your subconscious mind hears every word I say . . And your mind understands exactly what needs to be done . . that will be of the greatest value to you . .

When I was a child . . we used to play a game that illustrated how easily . . we could be released from tension . . stress and anxiety . . I'll tell you about the game because . . it will enable you to continue progressing . . in all areas of your life . . Physically . . mentally . . emotionally and . . spiritually . .

To play the game . . each of us would take a piece of chalk . . And each of us would draw a square on the sidewalk . . big enough . . to stand in . . Then, one of the children would be 'it' . . and would chase the rest of us . . until we got caught . . Or, until we ran and jumped inside our square . .

Once we were inside of our square . . we were safe . . The person chasing us wasn't allowed to catch us . . And we were not allowed to get out of our square . . until the person who was 'it' gave us permission to get out . .

We had a lot of fun, playing that game . . as young children . . But it would have been silly if we had taken the game so seriously . . that we let those chalk marks on the sidewalk become . . real walls . . that we could never go beyond . .

Suppose I was inside the chalk marks one day . . and the person who was 'it' went home . . forgetting to give me permission to get out . . . It would not have been sensible for me to have remained inside those chalk walls . . the rest of my life . . just because someone forgot to give me permission to leave . . Nor is it sensible for you to continue being overweight . . Experiencing that physical problem . . because of impressions . . ideas or thoughts . . from other people . . that absorbed into your mind from sometime in your past . . You make your own choices . . And only you . . are responsible . . for yourself . .

Beginning right now . . your subconscious mind . . and all levels of your inner mind . . are realizing that there is no GOOD reason for you to be overweight . .

In your mind now . . you can go anywhere you wish . . you can be in any type of situation . . Do anything you want to do . . Or be anyone you want to be . . (pause) You don't even need to listen to my voice because . . your subconscious mind will hear everything I say . . Your subconscious mind is cooperating while your conscious mind continues relaxing . . not needing to do anything of importance . .

You have altered your rate of breathing . . You are now breathing more easily and freely . . Your heart is pumping blood through your circulatory system more perfectly . . And your blood pressure has come down . . to correspond with the relaxed condition of your body . . And without any conscious effort by you . . your muscles and nerves are now more relaxed and steady . .

So there is nothing really important for your conscious mind to do . . All of these activities are controlled by your subconscious mind . . Your subconscious mind is cooperating by causing . . all of your body processes and activities . . to keep functioning more perfectly every day . .

You are continuing to experience more peaceful . . physical relaxation and comfort . . Notice how good you are feeling now . . It feels wonderful, doesn't it . .

You will find that you are automatically reducing your body weight down . . to the weight level where you want it to be . . as rapidly as your system is ready for your body to reduce . . And your body is healing in a very pleasant way, isn't it . . In a way that is very pleasing . .

Your subconscious mind is causing you to experience very pleasant changes . . And you are allowing your subconscious mind to take whatever time is needed . . to get rid of all of the excess fats and fluids from your body . . To heal your body completely and perfectly . .

Continue relaxing now and in just a moment . . I will give you some additional suggestions . . that will enable you to continue improving . . in all areas of your life . .

PROCEED WITH CONFIDENCE PRESCRIPTION FOLLOWED BY WEIGHT LOSS PRESCRIPTION

20. (Induction)   NOTES . . .

It is your God-given birthright to be healthy . . God did not create anything with the intention of . . having it work incorrectly . .

You were created with an immunity system . . that knows how to function properly . . However, because of misinformation that has gone into your mind . . your immunity system now experiences some difficulty in functioning correctly . . even though it does still know . . how it should be functioning . .

Each part of your body has a specific purpose . . Your heart pumps the blood through your circulatory system . . Your digestive system processes food and provides you with the nutrition . . strength and energy . . where it is needed in your body . . Your elimination system cleanses waste products . . and impurities . . out of your body . . Your glands, your organs, your muscles, nerves, ligaments, tendons and bones . . and all other parts of your body . . Each has specific purposes . .

In a like manner, your immunity system has the important job of . . keeping your body immune . . or protected . . from various diseases and illnesses . . and just as you want all other parts of your body to function properly . . you want your immunity system to do its job perfectly . .

There is a tree in Africa . . that is very special to a particular kind of ant . . The ants spend their entire lifetimes . . living on that tree . . They build their nests from its leaves . . They drink only the sap produced by the tree . . and they eat of the berries that grow on the tree . . They never leave the tree because it provides everything needed . .

If any other insect tries to crawl on the tree . . the ant guards send out an alarm . . and all the other ants come running . . They attack the foreign insect and destroy it . . or drive it away . . This way, they protect the tree from any invaders . . They save the tree and the tree saves them . .

There is a sense in which the human body is comparable to that tree . . and to the ants who live there . .

Our body has a built-in immune system . . It is designed to keep foreign substances out of our body . . It is designed to keep us free . . from all illnesses and diseases . . It is designed to keep our body temperature stabilized . . and to keep us healthy . . at all times . .

If you have a stone in your shoe . . it will probably cause you discomfort . . when you walk . . The best way to get rid of that discomfort is to . . take off your shoe and get the stone out . . And that is the very same way your body reacts . . Any time a foreign substance gets into your system . . that does not belong there . . your system immediately sends troops to that area . . and the foreign substance becomes surrounded . . and is carried out of the body . . through the natural process of the elimination system . .

The immune system is always on guard . . against anything that enters the body . . that could be harmful . . It is known immediately if something is wrong . . and where something is wrong . . and exactly what . . is wrong . . The body processes begin working at once . . to make proper corrections . . and to fix the problem . . It is normal and natural . . for your body to keep your immune system functioning perfectly . . Automatically eliminating any organisms . . that your body does not need . . Your immune system knows how to perform perfectly . . at all times . . The white blood cells do their job perfectly . . overcoming any invading bacteria or virus . . that attempts to enter your body . . in an easy, natural way . . through the normal processes of your elimination system . .

In every way, your mind and body . . are doing their job perfectly . . healing your body . . keeping your body functioning properly . . Let your body take care of itself . . with the same amazing capabilities . . as those ants in Africa . . taking care of their tree . . Automatically doing all of the things needed to heal and to protect . .

Your subconscious mind has the important task of directing . . all of the various activities . . taking place in your body . . and any time a part of any system . . such as your immune system . . is not functioning correctly . . your subconscious mind reviews, explores and examines . . the information in your mind . . and can realize that your mind understood that information . . from the level of understanding you had . . at the time it went into your mind . . And can understand it now . . from a more knowledgeable . . more mature point of view . . and will get the misunderstanding . . corrected . .

And then your mind will work out the solution to the problem . . and cause you to experience changes . . that will heal your body . . including your immune system . . completely and perfectly . .

Scientists have discovered that your entire body . . is in a constant process of developing new cells . . to replace those that have been damaged . . or those that have completed their mission . . These new cells are pure and perfect . . They are pure energy . . And the scientific fact is . . that your immunity system . . is made up of cells that can be replaced . . with new and perfect cells . . that do function properly . .

Permitting yourself to be hypnotized lets your subconscious mind know that you are determined . . to achieve the complete healing . . of your immunity system . . and of your entire body . .

AIDS has controlled your life long enough . . and you are determined that you are going to overcome this problem . . for now and forever . .

I am going to give you some suggestions now . . that will be of great benefit . . to increase the process . . of the complete healing of your immunity system . .

I want you to visualize that radiant, blue light . . coming down onto the top of your head . . That radiant, blue light is pure energy . . from the astral realm . . shining directly onto your head . . pouring energy onto your brain . . You can see your brain glowing now . . vibrating with the energy . . A soft, blue glowing ember . . softly radiating around your brain . . slowly emanating from your cranial mass, into your nervous system and . . blood system at the top of your spine . . Filtering its way downward . . through your spinal column . . You can watch the blue glowing energy . . permeating, all throughout your entire body . . from the top of your head . . all the way down to your toes . . The energy flows . . wrapping itself around your rib cage . . entering every gland and organ in your body . . It has entered your blood stream . . reinforcing the production of white corpuscles . . bringing up their numbers to their proper count . . Your immune system has been weak in certain of the organs and glands of your body . . but the astral flow of blue energy will prime your system . . and rejuvenate any shortfalls you have had in the past . . Your immune system is gaining in the power . . and in the strength . . to replace any dysfunctional cells . . everywhere they are needed . . throughout your body . .

I want you to travel now . . on a complete tour . . through your body . . where ever you want to go . .

Follow the blue glowing light . . through your blood veins . . your glands . . your various organs . . follow the flow of energy . . and be sure it saturates everywhere it is needed . . If there are any organs or glands that you are aware of . . needing special attention . . go there . . concentrating . . to be sure they are permeated with the energy . . For this energy is powerful . .

It is the healing power given directly from God . . and it cannot fail . . because failure is impossible . . at the level of the soul . . (Pause)

Now, I want you to use your imagination . . Imagine your body as being healthy, strong . . and in perfect physical condition . . Imagine your immunity system . . functioning perfectly . . Think of your skin as healthy, smooth and youthful looking . . Think of your circulatory system . . functioning properly . . Producing a sufficient amount of white blood cells to keep your immunity system healthy . .

Get all of these ideas of a healthy, glowing body, in your mind . . Your mind is accepting that image . . and is causing you to experience the changes needed . . to heal your immunity system . . and the rest of your body, perfectly . .

In the past, you have had some doubts . . but those doubts are fading away rapidly . . All doubts are being replaced with a strong sense . . and a feeling of confidence and sureness . . that the healing processes in your body are already beginning to take place . .

It may take a week or two . . or even three weeks for your immunity system to be completely healed . . and functioning perfectly . . But you will be pleased as you notice yourself improving . . more and more each day . .

You may not understand the processes your subconscious mind is using . . to cause your immune system to be healed and function properly . . But that's okay . . You can be pleasantly surprised and very happy . . as you become more and more aware . . of the progress you continue achieving . .

At this very moment, your system is making comfortable adjustments . . Your system is now synthesizing proteins, nutrients and other chemicals and substances in your body . . Rejuvenation is now taking place . .

Your expectations are, naturally, increasing . . and you will be sensing the pleasant changes taking place within you . . You can feel pleased and proud of what you are accomplishing . . The feeling of knowing that it is happening . . gives you a strong sense of satisfaction and contentment . .

When your subconscious mind knows the changes have started . . and the healing processes have begun . . to heal your immunity system . . your subconscious mind will cause one of the fingers on your right hand to raise up . . toward the ceiling . . and remain there until I tell it to go back down . .

(Pause and wait for response. After getting response, tell finger to go back down, then tell client he is doing very good.)

EMERGE - -
You are responding very well to these suggestions . . Now, I want you to rest a few moments . . while your subconscious mind continues to absorb . . all it has been instructed to do . . (Pause)

Now, I am going to begin my count from ONE up to FIVE . . When you hear the count of FIVE . . you will be wide awake and alert . . Feeling refreshed and wonderful . . You will remember everything we have talked about today . .

ONE - Beginning to emerge now . . Move your fingers and toes . . just a little . .

TWO - Waking more now . . Coming up . .

THREE - Your arms and legs are still asleep . . move your arms and legs now . .

FOUR - Take a deep breath now and . .

FIVE - Open your eyes . . feeling good . . feeling wonderful . .

It has been found that those who have been diagnosed . . as having AIDS or ARC . . can overcome the problem . . Those who have overcome the problem . . have revealed about eight different characteristics, about themselves . .

Number one . . they are realistic . . they accept the AIDS diagnosis . . but they do not take it as a death sentence . .

Second, They have a fighting spirit . . refusing to be helpless and hopeless . . and . .

Third . . they have changed their lifestyles . .

Fourth . . They are assertive and have the ability to either avoid . . or to get out of, stressful . . and unproductive situations . .

And the Fifth characteristic is very important . . They are tuned in to their own psychological and physical needs . . and they take care of them . .

A Sixth characteristic they have revealed . . is being able to talk openly about the diagnosis of A.I.D.S. . . or A.R.C. . .

And Seventh . . they accept a personal responsibility for their own health . . and they think of their treating physician as a collaborator . .

And, finally, they become involved in helping to work with others who also have AIDS . .

The fact that you have permitted yourself to be hypnotized . . means that you are realistic . . You have accepted the AIDS diagnosis . . but have not taken it as a death sentence . . and that you have a fighting spirit . . You refuse to be one of those who are helpless and hopeless . .

Therefore, your subconscious mind . . will cooperate with the suggestions I give you . . and will increase the numbers of white cells in your blood system . . and will rebuild your immune system . .

(Metaphor)

I read a story once . . that your subconscious mind can listen to . . therefore, increasing your chance of full recovery by many, many years . .

According to the story . . After God created the world . . He was in the process of setting up the life spans of each creature he had created

. . on the Earth . . And the Ass came to him, asking . . "Lord, How long am I going to live ?"

"Thirty years", answered God . . "Is that all right with you"?

"Oh, Lord", replied the Ass, "That's such a long time . . Just think about the hard life I lead . . From morning to night . . I carry heavy loads . . drag sacks of grain to the mill . . so that others can eat bread . . and I receive nothing in return but kicks and blows . . and it's so hard to remain cheerful . . Please, Lord . . I beg you to relieve me of part of that long life" . .

God took pity on the little Ass and shortened his life span by eighteen years . . The Ass thanked God and went away . .

Next, a Dog appeared . . and God asked the dog . . "How long do you want to live . . Thirty years was too much for the Ass . . Would you be content with that ?"

"Oh, Lord, Please consider how much I must run . . My feet will never be able to hold up that long . . and my bark won't hold up either . . And my teeth for biting will be long gone by then" . .

God saw that the Dog was right . . and so, He shortened his life span by twelve years . .

Next came the Monkey . . "Certainly, you'll want to live thirty years, won't you"? asked God . . "You don't have to work like the Ass or the Dog . . and you're always in a cheerful spirit" . .

"Oh, Lord", said the Monkey, "It just appears that way . . but it's not really so . . I'm always expected to perform pranks and make funny faces . . Yet, whenever I'm handed an apple and I bite into it . . it's always sour . . I'm only putting on a front, you know . . acting happy . . I'll never be able to endure for thirty long years" . .

So, God was merciful and took away ten years of his life span . .

And, finally, Man appeared . . He was joyful . . He was healthy . . Full of energy and vitality . .

And God said to Man, "Surely, you will want to live thirty years" . .

Oh, Lord", Man replied, "Thirty years is way too short . . Why, I'll just have my house, and I will have planted some trees, and I will

71

just be getting a good start on my career . . I'll just be getting ready to enjoy life . . and then I'll have to die ? . .

Please, Lord", he implored, "You've got to give me more time" . .

"Okay", God agreed . . "I'll add on the eighteen years from the Ass" . .

"But . . that's still not enough", said the Man . .

"All right then, I'll add on the twelve years from the Dog" . .

"Still too little", said the Man . .

"Very well, then", said God, "I'll give you the ten years from the Monkey. Now, how's that ?" . .

Man accepted what God dictated . . but was disgruntled . . Still not satisfied . . And has been working hard ever since . . to increase his life span . . And the great thing is . . he is succeeding . .

It has been found that . . man's own mind has the power to cause disease and illness . . But it also has the power to cure any kind of disease or illness . . including AIDS . .

One of the most important steps in being cured . . is to learn to be relaxed . . We live in a world with other people . . and most of those people are tense . . anxious . . and going through some kind of stress . . But by learning how to relax . . as you are doing now . . in these sessions . . you are achieving your emotional stability . .

Being more relaxed . . causes your nerves to continue becoming more steady . . and enables the processes . . and activities of your body . . to function properly . . and causes the white blood cells in your immune system . . to increase . . and rejuvenate . . and rebuild your body's immune system . .

Your subconscious mind understands . . that the chemical activities of your body . . are controlled by small substances called Hormones . . in your blood stream . .

Your Thyroid gland produces something called . . Thyroxin . . and that directs the rate . . at which your body processes work . .

Your mind understands that now . . and is causing your Thyroid gland to increase the speed . . at which your body processes produce white blood cells . . to rejuvenate your body's immune system . .

Your body is a complex organization of glands . . blood vessels . . nerves . . organs . . brain cells, muscles, ligaments and bones . . And you also have a mind that knows exactly . . how to stimulate your body responses . . And coordinate every cell . . every atom and every molecule in your body . . And cause them to function exactly the way . . they were intended to function . . Organs, blood vessels and all tissues in your body . . will become stronger and healthier each day . .

As you become more attuned to relaxation . . you will be more at ease . . going about your daily activities . . And you will continue to be calm and in control . . of every situation and circumstance . . in which you find yourself . . Each day, you will find . . you are more emotionally calmer . . Your nerves will be more relaxed and steadier . . and you will be more at ease in everything you do . .

Take a few moments now to pay attention to the relaxed feeling all over your body . . Memorize it as completely as you can . . Store into your memory, the entire feeling of your whole body in complete relaxation . . You enjoy this peaceful feeling . . and you look forward to re-experiencing this wonderful, restful state of mind in the future . . Each time you are hypnotized . . you will go into a deeper level of hypnosis more quickly and more easily . . (Pause)

In a few moments, I will count to five (5) . . and at the count of 5, you will open your eyes . . You will feel wide awake . . and you will feel wonderfully better for this long and relaxing rest . . You will feel completely relaxed . . both mentally and physically . . You will be more refreshed and more invigorated than you have ever felt in your life . . You will be totally free from all feelings of stress or anxiety . . You will always find hypnosis to be relaxing . . refreshing . . and invigorating . . An experience you truly enjoy . .

Now, the counting begins . . On the count of 5, your eyes will open and you will emerge, feeling wonderfully refreshed and completely relaxed. As though you were awakening from a long nap . . Here we go . .

1 - Coming up now . . Energy and vitality flows through your body . . You are clear from head to foot . . Refreshed, physically, emotionally . .

2 - Rising up now . . coming to the surface . .

3 - Feeling wonderful - wonderful . . for you truly are a wonderful person . .

4 - Your eyes are ready to open as you return to a waking state . .

5 - Open your eyes now, feeling refreshed and alert.

Now, I want you to sink deeper and deeper . . into relaxation . . Deeper and deeper . . Relax and just let your body completely immerse in the velvet world of complete . . relaxation . . All of the sounds fade away . . far into the distance . . and you hear only the sound of my voice . . Going deeper and deeper . . and deeper . .

There are five steps . . in the elimination of an alcoholic problem . . The first step is . . relaxation . .

You must obviously be relaxed . . so that adequate communication can take place . . between yourself and the hypnotherapist . . Therefore . . If for any reason, you are not completely relaxed . . I want you now to completely relax . . Let go of everything . . Let your arms and your legs just relax . . Let it go . . And let your entire body completely relax . . Relax . . Let yourself go completely . . all over your whole body . . Let yourself float in complete, comfortable relaxation . . Let yourself relax . . more than you have ever done before . .

The second point is . . realization . . You are going to be brought to realize. . . some of the causes for your drinking problem . . and understand them completely . . First of all . . in almost every case of a drinking problem . . the person with the drinking problem . . including yourself . . first formulated the problem in his (or her) own mind . . and it stemmed from the deficient Father figure or . . deficient authoritarian figure . . Maybe your own Father was an alcoholic . . or at least, a heavy drinker . . Or, maybe it was your Mother who . . on frequent occasions . . accidentally placed you in a trance-like state . . screaming at you that you were nothing but a bum . . that you're no good for anything . . and that you'll always be nothing but a bum . . just like your Father . . Or a no good drunk . . just like your Father was . . If this never happened to you . . a very similar suggestion has been planted in your subconscious mind . . from somewhere in your childhood . . Your problem may have stemmed from multiple causes . . but you recognize the deficient Father figure in your early upbringing . . You also may recognize a domineering Mother figure . . who gave you everything . . but depleted you of learning responsibility and . . taught you well how to . . manipulate people to have things only your way . .

Whatever it is . . someone in the position of authority has let you down . . and your mind has picked up on this . . causing it to become an integral part of your personality . . even though you do not say so . . And if one of the main causes for alcoholism . . is a deficient Father figure then . . obviously, the formation of a Father figure . . should promote a cure . . However, without there having been a prior insertion of an adequate Father figure . . then we can assume that a vital part of the cause for the problem . . is based on . . a deficient Father figure . .

The second most frequently observed cause of alcoholism . . which appears in over 95% of all cases . . is a great deficiency of Ego . . The alcoholic always says, "I'm no good . . I'm just a bum." . . And if you argue with him when he is drunk . . and you tell him . . "Oh, you're all right." . . He'll say, "No, I'm not. I'm just a bum." Somewhere in his past, an alcoholic has nearly always been kicked. Certainly, nothing is more damaging to the ego for an individual . . than physical abuse from the foot of another individual . . Since emotion dominates the mind . . and, of course, being physically kicked would be fraught with emotions . . it is easy to understand how other suggestions . . of heavy ego damage . . can be implanted in the subconscious mind . . as, at times such as this . .

And so, you are receiving a number of suggestions . . as far as realization goes . . First, you will realize how you came to be . . an alcoholic . . How you had to accept . . a deficient Father figure . . and why the Father figure in your life does not, necessarily, describe you . . You are NOT like your Father . . You never were your Father . . and you are not responsible . . for the choices he made . . in his life . .

Regarding your deficiency of ego . . We are going to work on that and build it up . . From this moment on . . you are going to think well of yourself . . in every way . . You are going to be surprised and amazed . . at what a better person you are going to become . . Not because of what you do but . . because of what you are . . Your composition . . your make up . . the fact that you ARE . . and not who you are . .

From this moment on . . it is imperative that you become completely re-educated . . and to get rid of your old habit patterns . . You finished with realization . . and now, comes re-education . .

From this moment on . . you have NO compulsion to drink . . That has been removed . . You'll be surprised and amazed at how much better you'll feel . . You have lost all desire to run into a bar . . or to buy it at the grocery store . . And you no longer need your drinking friends or associates . .

The bottle is gone for you . . You are no longer interested in alcohol . . in any form . . And all of the suggestions you have heard . . will take complete and thorough effect on you . . from this moment on . .

The fourth point in hypnotherapy for the alcoholic is . . rehabilitation . . That consists of breaking the habit-pattern and . . strengthening the ego . . Think of the habit-pattern as being only a part of yesterday . . And yesterday's habit-pattern, with regard to alcohol, is gone . . And . . your damaged ego . . has been repaired . . This is a dynamic way for treating the alcoholic . . for you to recognize that your drinking was merely a pattern . . and that alcohol, to you, is very distasteful . . You have NO desire for it in any form . . and should you ever taste it . . it will be VERY distasteful to you . . Your ego is strengthened and these suggestions are being firmly reinforced . . Which is the fifth point . . And they will continue to be reinforced . . over and over again . . until you have won . .

Now, I want you to go deeper and deeper . . to relax yourself a little longer . . Deeper now . . Go deeper . . Just relax a little longer . . while your subconscious mind takes over . . sorting through the meaning of it all . . (Pause)

When you awaken . . you will easily remember everything I have said to you today . . you will feel refreshed and alert . . and you will feel a much stronger awareness for attaining your goals . .

I am now going to count to five and at the count of five . . you will feel wide awake . . alert and refreshed . . you'll be completely relaxed and invigorated . . with the knowledge you have gained . .

One . . Coming up now . . Feel the energy and the vigor flow through your body. Head to foot, you feel refreshed . . physically and mentally . .

Two . . Rising up now . . Coming to the surface . .

Three . . Feeling wonderful . . For you truly are . . a wonderful person . .

Four . . More alert . . More and more aware . . you feel vigorous . . energetic.

Five . . Open your eyes now . . feeling refreshed and awake . .

As you go deeper and deeper into relaxation . . all of the sounds fade into the background . .

Deeper and deeper . . Relax and just let your body completely immerse in the velvet world of complete relaxation . . All of the sounds fade away . . far into the distance . . and you hear only the sound of my voice . . Going deeper and deeper . . and deeper . . Listen carefully to the sound of my voice . .

We are going to remove a number of negative suggestions . . which have been in your mind for some time now . . We are going to remove them completely . . And as you carefully consider them . . we are going to simply dissolve them . . Throw them out of your mind completely and forever . . Nothing disturbs you and nothing bothers you . . You are completely relaxed . . and nothing will distract you from listening to the sound . . of my voice . . or from completely accepting . . everything I tell you . . For your subconscious mind understands that . . everything I tell you is the absolute truth to you . . And we are going to remove all suggestions from your mind . . that have been detrimental to you in the past . .

The first suggestion you have had in your mind was that, somehow . . you thought alcohol was of some value . . of some use to you . . Drinking alcohol has never been of any use to you . . It has never given you any benefit . . It does not make you relax . . It does not help you to sleep well . . It does not do anything to help you . . The fact is . . it ruins your efficiency . . It robs you of your ability to make sound judgments . . and it makes you look foolish in front of your friends and relatives . . Consequently . . you are through drinking alcohol for any reason . . The suggestion in your mind that alcohol has ever been beneficial to you . . in any way . . will be completely removed from your mind . . I am going to count to five . . and that suggestion will be completely removed from your mind . . Never . . never . . to return . . One . . Two . . Three . . Four . . Five . .

The next suggestion that you may have accepted . . is that alcohol is a good means of punishing yourself . . In the first place . . you are through punishing yourself . .

And in the second place . . you are through using alcohol as a means to do it . . You are through punishing yourself . . and you are through using alcohol . . as a means to do it . . The only reason anyone ever punishes them self is because . . deep in their mind . . they feels guilty . . and you will no longer allow yourself . . to feel guilty . . And so, we are going to remove the feelings of guilt . . whatever it is caused by . . We will eliminate the need for you to punished yourself . . and there will no longer be a need for alcohol . . to be used as a means of achieving that punishment . . One . . Two . . Three . . Four . . Five . . The punishment and the guilt are gone from your life . .

Alcohol, to you, is a poison . . and a lousy, inefficient poison at that . . Just enough poison to make you sick and ineffective . . But now, you are through poisoning yourself . . You are through using alcohol . . for any reason . . And so, that need to poison yourself with alcohol . . is permanently removed from your mind . . One . . Two . . Three . . Four . . Five . .

Now, we are going to remove any and all connections . . that alcohol has in your mind . . the only kind of alcohol that you care about . . or know anything about . . any more is . . rubbing alcohol . . and the only use to which you put the rubbing alcohol . . is to rub it on your skin, if necessary . . It is wonderful for that . . It makes a nice back rub . . and that is all it means to you . . As a beverage . . it is completely out . . And so, you remove all connections in your mind . . that have to do with alcohol . . as a part of your life . . You don't even think of it . . you don't ask for it . . You don't desire it in any form . . Even if offered to you . . you refuse it . . because you know it is disgusting . . foul tasting . . and vomit producing . . One . . Two . . Three . . Four . . Five . . All connections to alcohol . . in your mind . . have been removed . .

And so, all these negative suggestions you had acquired . . are now removed from your mind . . And all of the positive suggestions which I have given you . . will now replace them, at the count of five . . One . . Two . . Three . . Four . . Five . .

From this moment on, you are free . . Free from the specter of alcohol . . Free from its entangling, octopus-like tentacles . . Free from its degrading, self-punishing nature . . Free from its ruination . .

Free from its ability to wreck your life . . You are completely free now . . Because . . all of the connections in your mind . . with alcoholic beverages . . have been completely removed . . The wires have all been pulled out . . and you are unable to restore them . . Just imagine a big, telephone switchboard in your head . . and we have pulled out all of the wires connected to the hole marked 'Alcohol' . . so that, even if something does get plugged into it . . nothing will happen . . You don't want it . . You don't buy it . . You don't drink it . . and if offered, you would refuse it . . It is disgusting to you . . Tastes foul . . has a terrible affect on your mentality and makes you sick to your stomach . . to even think about it . . It is completely gone from your life . . One . . Two . . Three . . Four . . Five . .

Now, you are going to be completely successful . . in every way . . And surprised and amazed at the self-control and self-discipline . . and confidence . . that you have in yourself . . knowing that you have licked the problem . . and that it will stay that way . .

Now . . I want you to go deeper . . Deeper . . and relax . . Deeper and deeper . . Your mind concentrates only on my voice . . and you go deeper . . Completely relaxed now . . Just relax . . (pause)

In a moment . . I am going to count from Five . . down to One . . When I get to the count of one . . you will be wide awake . . feeling revitalized . . and you will remember everything we have discussed today.

Starting with Five - You are beginning to come up now . .

Four - Your senses are awakening . . Your mind is becoming more alert . .

Three - You are feeling more alive . . more alert . . Feeling wonderful . . after a long rest . .

Two - Feeling wonderful now . . Your fingers and hands want too stir . . Take a deep breath . .

And One - Open your eyes now . . You are alert and aware of everything around you . .

You are very deep now . . And as you go deeper and deeper into relaxation . . the sounds have faded away . . Deeper . . Deeper . . Relax and hear only the sound of my voice . . Relax . . Relax completely . . Let everything go as you sink firmly and comfortably . . into complete relaxation . . Nothing will disturb you . . Nothing will penetrate your mind . . but my voice . . Just relax . . relax . . You sink deeper and deeper with every breath you take . . Deeper . . Complete relaxation . .

In the past, Alcohol . . may have been something that meant life . . in your mind . . You may have accepted a suggestion . . that somehow . . alcohol saves lives . . or alcohol protects you from being injured . . Or would keep you warm on a cold night . . That, somehow, alcohol was good for you . .

But that was yesterday . . Yes, all that was yesterday . . Alcohol never saved you from injury . . and it never saved your life . . To some people . . Alcohol is a medicine . . so terribly necessary . . And those suggestions may have been good suggestions . . at one time . . but they have outlived their usefulness . . And if any of those suggestions are present . . to any degree . . in your mind . . they are completely removed . . as of now . . And this suggestion . . to remove them . . has a complete and thorough presiding effect . . upon your mind . . body . . and spirit . .

Now, to other people . . alcohol means DEATH . . It is used as a way of punishing oneself . . It is a poison . . and some people want to poison themselves . . It is a method of slow, suicide . . How nice . . Well, you don't need that either . . If alcohol ever meant death . . or suicide to you . . and you had a need to punish yourself . . those needs are now gone from your mind . . as we remove those suggestions from your thinking . .

The truth of the matter is . . alcohol is just that . . Alcohol . . It is not life . . it is not death . . It is not anything to you . . anymore . . It is nothing . . It merely represents a very bad habit that you don't need in your life anymore . . You don't need it . . Nor do you want it . . You have lost all of your desire for using alcohol, ever again . .

You are only interested in life and good health . . You are interested in coffee and tea . . hot or iced . . and especially, when it is good . . Unless you are limiting your caffeine intake . . in which case . . the last suggestion for coffee and tea is removed . . There are many other beverages that you like . . and you can drink . . There is milk and cocoa . . and many soft drinks . . or athletic drinks . . a number of which I know you enjoy . . But the one that will do you more harm than good . . and the one you care nothing about anymore . . is alcohol . . Stay away from that one . . Alcohol may have saved your life . . or protected you . . or it was a means of self-punishment . .

But that was yesterday . . When you ran yourself down and . . lost your ego . . That was yesterday . . When you thought so little of yourself . . That was yesterday . . When you made yourself into a failure . . When you were a complete fool in front of your friends and relatives . . Yes, that was yesterday . .

But this is not yesterday . . This is today . . And today is when you put alcohol aside forever . . And with that alcohol . . goes all of the other means of self-punishment . . All of the fears . . the anxieties . . the throbbing head . . the sickness in your stomach . . All of it . . You do not need any of it . . Today is the day you become successful . . the day you begin to care about yourself . . The day you will change your life forever . . with no regrets . .

Today is the day you have waited for . . the day in which you will strive toward the goals . . you have wanted to accomplish . . Today is the day in which you will have . . a nice, clean cut appearance . . In which you feel proudly sober . . and can think straight with reason . . and can make decisions based on good judgment . . and past experiences . . Today is the day in which you start loving yourself . . and appreciating yourself . . for the really good and wise . . and intelligent individual . . that you truly are . . Today is the day . .

Today is the day in which you turn yourself over . . and turn your life into something higher . . than just yourself . . Not only to a higher principle . . but to a higher power . . Let that power run your life . . Today is the day you will bury . . all of your past mistakes . . and make something out of yourself . . Today is the day that you wipe failure . . out of your book of life . . and replace it with success . . And that 'success' is going to become so meaningful to you . . in a very personal way . .

To be completely succinct about this . . today is the day you throw alcohol away . . You throw it away for good . . You do not need it and you will never need it . . You cannot want it . . and you will never want it . . You cannot desire it and . . you do not have any desire for it . . You are through with alcohol . . You do not need it . . You do not want it . . and you cannot drink it . . You know how it tastes . . You know how it makes you act . . and how it makes you feel . .

From this moment on you are going to enjoy life fully in every way . . You will feel happy . . Live, laugh, love and be happy . . For that is what today means to you . . Now, all of these suggestions take complete and thorough effect upon your mind . . body and spirit . . as you sink deeper and deeper . . into full and complete relaxation . . And they seal themselves into your subconscious mind . . And they reinforce themselves . . over and over again . . Relax now . . Just relax completely . . (pause)

I am going to give you a period of silence . . for all of this to take effect in your subconscious mind . . and that period of silence begins now. (Pause)

In just a moment now . . I am going to count to five . . When you hear the number FIVE . . you will awaken . . feeling happy and content . . refreshed and alert . .

One - Your mind is back in reality now . .

Two - You are coming up quickly . . feeling rested and refreshed . .

Three - Your body is wanting to stir . . Move your toes and your fingers . .

Four - Move your arms and your legs . . Take a deep breath now . .

Five - Open your eyes and breathe deeply . . How do you feel ? . .

As you go deeper and deeper into relaxation . . all of the sounds fade away into the background . . Going deeper and deeper . . Relax and hear only the sound of my voice . . Relax . . Relax completely . . Now, allow yourself to go even deeper . . deeper relaxed . . completely relaxed . . Every muscle and every fiber of your being . . completely relaxed . . Just let it all go . . relax . . just relax . .

To an individual who has had a drinking problem . . Alcohol is poison . . It is poison in two ways. First of all . . it is poison because it breaks down the very will power . . the very . . ego . . the very faith in oneself . . that the individual has been able to build up . . And so, it is a PSYCHOLOGICAL poison because . . having once conquered the alcohol problem . . if you ever allow it to get back into you again . . then you begin thinking negatively about yourself . . All of the bad thoughts you had about yourself before . . Namely . . Well, I really am no good anyway . . I really didn't lick it after all . . And so on . . You see, it really is a psychological problem, isn't it . .

Now, in addition to that . . for anyone who has ever had an alcoholic problem . . it is a PHYSICAL poison . . It actually does poison your system . . because you are allergic to alcohol . . Just like other people are allergic to other things . . And so, when you are allergic to something . . even penicillin . . it is poison to you and you must never take it . . The same is true with alcohol . . When you are allergic to it . . you must never take it . . You are through with it . . or you will die because of it . .

Now you know . . that you are allergic to alcohol . . and alcohol is a poison to you . . Usually, the reason why one is drawn to alcohol is not for most of the reasons people prescribe . . "That it makes me feel good" or "I like the taste of it" . . and other things . . You have heard them . . On the contrary . . almost every person who has had a problem with alcohol will tell you . . just the opposite . . "I do not like it . . It is ruining my life . . It is terrible" . . And, if that is true . . why are they drawn to it ? . . For precisely that reason . . Because it IS a poison . . and because, they . . in their subconscious minds . . feel the need to commit suicide . . And so, they do the slow, torturous way out . . They, literally, drink themselves to death . .

And that is why it is so important . . that the underlying cause of the problem be completely removed . . So that you will never have to punish yourself again . . with alcohol . . And that is why we removed all of those underlying causes . . No, you do not need to punish yourself anymore . . because you realize that you were not guilty of anything . . to begin with . . And if you were not guilty . . you have no reason to punish yourself . . Besides, that is God's domain . . And you have no right taking it over . . He does the judging as well as the punishing . . according to His laws and His ideals . . And now, since you are through punishing yourself . . you are also through poisoning yourself . .

And alcohol IS a poison . . It is important that you recognize it as a poison . . And you are leaving all poisons alone . . because you do not need poisons in your life . . anymore . . You do not need to poison yourself . . You do not need to punish yourself . . You are through with all of that . . From now on . . you are going to appreciate yourself . . It is what you are going to do . . Appreciate yourself for the God-given talents that you are blessed with . . For the fact that you have a good life . . and for all the good you can do with that life . . For yourself . . and for those who love you . .

In talking about alcohol . . we often say . . "He certainly got stiff" . . But that is the same term we use for . . a corpse . . We say . . "Gee, He's dead drunk" . . Interesting, isn't it, how 'DEAD' and 'DRUNK' go together . . You are through with alcohol . . You do not even smell it . . You are just beginning to appreciate yourself . . to value yourself . . your mind . . and your body . . and to make them really work for you . . to be the person that you truly want to be . .

You are going to make yourself happier . . and you are going to make others happy . . by staying sober . . By avoiding, completely . . like the plague . . any compound which you are allergic to . . And alcohol, especially . . For you are most allergic to that . . You have won a great victory . . in forever placing alcohol behind you . . For, in so doing . . you have now placed a beautiful future before you . . And no matter what may befall you . . good, bad or indifferent . . it is so much better and happier . . and easier for everyone . . for you to face your future sober . . than as a drunk . .

Indeed, you are going to have twice the fun, sober . . than you ever had . . as a drunk . . Because drunk . . you never had any fun . . You were only using alcohol as a means to punish yourself . . To poison yourself . . To get rid of yourself . . To 'stiffen' yourself up . . and to be 'dead drunk' . . perhaps in a ritualistic preparation . . And you almost succeeded in that . .

But you have removed all those thoughts from your mind . . and you are now on a course to build yourself up . . From now on, you are going to appreciate yourself . . compliment yourself . . and take good care of yourself . .

You are going to feel wonderful . . and you are going to be wonderful . . because you truly are . . a wonderful person . . You are going to build yourself up . . more and more . . and more . . with every breath you take . . as you go deeper and deeper . . deeply relaxed . . deeper and deeper, as you relax . . You are going to remember . . everything you have heard in these past sessions . . And all of the suggestions you have received . . will be reinforced in your mind, again and again . . every single day of your life . .

I want you to relax now . . Go deeper and just relax . . as your subconscious mind takes over . . absorbing . . ratifying . . and instilling within itself . . everything you need . . to help you be the person . . you are to become . . And may God be with you . . wherever you go . . (pause)

I will give you another moment of silence . . (pause)

I am now going to count to Five . . and at the count of Five . . you will feel wide awake . . alert and refreshed . . You'll be completely relaxed and invigorated . . with the knowledge and satisfaction of your accomplishments . .

One . . You are coming up now . . you feel the energy and the vigor flowing through your body . . From head to foot, you are feeling refreshed . . both physically and mentally . .

Two . . Rising up now . . Coming to the surface . .

Three . . Feeling wonderful . . wonderful . . for you are, truly, a wonderful person . .

Four . . Now you are more alert . . more and more aware . . You feel vigorous . . energetic . . and so relaxed over your entire body . .

Five . . Open your eyes now . . Refreshed and awake . .
Congratulations . . You have completed the Four Session Program . .

I am going to give you some suggestions now . . for your subconscious mind to absorb . . These will be very beneficial . . in helping you to overcome this problem you are having . .

The word, "Allergic", has been misused and improperly used . . by many persons for many years . . For example . . people often use the word, allergic, when they talk about something they dislike . . and they often use it when they are talking about a certain characteristic . . or physical feature . . that they do not like . . But medically, the words, "Allergy" or "Allergic", pertain to a condition, or to a sensitivity . . to some substance . . Usually, it is caused by a protein, which is called, an "Allergen" . .

A person who is allergic, will react in a way that is different . . from the way others react . . when they eat . . inhale . . or touch the allergen . .

An allergy is actually a very normal, protective reaction of the body . . However, there are times when the allergy is being misused by the body . . I will explain what I mean by that . . If a person inhales a harmful irritant or bacterial toxin . . it is normal for a watery secretion to come out of the nose . . or the eyes . . That is the normal way the body reacts . . to cleanse the harmful irritant . . or bacterial toxin . . out of the body . . Thus, keeping it . . in its healthy condition . .

That is a natural reaction to a natural allergy . . But it is not normal . . and can be very distressing for a person's nasal, to drip . . just because they get near grass . . or too near a dog or a cat . .

The reason some people become allergic while others do not . . has been a mystery for many years . . The medical profession has been baffled as to the reason . . some people develop a runny nose or hay fever . . because of night air . . or because of rainy weather . . or from breathing the same dust that other people breathe . . And yet, most people are not bothered by any of these things . .

In recent years . . studies have revealed that thoughts . . or ideas . . in a person's mind can cause allergic conditions to develop . . By saying that thoughts or ideas in the mind causes . . allergenic conditions to develop . . does not mean a person wants to have those allergies . .

People do not want to have hay fever or asthmatic attacks . . But it is the thoughts or ideas which create misunderstandings . . in the subconscious level of the mind . . that causes those conditions to develop . .

Tension and stress have also been found to cause asthma . . eczema, hay fever, hives . . and other types of allergic reactions . . Emotional factors, anxiety . . and even grief . . are often found to be the cause . . of those conditions . .

In most cases involving allergenic conditions . . it has been found that the situation . . or circumstance . . which caused the condition to develop . . has changed . . But the person continues to have the allergy because . . it has become a learned response in the mind . . In other words . . the subconscious level of the mind causes the allergic condition to continue . . merely because it has become a habit . . However . . anything the mind has caused . . the mind can also cure . .

Your subconscious mind is, now, understanding what I have been telling you . . and is causing all of your body processes . . to function properly . . and to cleanse all impurities out of your body . . and eliminate the allergic symptoms you have been experiencing . .

You are going to experience a change in your life . . because, right now, your mind is releasing those thoughts, ideas, imprints and impressions . . that caused the allergies to develop . .

The usual pattern of being allergic will never be the same again . . Beginning right now . . Your subconscious mind is with the understanding . . that you want to be rid of all unnatural allergies . . And allergies will never control your way of life again . .

In going through various experiences . . during your normal, every day living . . your subconscious mind has received information . . that caused you to develop the habit . . of being allergic . . But your subconscious mind is now understanding . . that the information you received . . was erroneous . . It was misunderstood . . and you want it to be understood correctly now . . from a more knowledgeable . . more mature . . point of view . . You want it to be changed and corrected and . . you want the processes of your body to function properly . . and cleanse out all impurities and substances . . which have any allergenic elements . . from your body . . through the natural processes of your elimination system . .

Your subconscious mind will now cause you to become desensitized . . to all substances and conditions which . . in the past . . have caused you to suffer with allergic reactions . .

You now, refuse to maintain those unnatural allergies . . Your subconscious mind is now getting rid of the habit . . of responding to the situations and conditions . . that caused you to experience those allergies in the first place . .

You are continuing to relax even more peacefully now . . and your subconscious mind is accepting . . all of my suggestions . . and is improving your health . . And is enabling you to live your life in a more peaceful . . more calm, more relaxed way . . with no allergenic conditions . .

Each day, these suggestions will become even more effective . . you are learning to use these principles of relaxation . . which you are now experiencing . . in all phases if your daily life . . And they will keep you calm and relaxed . . at all times . .

In every situation or circumstance . . that comes up in your life . . you will remain calm and relaxed . . Your nerves will be relaxed and steady . . and you'll be able to do everything in a relaxed way . . You will be able to cope with . . every day changing circumstances . . in a loving, peaceful way . .

Regardless of what comes up in your life . . you will be in control of your emotions and feelings . . That is what will cause the allergenic reactions . . to keep fading away . . more and more . . And soon they will be gone from your life completely . .

Now, I am going to count from 1 to 5 . . and on the count of 5 . . you will open your eyes . . to an alert, waking state . . feeling clear of mind, relaxed and wonderful . . for you are, truly, a wonderful and confident person . . I will begin . .

One.   You will remember everything with complete understanding . .
Two.   You are now connected to your inner supporting strength . .
Three. Everything I have told you is true . . and is already happening . .
Four.   Beginning to be more aware of your body now . .
Five.   Let your hands and feet move a little . . Stir and stretch as you open your eyes, feeling clear, rested and wonderful . .

ANGER - CONTROL

You are now in a pleasant state of relaxation . . Continue to relax as I talk to you . . about how you can develop more control in your life . .

A woman came into my office to be hypnotized . . for overcoming a problem of anger . . She was experiencing anger towards her friends . . towards her neighbors and towards her loved ones . . She was also experiencing arthritis . . but didn't realize that it was her own mind . . that had caused her to develop arthritis . . as a result of her continuous inner anger . .

After discussing her problem, she said, "I'm going to stop giving everyone a piece of my mind and start speaking from my peace of mind".

Much useful energy that could be used for creative thinking . . creative doing and creative living . . is wasted, when tempers get out of control . . It merely causes adverse situations . . to become worse . . It is a waste of energy . . No one benefits from it . . However, if we learn to be loving and kind . . we remain peaceful, regardless of what goes on around us . .

Each morning, when I come to the office . . I stop for a few minutes at a little pond on the way . . It has a fountain and there is continuous flowing water into the pond . . And in the pond, there are a number of different kinds of colored goldfish . . In the calm, I listen to the gentle sounds of the water . . splashing its way from the fountain, into the pond . . And I see, in this peaceful activity, my need to be peaceful in all situations . . The water flows into the pond, continuously . . without being anxious, worried, fearful or hurried . . When I leave the pond, I bring this peaceful tranquility with me . . It enables me to live my life with a wonderful feeling of complete peace . . flowing through me, at all times . .

Whatever has been the cause for you to develop anger . . the subconscious part of your mind is realizing . . that you are the only one . . who is hurt by your anger . . emotionally and spiritually . . Each of us is an individual . . And each individual has beliefs that differ . . from every other person . . Each person makes his own choices in life and commits to his own actions . .

We cannot control the actions of another person . . The only control we have is over ourselves, in the way we let another person's actions affect us . . We cannot change another person's actions . . However, we can change the way we allow ourselves to respond to those actions . .

No matter how we may want another person to think or to speak . . Regardless of how we may want that other person to act . . we cannot change that other person . . Any more than we can change lemonade into root beer . . or lead into gold . . We may want every person to be loving, kind and generous . . but we cannot make anyone become that way . . We can do our best to influence them but . . the only one we can really change is the one . . inside our own body . .

It is important to learn to accept people as they are . . By doing that . . and by not expecting everyone to be the way we want them to be . . it enables us to enjoy life as it comes to us . . As it truly is . . By accepting people as they truly are . . we begin noticing their good qualities . . their good attributes . . and their good achievements . . which are deserving of praise . . And we become more and more willing to provide that praise . .

In the future . . if you feel that another person is taking advantage of you . . you will think of water . . Think of that peaceful fountain, flowing into the pond with the goldfish, swimming peacefully . . You will remain calm and relaxed . . You will speak up in your own defense . . with clarity . . but with kindness . . Without being offensive . . or feeling offended . .

Each day your confidence will continue to increase . . and you will become more sensitive to the emotional needs of those around you . . By doing so, you will attract many people who will look upon you as a friend . . to whom they can come for advise and comfort . . And there will be many of whom you, too, will look upon as friends . . Every day will keep becoming happier and more enjoyable . . For you will be enriching the lives of those around you, in so many ways . .

By making this connection to your subconscious mind . . you are enabling yourself to gain more confidence in yourself . . Confidence that says you will not only control your bursts of anger . . but you will stifle them completely . . Within yourself, you are realizing that you are, indeed, an outgoing, kind and friendly person . . These are attitudes and characteristics which you already possess . .

And the subconscious part of your mind . . is causing you to freely express those attitudes and characteristics . . in an appropriate and welcome manner . .

As time continues, the pleasures of your relationships with others . . will keep increasing . . And they will cause you to discover new depths of appreciation for life . . and the lives of those around you . . And they will increase your ability to experience a far more satisfying life . . From now on your life will be much richer and far more rewarding . . than you have ever experienced it to be . .

EMERGE

I am going to count from 1 to 5 now . . and on the count of 5 . . you will open your eyes . . to an alert, waking state . . You will feel clear of mind, relaxed and wonderful . . for you are a wonderful and confident person . . Relax . . as I begin . .

One.   You will remember everything you have experienced with complete understanding . .

Two.   You are now connected to your inner supporting strength . .

Three. Everything I have told you is true . . and is already happening . .

Four.   Beginning to be more aware of your body as it fully awakens and wants to stir . .

Five.   Let your hands and feet move now . .   Stir and stretch . . as you open your eyes   . .

You are very deep now and you continue drifting . . into a deeper hypnotic state . . You are beneath the trees . . deep in the forest . . You are walking along a path . . through the woods . . as you continue moving into the deepest . . hypnotic state you can . . Deeper . . Deeper still . .

Enjoy the beautiful trees . . and the scenery . . in the woods . . The creek is home for many fish . . in its sparkling waters . . surrounded by huge boulders . .

Beside the path in front of you . . there is another huge boulder . . about waist high . . Leaning against the boulder is a large, 25 pound hammer . . with a long handle . . Nod your head when you can see the hammer . . (Pause for response.)

As you are walking over to pick up that hammer . . you are aware that the boulder represents . . all of the pent up anger you have been feeling for a long time now . . It symbolizes all of the frustrations . . All of the resentments . . the hostilities . . Everything that has been boiling up inside you . . for so long now . . You have kept them hidden deep inside you . . You have done well . . But now you understand . . that it has all accumulated there . . in that massive stone, in front of you . .

(If the frustration and anger was caused by a particular person, suggest that the stone be a sculpture of that person , or of himself.)

You are picking up that hammer now . . and you are beginning to smash the boulder with that big hammer . . Hitting it harder and harder . . again and again . . Getting rid of all that frustration and anger that has built up inside of you for so long . . Hit it again now . . That's it . . Hit it again ! You are free to smash that boulder as long as you need to . . To get rid of all that frustration and anger . . Each time you swing that hammer down . . pieces of it will break off and crumble . . And you will keep hitting it until it is completely demolished . . Now, hit it again . . Hit it harder . . Get rid of all the anger . . Keep hitting that boulder . . You are eliminating all of that anger from your system . . Pound on it until it is completely shattered . .

And by the time it is shattered into dust . . you will have gotten all of those feelings of frustration and anger . . out of your system . .

Those feelings will be gone from your life forever . . Keep it going . . Hit it again now . . (pause)

When you feel you have eliminated all the frustration and anger within you . . lift up one finger on your right hand and leave it there until I tell it to go back down . .

(After finger has lifted - continue with the following suggestion.)

You can drop the hammer now and . . continue your walk along the path through the woods . . Just ahead, you see a beautiful meadow . . with wild flowers in bloom . . And there is a nice, gentle brook . . flowing through the meadow . . with big, brown trout swimming in it . . The sun is shining comfortably . . and a soft, gentle breeze is blowing . . You follow the stream until you notice a large shade tree nearby . . You walk to the tree and sit underneath it . . Leaning your back against the large tree . . and watching the water flowing gently by . . your subconscious mind is now reviewing all of the events . . that had caused your frustration and anger . . and what brought you to this point in your life . . You continue watching the flowing water . . Your subconscious mind is making sure it understands . . all of the causes and all of the affects . . And it will work out the solution completely . . and permanently . .

When your subconscious mind fully understands . . what has been causing the anger . . and knows how to resolve the problem . . so that it will be permanently overcome . . one of the fingers on your right hand will lift up toward the ceiling . . And your finger will remain up . . until I tell it to go back down . .

I want you to take notice of your toes . . on your left foot . . In a moment, you will become aware of a tingling sensation in your toes . . When you notice that feeling . . one of the fingers on your left hand will lift up . . and will remain up . . until I tell it to go back down . .

(Wait for response, then tell finger to go down.)

Good . . Your subconscious mind is responding well . . to everything I say . .

Now, I want you to notice how the tingling sensation is spreading . . through your foot . . and when it has spread up to your ankle . . a finger on your left hand will lift up again . . and will remain up . . until I tell it to go back down . . And after I tell your finger to go back down . . you will notice that pleasant . . tingling sensation . . moving up your leg and spreading into your . . whole body . . Those enjoyable sensations are coming . . from your own good feelings about yourself . . They are coming from the good experiences . . recorded in your subconscious mind . . and are increasing your feelings of respect and love . . for yourself . . and for others . .

Now, you are feeling very good about what you have accomplished . . You have desensitized yourself from any anger or frustration . . You have depleted all of that anger from your psyche . . your inner self . . It is now gone from your life completely . . and you have come to realize . . that you are indeed, a loving . . caring person . . and you will keep feeling better about yourself . . as each day passes, from now on . .

You are continuing to relax even more now . . and your subconscious mind is accepting . . my suggestions . . and is improving your mind set . . and is enabling you to live your life in a more peaceful . . more calm, more relaxed way . .

Each day, these suggestions will become even more effective . . you are learning to use these principles of relaxation . . which you are now experiencing . . in all phases if your daily life . . and that will keep you calm and relaxed . . at all times . .

In every situation or circumstance . . that comes up in your life . . you will be calm and relaxed . . Your nerves will be relaxed and steady . . And you'll be able to do everything in a relaxed way . . You will be able to cope with . . every day changing circumstances . . in a loving, peaceful manner . .

Regardless of what comes up in your life . . you will be in control of your emotions and feelings . . And that is what will cause the angry outbursts and reactions . . to keep fading away . . more and more . . And soon they will be gone from your life completely . . Now continue to relax, for just another moment . . (pause)

Now, I am going to count from 1 to 5 . . and on the count of 5 . . you will open your eyes . . to an alert, waking state . . feeling clear of mind, rested and wonderful . . for you are a wonderful and confident person . . I will begin. . .

One.   You will remember everything you have experienced with complete understanding . .

Two.   You are now connected to your inner supporting strength . .

Three. Everything I have told you is true . . and is already happening . .

Four.   Beginning to be more aware of your body as it fully awakens and wants to stir . .

Five.   Let your hands and feet move . . Stir and stretch as you open your eyes, feeling clearly inspired, rested and wonderful . .

010 Prescript.   ANGER - TEMPER CONTROL
(Follow Relaxation)

You will continue drifting into a deeper . . and more peaceful state of relaxation . . Drifting deeper now . . DEEPER . . DEEPER . . and DEEPER . . All other sounds are in the far distance . . except for the sound of my voice . . There may be times when you don't hear my voice . . and that is okay because . . your subconscious mind is aware of everything I am saying . . As you go DEEPER . . and DEEPER into a restful state of complete relaxation . . It is so peaceful . . as you sink down deeper and DEEPER . . into a blissful state of relaxation . . Going just a little deeper . . with every breath you take . . It is so good . . to be calm . . and sedate . . So peaceful here . . Just relax . . (Pause)

Now, I am going to talk to you . . about a problem you are having . . Then, we're going to make some adjustments . . to get you to a level . . where your actions will be more acceptable . .

How many times have you heard someone ask . . "Why don't you control your temper?" . . The one thing that is even more important . . than controlling one's temper . . is finding out why the temper needs to be controlled . . Every one of us has a temper, of some sort . . We use the word, 'temper' in connection with steel . . And then, we say, we should be tempered . . And we talk about an 'even temper' . . What does that mean ? . . Simply put, it means, we don't allow ourselves . . to get out of control . . So, what is, 'control'? . . Basically, it's a state of reason . . And when the emotions get too strong for the state of reason . . then we lose control . . Obeying only our emotions . . And we are said to have 'lost our temper' . . So, temper is a good thing . . Tempered steel is stronger . . It's when we lose the temper, that the troubles begin . . And we DON'T want to lose . . the temper . .

And so, we wonder why it is that, occasionally . . we do lose our temper . . We lose our temper because . . we allow an emotion . . to get out of hand . . And how does that happen ? . . An emotion gets out of hand, not because of what's happening around us . . but because the event we are involved in . . triggers an emotional memory from our past . .

96

For example, if you had a reason . . a long time ago . . to really hate someone . . To get mad enough to want to fight . . but you couldn't fight them . . and win . . And you were beaten down . .

Another example . . What if you were in a bad car accident . . and you wanted to lash out at the person who smashed your car . . and cost you so much money . . But you can't lash out at them . . You couldn't, at the time, and you can't now . .

So, when an opportunity comes . . the trigger mechanism fires you off . . You can lash all the hostility at this new individual . . and take it out on them . . instead of on the individual that you really wanted to express the hostility toward . . Maybe you became raging mad at your parents . . or your friends . . or the boss . . So, along comes a waitress or a telephone operator . . Someone you are in contact with, that you have the edge over . . And that you can either verbally . . or physically beat up on . . Someone who can't talk back to you or can't give you any trouble . . Perhaps, someone much younger than you . . Someone you can dominate your power over . .

And so, you have found an outlet for your temper . . For your hostility . . Because, here is a place where you are safe . . Where you won't get hurt . . and you can let the hostility out . . And so, the hostility is vented, at last . . and you have lost your temper . . once more . . So, now what ? . .

One of the ways to prevent this . . is to control it . . One of the ways to hold it back is to say . . "I'm not gon'na let that happen" . . But that's like slamming the lid down on a boiling tea kettle . . It only makes it worse the next time . . And you have found that to be true . . haven't you . .

Now, another good method for controlling the loss of your temper is . . when it is eminent that you will lose your temper . . you will picture in your mind . . the real person or situation where you first felt the hostility . . The real person you are mad at . . and you'll say to yourself . . "Wait a minute . . I'm not mad at this individual, confronting me now . . The only reason I'm losing my temper now . . is because of the trigger that reminds me of the incident, in the past . . when I wanted to express my hostility, but couldn't" . . That is what you will say to yourself . . And it will prevent a great many losses of temper . . Especially fortunate . . in unfortunate circumstances . .

But, there is yet another important area . . And that area . . which allows for the possibility of control . . involves releasing hostility in other ways . . Like letting steam out of the boiling tea kettle, rather than holding it back . . We're going to add an escape valve . . so you can let off a little steam now and then . . Now, there are many ways you can do just that . . while causing no harm to anyone . . I can't say exactly how you can do it . . but I will propose a suggestion, which is . . You are going to find particular ways . . of letting off steam . . And you're going to let it off . . so that you don't 'blow up', as you have in the past . . And as you're threatening to do in the future . .

One thing you can do is to put up a punching bag . . and punch the hell out of it . . whenever you feel frustrated . . You can label that punching bag, anything you want to . . Hang a sign on it . . or a picture . . and get it out of your system . .

Another thing you can do . . Every morning, for a period of five minutes . . let your hand form into a fist . . A very tightly, clenched fist . . Then squeeze it hard to drain all the hostility out of your system . . Do this every morning . . before you leave your house . . Set another five minute period for noon . . and once again, in the evening . . So that, three times a day . . you're draining off your hostility . . Hostility that you don't need . . and which you may, otherwise, take out on innocent people, who cannot defend themselves . . This is a much better way to control your anger . . Your temper . . For this eliminates the emotion behind the temper . . Behind the action . . And it takes away the power . . Takes away the power from behind the hostile feelings . . So there is no more pressure . . pushing you to express yourself in such a hostile manner . .

All of these suggestions take complete and thorough effect . . upon your mind . . your body and your spirit . . and seal themselves into the deepest part of your subconscious mind . . Making you feel calm, serene, relaxed, comfortable . . and feeling wonderful . . in every way . .

Now, sleep deeply . . and let all these suggestions seal themselves into the deepest part of your subconscious mind . .

Now, I want you to go deeper . . Relax . . DEEPER and DEEPER Relax . . And let all these suggestions . . take effect immediately . . and seal themselves into the deepest part of your subconscious mind . .

Now, sleep . . deeply . . I am going to give you a period of silence . . for this to occur . . That period of silence . . begins now . .

(Pause - Three to Five minutes)

We are completing our session for this time . . And so, in a moment . . I will resume my count, from one to five . . and you will return to your normal, conscious state of mind . . When you hear me count out the number, five . . you will open your eyes, feeling wide awake, alert and feeling good about your accomplishments . .

Here we go now . .

ONE . .
TWO . .
THREE . .
FOUR . . and . .
FIVE . . You may open your eyes now . .

ANXIETY - ELIMINATE

You are responding nicely to the suggestions and recommendations I am giving you . .

Now, I want you to use your imagination . . Imagine yourself standing at the top of a flight of steps . . You notice there are ten steps leading down . . to a beautiful garden at the bottom . . There is a path leading through the garden . . It crosses a lawn . . and leads to a little cottage . . The cottage is light green in color . . trimmed in white . . and has an old fashioned thatched roof . . This is your little cottage . . The neighbors are very friendly . . but respectful of your wishes when you want solitude . . And so, you look forward to coming here . . to your home . . whenever you can . .

In a moment, you will walk slowly down the steps . . as I count from TEN down to ONE . . You'll take one step at a time . . as I say each number . . As you slowly descend the steps . . and walk the path through the garden . . and across the lawn . . to the cottage . . you'll allow yourself to feel that you are leaving the ordinary, everyday world . . and are finally returning home . . You will become more calm . . and more relaxed . . with each step you take . . And you will continue to feel more peaceful . . and more at ease . . When you reach the bottom step and walk the path to the cottage . . other sounds and noises will fade . . farther and farther away from you . . The ordinary world will completely disappear . . as you reach for the door and open it . .

When you go through the door of the cottage . . you will find yourself in a beautiful living room . . full of luxurious furnishings . . You will sit down in the soft, velvet lined recliner . . and feel yourself drifting into a deeper, more peaceful, more comforting state of relaxation . . You will experience wonderful feelings . . and sensations, moving through your entire body . . You will enjoy complete peace of mind . . (Pause about 15 seconds)

You are patiently waiting at the top of the steps . . and so, I will begin counting now . . and you will go down one step . . with each number I say . .

TEN . . NINE . . You are becoming more tranquil and serene . . EIGHT . . Outside noises and sounds are fading away . . SEVEN . . You are only aware of my voice and the soothing sounds coming from the tape player . . SIX . . FIVE . . You are leaving the events of your ordinary, everyday life . . further and further behind you . . FOUR . . You are getting near the bottom of the steps now . . THREE . . You will soon be on the path leading to the cottage . . TWO . . ONE . . You are on the bottom step now . . so you may begin your walk up the path to the front door of the cottage . . When you get to the door . . open it and go inside . . closing the door behind you . .

What a wonderful feeling . . so calm and so . . relaxing . . You feel as though a very big load has been lifted from you . . and you feel an overwhelming excitement . . stirring inside you . . Oh, such pleasurable relief . .

Walk into the living room now . . and go to that luxurious, soft and comfortable recliner . . Rest yourself in it . . As you bask in the recliner, you feel even more calm and . . more at ease than before . . Feel yourself absorbing the peacefulness . . the stillness . . and the sheer beauty of the furnishings . . in this room . . This is your room . . Your ambiance . . It is just the way you want it to be . . The grand paintings on the walls . . The gentleness of the lighting . . So relaxing . .

Now, I would like you to concentrate on the word . . PEACE . . As you concentrate on the word, peace, . . you'll notice a soothing feeling of calmness . . moving through your entire body . . PEACE . . PEACE . . Now, you are beginning to feel as though you are floating away . . on a soft, fluffy, white cloud . . Floating out . . somewhere beyond space and time . . Gently floating . .

You are now very comfortable, relaxed and totally at ease . . You are experiencing perfect peace of mind . . And in the future . . you can enjoy this same perfect calmness and respite . . any time you want it . . All you will need to do is to sit or lie down in a comfortable position . . close your eyes and imagine yourself in this . . cozy little cottage with the fireplace . . Then count backward in your mind from TEN down to ONE . . By the time you reach the number ONE . . you will be completely relaxed . . calm and at ease . . And you will know peace with the world . .

And you can remain in that state for as long as you desire . . When you are ready to return to a wide-awake and alert state of mind . . you'll only need to open your eyes . . Whenever you do this . . you will always feel rested and refreshed . . Full of energy, strength and vitality . . after relaxing this way, for only a few minutes . .

You will remember everything I have said to you today . . and you will greatly benefit from everything I have told you . . Continue now, to relax, for just a little longer . . (Pause)

In just a moment we will be concluding this session . . I will be counting to FIVE for you to awaken . . You will come up to a wide-awake, fully alert state, when I say the number FIVE . .

ONE - Feeling so good . . feeling wonderful . . all over . .

TWO - Your hands are tingling and your legs are feeling a bit numb yet . . Get the feelings back into your body . .

THREE - Coming up now . . More alert . . More aware . . Stirring into conscious awareness . .

FOUR - Gently inhale now . . Breathe out . . and . .

FIVE - Open your eyes now and focus on your surroundings . .

012 Prescript.   ANXIETY - OVERCOME

Follow Relaxation :

(This technique can be used to help clients be released from many different types of problems ; physical - emotional - mental.)

Important - Discover if client is right handed or left handed -

You are continuing to relax . . letting go completely . . Feel yourself responding to the idea of relaxation . . And keep feeling more comfortable . . more peaceful . . and more at ease . .

It may now be feeling like your body is going into a deep . . peaceful sleep . . But your subconscious mind is ever aware . . of everything I say to you . . and will enable you to respond . . If I tell you to talk . . you'll be able to talk easily . . If I tell you to move . . you'll be able to move easily . . Your conscious awareness keeps narrowing down . . while your subconscious mind is concentrating on every word I am saying . .

You continue to get drowsier and more relaxed . . and it is easy for you to respond to the suggestions I have for you . . In a moment, I am going to count from Five to One . . and when I reach the count of One . . you will recall a very happy, very pleasant and enjoyable experience . .

You are continuing to relax . . and to wait . . And your subconscious mind will cause you . . to recall clearly and vividly . . one of the most pleasant . . most enjoyable experiences of your life . . It may be something that happened in your early years . . before you started school . . Or it may be something from your early grade school or junior high school days . . It may be from something that was very important to you . . A time when you felt confident . . needed, loved, accepted, healthy and happy . .

As soon as you begin to recall that experience . . I want you to form your right hand (dominant) into a fist . . as a symbol of confidence and determination . .

You can trust your right hand . . and you can keep that confident feeling of trust . . by keeping your right hand clenched . . while you are remembering that happy experience . . mentally . . emotionally . . spiritually and, perhaps . . physically . . in the privacy of this room . . You will enjoy remembering that happy experience . . as soon as I count from Five . . down to One . .

103

When you finish recalling and reliving that happy experience . . you will open your right fist . . and then I will give you some additional suggestions . . that will be helpful to you . .

FIVE . . You will recall a happy, pleasant experience . . as I reach the count of one . . FOUR . . THREE . . You will close your right hand into a fist . . when you begin to recall that happy experience . . TWO . . ONE . .

(Wait for Client's right hand to close and open before proceeding. It may take 5 to 10 minutes.)

You are responding quite well . . Relax for a moment now . . then we will proceed . . (pause)

The next time I count from FIVE down to ONE . . you will recall a very unhappy and . . unpleasant experience . . An experience that has been responsible for causing you that problem . .

And even though it will be an unhappy, unpleasant experience . . you will remain calm and relaxed . . And you will recall . . just enough of that experience . . to enable you to understand . . what it had to do with causing your present problem . . You will allow the stress, the strain . . the tension or anxiety . . or whatever nature it may take . . be it physical or emotional . . to develop just long enough for you to recognize it . . At the same time . . you will recognize the connection with the problem you have been experiencing . .

As soon as you begin recalling that . . unhappy, unpleasant experience . . I want you to close your left fist . . and keep recalling that experience . . until you understand all the causes and the affects . . and until you feel . . you have taken all of the distress you can stand . .

When you feel you have stood all of the distress and conflict you need . . you will open your left fist and . . let it all go . . As soon as you open your left fist . . you will be released from all stress . . From all anxiety and tension . . And from all other problems that have been caused by . . that unsavory experience . .

As you are recalling that experience . . you will be bringing all the tensions . . all the problems . . and all of the difficulties . . caused by that experience . . down through your left shoulder . . arm and forearm . . and into your left fist . . You will lock them tightly into your left fist . . and will keep them there . . until you are sure they are all in your left fist where you put them . .

When that unhappy, unpleasant experience happened . . your mind understood it . . from the level of understanding you had . . at that time . . But now . . you have a more mature . . more calm . . more knowledgeable understanding . . And your mind can use that understanding . . to resolve your problem . . in a way that will be beneficial to you . .

When I count from Five down to One . . your subconscious mind will permit you to review . . explore and examine . . what has been causing that problem . .

As you are recalling that experience . . all the tension . . anxiety . . stress and strain from that experience . . will funnel down through your left shoulder . . arm and forearm . . and into your left fist . . When it is all locked up in your left fist . . you will realize that you can remove it . . and be rid of it forever . . All you have to do is open your fist . . When you open your left fist and . . let it all go . . you will feel a big load being lifted from you . . You will feel a strong sense of joy and relief . . And an overwhelming sense or renewed confidence . . You will be free from all the tension . . All the anxiety . . All the stresses and discomforts . . And all problems that have been caused by that experience . . Because you won't need them anymore . .

They will have served their purpose and you will not need them anymore . . So you will then squeeze your right fist . . Your right fist is your strong . . capable, confident, determined and happy fist . .

As soon as you squeeze your right fist . . your left fist will relax and open . . And all of the problems caused by that unhappy . . unpleasant experience . . will fade away rapidly and be gone completely . . by the time you awaken from your hypnotic state . .

I'm going to count from Five down to One now . . and you will recall that unhappy, unpleasant experience . . that has been causing you that problem . .

Five . . Four . . Three . . Two . . One . . (Wait for left fist to squeeze closed - then open. Wait for right fist to close tightly.)

Now, that terrible experience is past . . You are feeling relaxed and calm . . Continue relaxing for a moment . . then I will give you some additional suggestions . . (pause)

(Go to another prescription such as, Self Confidence - Building , etc.)

ANOREXIA - OVERCOME

(Have client get numbness in hand, according to suggestion. Continue by having client 'lock hands' together. Each session with client, have him or her respond to some suggestion which demonstrates how the subconscious mind controls the body . . i.e.. arm becomes rigid, etc.)

You are realizing more and more . . that the unconscious level of your mind . . controls every part of your body . . You got numbness in your hand without any conscious effort . . You responded to _____ without any conscious effort . . And you are realizing that the power of your unconscious mind . . can and will . . enable you to accomplish any goal . . that is necessary or desired . .

Notice that you are continuing to become more relaxed . . You are feeling more comfortable and at ease . . You are becoming more confident . . that you are . . overcoming your problem . . in an easy, natural way . . You will soon be eating and digesting food easily and comfortably . . You will eat the amount of food your body needs . . to keep you healthy . . and to increase the weight of your body . . to a normal level . . And then your body will remain at a normal level . . You will enjoy eating the right amounts of food needed . . to provide your body with proper nutrition . . And to always keep your body healthy and strong . .

Your subconscious mind is causing you to have . . stronger and stronger desires and urges . . to eat the amounts of good foods . . needed by your body . . to increase the weight of your body . . to a level that is perfect . . and healthy . . You will notice that you feel hungry . . each time your body needs food . . and you will enjoy eating the amounts of food . . your body needs at that time . . Eating the amounts of food needed by your body . . will be a pleasant, enjoyable experience for you . . And you will notice your health improving . . more each day . . Food will become a source of comfort because . . you will realize that in eating . . you are getting well . . You will gradually eat a little more food each day or two . . until you are eating the perfect amount of food needed . . to keep your body healthy . . and at a perfect weight level for your height . .

Now, I want you to imagine . . that you are sitting comfortably . . in your living room . .

And you have just put a new video . . into your video player . . You are feeling excited about seeing it . . It's about ready to begin . . You notice that it is a film showing your life . . but it is going backward . . from the present time . . back to your early childhood . . Begin watching your life-video now and . . if you see anything upsetting . . one of the fingers on your right hand will lift up immediately . . and you will tell me about it . . If the event is too traumatic . . you will be able to turn the video off . . and tell me as much about it . . as you are willing for me to know . .

(If client turns off video, ask the client's subconscious mind if it is okay to get the answers by having the subconscious mind cause the finger to lift up - to answer the questions. If such is the case, one of the fingers on the right hand will lift up - and remain up - until you tell it to go down.)

The video, going back to your early childhood . . is beginning now . . and you will tell me if you see anything upsetting . . realizing . . that you now have a more adult-like . . more mature understanding about the problem . . than you had at the time that it occurred . . And this will enable your subconscious mind to work out the solution . . in an easy, natural way . .

AD LIB through experience, then - EMERGE -

You are relaxing deeply now . . and I am going to give you suggestions . . that will help you . . with your situation . .

There have been numerous research projects conducted . . to discover the causes of arthritis . . and what can be done to cure it . . It has been found that . . one of the major physical causes of arthritis . . is calcium deposits forming between the bones . . And it has also been found that certain . . emotional states . . can cause the body to build up those calcium deposits as well . . Research conducted with hypnosis has revealed . . that getting the mind to review and examine the causes . . enables the subconscious level of the mind . . to work out a solution . . And to resolve the problem causing the arthritis . . That allows the bodily processes to function properly by . . cleansing the arthritic condition out of the body completely . . You have natural chemicals and fluids in your body . . that will dissolve calcium deposits . . and cleanse them out of your body completely . .

Thomas Edison discovered . . many years ago . . that every cell of the body . . can be influenced by the mind . . In fact . . through his research . . he found that 'every cell of the body, "thinks" . . and your own subconscious mind can send instructions . . to all of the cells in your body . . and regenerate every chemical needed to heal and to restore . . all parts of your body . . to a vibrating, healthy condition . .

Your subconscious mind is deciphering and accepting . . the suggestions and instructions I am giving you . . and is stirring the natural functions of your body to action . . Causing them to begin working immediately . . They are influencing your thoughts . . your feelings and your actions . . in a positive . . helpful way . . Even after you awaken from the hypnotic state . . these suggestions and instructions . . will continue influencing you . . just as strongly . . just as surely and just as powerfully . . as they do while you are hypnotized . . And you will be pleased with the improvements . . in your physical condition . .

Your subconscious mind is causing the processes of your body . . to function properly . . Each time you move your fingers, your hands, your arms, your legs . . or any other part of your body . . the natural fluids in your body . . will penetrate the places where calcium has been deposited . . And those natural fluids of your body . . will lubricate your bone joints . . and will cause calcium deposits to dissolve . . And you will notice your body feeling more comfortable . . as each day goes by . .

Your bones will continue becoming more normal in size . . and all of the joints in your body . . will move more easily . . and more freely . . You will notice the improvements . . as your body continues feeling more comfortable . . more calm . . And you will be able to do everything . . in a more relaxed way . .

The calcium deposits are dissolving and soon . . you will be able to move your fingers . . your hands, your elbows and shoulders . . and all other parts of your body . . easily and comfortably . . Your body healing processes are working . . right now . . and will continue working . . as your body continues to heal . . completely and perfectly . .

You will notice the improvements . . regardless of how slight they may seem to be, at first . . And you will be pleased with the progress you are making . . You will be confident that your body is being healed . . And you will be able to use all parts of your body . . freely and comfortably . . The healing processes of your body are all working properly . . because you want them to work . .

Your subconscious mind is obeying your thoughts and desires . . for your body to be healthy and strong . . Your body is responding . . and you will be happy as you notice the continuous progress being made . . in every part of your body . .

After you awaken from the hypnotic state . . you will feel wonderfully relaxed and refreshed . . You will feel peaceful . . relaxed and at ease . . These principles of relaxation . . which you are now experiencing . . will continue during your daily life . . and you will be more calm . . more relaxed . . in all situations and circumstances . .

Whether you are alone or with others . . you will feel . . relaxed . . I want you to continue relaxing for another moment or two . . in silence . . to allow your subconscious mind to absorb . . and resolve . . everything we have talked about today . . (pause)

You are now very comfortable, relaxed and totally at ease . . You are experiencing perfect peace of mind . . And in the future . . you can enjoy this same perfect calmness and respite . . any time you want it . . All you will need to do is to sit or lie down in a comfortable position . . close your eyes and imagine yourself in this . . comfortable state of mind . . Then count backward in your mind from TEN down to ONE . . By the time you reach number ONE . . you will be completely relaxed . . calm and at ease . . And you will know peace with the world . . And you can remain in that state for as long as you desire . . When you are ready to return to a wide-awake and alert state of mind . . you'll need only to open your eyes . . Whenever you do this . . you will always feel rested and refreshed . . full of energy, strength and vitality . . after relaxing this way, for only a few minutes . .

You will remember everything I have said to you today . . and you will greatly benefit from everything I have told you . . Continue now, to relax . . for just a little longer . . (Pause)

In just a moment we will be concluding this session . . I will be counting to FIVE for you to awaken . . You will come up to a wide-awake, fully alert state, when I say the number FIVE . .

ONE - Feeling so good . . feeling wonderful . . all over . .

TWO - your hands are tingling and your legs are feeling a bit numb yet . . Get the feelings back into your body . .

THREE - Coming up now . . More alert . . More aware . . Stirring into conscious awareness . .

FOUR - Gently inhale now . . Breathe out . . and . .

FIVE - Open your eyes and focus on your surroundings . .

As you are relaxing . . you are realizing more and more . . that your subconscious mind controls all of the activities and processes . . of your body . . So, your conscious mind can continue relaxing now . . There is nothing it needs to do at this time . . Your subconscious mind is receiving all that I say to you . . and is causing everything I tell you . . to begin working immediately . .

In just a moment . . when I tell you to begin . . I want you to count from TEN . . down to ONE . . slowly . . in your mind . . and notice what is happening to your RIGHT hand . . as your LEFT hand becomes completely numb . .

Begin counting now, silently, from TEN down to ONE . . and notice what is happening to your RIGHT hand . . When you reach the count of ONE . . lift your RIGHT hand up to let me know . . the numbness has begun to settle in your LEFT hand . .

(Note : After the client lifts the RIGHT hand up, pinch the LEFT hand with your finger nails, and ask, "What does it feel like I am doing" . . The LEFT hand should feel numb. If the response is good, then pick up the LEFT hand with your finger nails, pinching it tightly. Then have the client open his or her eyes and look at the finger nail marks. Then pinch the RIGHT hand to show that it is not numb and pinch the LEFT arm, to show that it is not numb.)

Now, you realize that your subconscious mind . . can cause changes in your body automatically . . So in just a moment . . I want you to count backwards again . . from TEN down to ONE . . slowly, in your mind . . and notice the normal feeling . . coming back into your LEFT hand . . as your blood pressure is stabilizing at around 120 over 80 . . When you reach the count of ONE . . lift up your LEFT hand . . to let me know the normal feeling is back . . (pause)

You are responding perfectly to everything I say to you . . Your subconscious mind is causing your entire organism . . your body . . to cooperate with everything I tell you . . And you will be pleased to have that relaxed feeling continue . . even after you awaken from the hypnotic state . . You have experienced how easily . . your subconscious mind . . can make your hand numb . .

Now, I am going to give you instructions . . that will enable you to get rid of any future pain by yourself . . In fact, the instructions

I give you . . will enable you to have complete control . . over your whole body . . So that, any time you experience arthritic pain . . or any pain . . anywhere in your body . . you will be able to instantly cause . . any part of your body to become pain-free . . just as easily as your hand became numb . . when I gave you instructions to achieve that . .

You are beginning to feel a sense of confidence . . and a sense of competence and sureness . . And that feeling of calmness will continue . . as you go about the activities of your daily life . .

Before I had you get the numbness in your hand . . you may not have realized . . that your subconscious mind controls your physical body . . And you may still have some doubts in your mind . . But those doubts are being replaced . . with a strong sense of confidence and sureness . . And before this session is completed . . you know that the problem you have been experiencing . . will be completely healed . .

(Use Magnetic Hand Demonstration to show the mind controls the body.)

NOTE : DEMONSTRATE TO CLIENT HOW TO MAGNETIZE HANDS. IF PAINFUL AREA IS AVAILABLE TO TOUCH, AND NOT AWKWARD, HAVE CLIENT PLACE MAGNETIZED HANDS (PALMS) ON TWO SIDES OF AREA. LEFT AND RIGHT OR FRONT AND BACK.

I want you to open your eyes now . . and look at your hands . . Place your hands in front of you . . palms toward each other . . Push your hands together, slowly . . until they almost touch . . but not quite . . Now, pull them slowly apart and FEEL the energy pulling between them . . When you can feel the energy pulling between them . . nod your head . .

Very good . . Now, as you feel the energy flowing . . place both of your hands on either side of the painful area . . (This may take some coordinating.) The healing energy is flowing between your palms . . Do not quite touch the body . . Separate your hands, slightly, until you feel the energy pulling . . then hold that position . . for a moment . . on two sides of the painful area . . (Pause 2 minutes)

And now, sit back again as you were . . Relax . . and close your eyes . . You are beginning to feel a healing warmth . . flowing through the tissues of your skin . . The healing processes of your body are taking effect, right now . . They are working . . and you are beginning to feel more comfortable . . more at ease and more calm . . Your entire body is becoming more relaxed . . All pain . . All discomfort . . and all swelling . . are diminishing . . Flowing out of your body . . easily and naturally . . As though they were being drawn out from your body . . through your magnetic hands . .

The healing processes of your body . . are functioning properly now . . and will continue working properly . . And are healing your body completely . . and perfectly . .

Your muscles, nerves, ligaments and tendons . . are relaxing, more and more . . All swelling is decreasing . . and all of your joints are becoming normal in size . .

You are continuing to feel more comfortable . . as all pain and discomfort . . leave your body . .

And your body heals itself . . perfectly and completely . . When the healing has been completed . . you will be able to do everything . . in a relaxed way . .

Your muscles are becoming stronger . . Yet, they are loose and flexible . . and are functioning easily and comfortably . .

Notice, as you hold your hands on the affected area . . that you continue feeling more comfortable . . and more at ease . . Now I want you to open your eyes again . . so that you can see to put the energy charge back into your hands once more . . Palms towards each other . . Push them towards each other and slowly, draw them apart until you feel the energy flowing between them . . Now, place the palm of one hand . . on your forehead . . and the other, at the back of your head . .

Hold them in place for a moment . . You are feeling emotionally calm and serene . . You are feeling peaceful and relaxed . . And you are beginning to experience . . some wonderful feelings and sensations, all through your body . . Just hold that position with your hands for another moment or two . .

Take a deep breath now and . . relax your hands . . Place them comfortably in your lap . . Even after you remove your hands . . you will continue feeling wonderful . .

And you will keep improving more, each day . . And you will be very happy to realize the progress you are making . .

When you awaken from the hypnotic state . . you will feel much better than you did before you were hypnotized . . You will feel calm and peaceful . . Relaxed and comfortable . . Rested and refreshed . . The processes of your body are functioning properly now . . and are healing your body perfectly . . Your body is responding to its own natural healing energies . . And you will soon be in perfect health . . Remember, too, that you can easily repeat these steps at home . . feeling free to share this healing power with a friend or loved one . .

EMERGE

I am going to begin my count now . . counting from Five down to One . . And when you hear me count out the number, One . . you will open your eyes . . feeling refreshed, alert and in control . . You will feel spiritually rested and peaceful . . as though you were just waking up from a long relaxing nap . .

One. You are feeling good . . Feeling wonderful . .
Two. Becoming more aware of your body as it wants to awaken and stir . .
Three. Move your arms and legs now . . Awareness is entering your body.
Four. Rising up now . . Coming to the surface gradually . . and . .
Five. Open your eyes and focus on your surroundings . . How do you feel ?

Most people don't understand what asthma is, but you have experienced it and you understand it better than most people . .

Most people think it is hard for you to breathe because you can't get air into your lungs, but we know that when a person has asthma, it is really just the opposite . . A person having an asthmatic attack has difficulty getting the air OUT of the lungs to let fresh air in. Isn't that right? (Pause for response.)

Since that is true, it will be easy to help you overcome the problem, so you will never have another asthmatic attack . .

Do you want me to show you how to always be able to breathe easily, so you will never have another asthmatic attack? (Wait for response)

Good . . It's very easy . . In order to always be able to inhale and exhale easily and comfortably . . all you need to do is to let all the muscles in your chest relax . .

It's easy to let all those muscles in your chest and lungs relax . . and I'm going to show you how easy it is . . Are you ready ? . . (Wait for response)

Okay . . Hold your right hand up and out, so I can touch it . . Now, close your hand and make your fist real tight . .

That's good . . Now, if you had a piece of hot metal in your hand . . and it was burning you . . what would you do to get rid of it ? Show me what you would do . .

Right . . You would open your fist . . It would be silly for someone with hot metal in their hand to close their fist tighter, wouldn't it . . So, you would just relax the muscles, open your hand and let that piece of hot metal go . .

When a person is having an asthmatic attack, it's just like tightening their fist . . The little muscles around the air sacs of their lungs tighten up, so they can't exhale . . And those little muscles hold the old air in so there is no room for any fresh air to get in . . So, all an asthmatic attack is, is holding those muscles around your lungs so tight that you can't breathe out . . Right ?

Okay, now, I want you to practice this so you will get rid of those asthmatic attacks . .

(Note : The following suggestions will cause the child to bring on an asthmatic attack, then release it. This will cause the child to realize that his mind starts it, and can also stop it.)

You are beginning to tighten up the muscles in your chest and around your lungs . . and it keeps getting more difficult for you to breathe . . Okay, tighten up all those muscles now . .

You are doing this because you know you will be able to make the asthmatic attack stop, as soon as I tell you to make it stop . .

It's really getting hard to breathe now, isn't it . . Your lungs are feeling very tight . . You are doing this the same way you have been doing it, every time you have had an asthmatic attack . .

(Note : Keep giving instructions for lung tightening and difficulty breathing, until client is actually having an asthmatic attack. Then suggest client relax and breathe easily and freely.)

Now you are aware that you have been causing your own asthmatic attacks . . But it really hasn't been your fault . . It's just that no one has ever explained this to you before . . Now that you know, you will be able to relax those little muscles that have been holding air in . . And from now on, you will always be able to breathe easily and freely . .

It's easy for you to get rid of those asthmatic attacks . . Just as easy as talking . . Notice how easily you are breathing now . .

Now, you know how easy it is to stop an asthmatic attack . . So I want you to have another attack now, so you will remember how easily you can stop it . .

All of those muscles are beginning to tighten up again . . It's going to be even harder for you to breathe this time . . You are having a really bad asthmatic attack . . The muscles get tighter . . and tighter . . And your breathing gets harder and harder . .

(Wait until it becomes severe.)

Now, I'm going to time you to see how fast you can get it to go away completely, so you can breathe easily again . . (Keep track of time.)

You did real good . . It only took you _____ (min. / sec.) to get rid of the attack . .

Now that you know how to get rid of those attacks, there is really no need to ever have one again . .

Do you think you will ever have one again ? (Wait for response.)

If you ever start to have another attack, you will remember what you do to get rid of it, won't you ?

(Wait for response.)

Aren't you glad we took the time to get rid of those asthmatic attacks ? Now you know you are smart enough to never have another attack . . You know all about asthma now, and you know you will never let it bother you again . .

That's all there is to it . . You can feel proud of yourself . . You have been able to get rid of it . . by yourself . . And you will never be bothered by asthma again . . Congratulations . .

EMERGE, as needed.

(Note : This Prescription is to be used along with other prescriptions, i.e., Improving Health, etc.)

In a moment, I am going to ask you . . to think of the numbers, 8, 7, 6, 5, 4, 3, 2 and 1 . . in your mind . . With each number you think of . . you will go a little deeper into relaxation . .

From now on . . each of these numbers will have an additional meaning for you . . and each time you think, hear, see or say . . any of these numbers . . the meaning of that number will keep getting stronger in your life . . Now, think these numbers, silently, to yourself . .

The number, eight, will help you to relax more deeply . . more peacefully and calmly . . Every time you think, hear, see or say the number, eight . . your subconscious mind will cause you to relax . . more calmly and peacefully . .

Seven, means that your entire organism of body, mind and spirit . . is cooperating to enable you to control . . the flow of energy from the ethereal realm . . into your body . . Providing you with the power for self-healing . . of your spirit, mind and body . .

Six, means that your confidence in your ability to be relaxed and calm . . at all times . . continues increasing . .

Five, represents your self-confidence, self-acceptance, self-reliance and self-esteem, which continues increasing . . Every time you think, hear, see or say . . the number five . . your self-confidence, self-acceptance, self-reliance and self-esteem . . will keep increasing . . and you will continue progressing in all areas of your life . .

Four, means that your subconscious mind is cooperating by causing your lungs to function perfectly . . enabling you to inhale and exhale easily and freely . . continuously . .

Three, provides you with more confidence in your own opinions and your own points of view . . and allows you the pride . . to feel good about those opinions . .

Two, gives you freedom . . from having any fears, anxieties or tensions in your life . .

And the number, One, means, the cells of your body . . are working in perfect harmony . . causing your metabolism, your hormones . . and all of your organs and glands . . to function perfectly . .

From now on and for the rest of your life . . any time you think, hear, see or say . . any of those numbers . . the meaning for that number . . will keep becoming more strongly reinforced . . in your mind . . and your mind will cause the meaning for that number . . to continue becoming more effective . .

Your subconscious mind is causing the meaning for each number . . to keep becoming stronger . . and to work more effectively . . So, I want you to repeat those numbers, to yourself . . from Eight, down to One, as you continue moving into a deeper hypnotic state . . and the meaning for each number . . becomes more deeply reinforced . . in your mind . . Count those numbers to yourself now . . from Eight . . down to One . . and connect their meanings to each number . . (pause)

Whenever you are confronted with any kind of unpleasant situation . . you will automatically become calm and relaxed . . You will use these principles of relaxation . . which you are now aware of . . and you'll be in control of your feelings rather than letting your emotions control you . .

The ability to be calm and relaxed . . is becoming more automatic to you . . and will enable you to handle situations that come up in your daily life . . in a loving, peaceable manner . .

Your self-confidence and self-reliance increases daily . . You will become emotionally calmer . . and will be able to handle situations more maturely . . And that will cause all allergic reactions to fade away . . more and more . . And soon, they will be gone from your life, completely . .

You will be sleeping better at night . . And each morning, you will awaken feeling rested, relaxed and refreshed . . mentally and physically . . You will maintain that feeling of relaxation, during the day . . while your body processes respond and continuously improve your health . .

All cells of your body are continuously functioning more perfectly . . cleansing all impurities out of your body . . You will continue feeling more clean, more pure and more refreshed . . as your elimination system keeps your body cleansed . . of all waste materials and impurities . .

Your subconscious mind is causing your body to function . . according to the perfect laws . . of God . . Your life will continue reflecting peacefulness and calmness . . and that enables all parts of your body . . to function in perfect harmony and attunement . .

Your subconscious mind is working out the solution . . to the problem . . completely and perfectly . . and is releasing you . . from the control of any . . unpleasant experiences from the past . . Your mind realizes that the past is gone . . Nothing is of the past . . but memories . . And that is not where you are . . You are living today . . for tomorrow . . Your mind refuses to recognize past memories . . as a way of life for you, today . . And your mind refuses to let those past memories . . cause you difficulties now in your present life . . You are becoming more free and complete . . with each passing day . .

Every part of your body . . All organs, glands, muscles, nerves and tissues . . your entire circulatory system . . your metabolism . . your intestines and elimination system . . Every system of your body, mind and spirit are working well . . in accordance with God's Laws of health, strength and vitality . .

Peace, poise and confidence are growing stronger within you . . You are becoming stronger, healthier and more secure each day . . And you will continue to be amazed and pleased . . with your improvements . .

Continue to relax a few moments longer . . then, I will begin my count . . from one to five . . When you hear the number five . . you will be wide awake, feeling refreshed and relaxed . . and ready for new challenges . . (Pause briefly)

One - You will remember everything you have experienced today . . You are feeling good now . . Relaxed . . In control . .
Two - Coming up now . . Move your fingers and toes a little . . Let the body awaken . .
Three - Move your arms and legs a bit now . . Feeling good . . Feeling wonderful . . For you are a wonderful person . .
Four - We're nearly there . . Take a deep breath now and . .
Five - Open your eyes . . Focus on your surroundings . . How do you feel?

It is your desire to excel in your ability as a baseball player . . You have chosen baseball as a sport . . in which you want to continue improving your talents . . skills . . and abilities . . You love the game of baseball and have a great enthusiasm for it . . It is so important in your life . . that you want to be an exceptionally . . outstanding player . .

Baseball has its own special brand of competition . . It is a team sport . . in which each player on the team contributes in his own special way . . As you know, each player plays a different position . . and needs to keep practicing so he can play the position perfectly . . Each player must also be able to hit the ball with exceptional ability . . and therefore, must continue improving his skills . . to maintain a high average in batting . .

To be an excellent baseball player, the top players in the game say . . there are several basic qualities and attitudes you must develop . . to help you to be outstanding in the game . . Knowing those qualities and attitudes . . by having them implanted in the subconscious levels of your mind . . causes you to continually increase your abilities . . to be the really outstanding baseball player you are capable of being . . As I explain about those important qualities and attitudes . . you can continue relaxing more completely and comfortably . . There may be times when I am talking to you and . . it may seem as though my voice is a long distance away . . However, that's okay because the subconscious levels of your mind . . will receive and accept everything I tell you . . and will cause you to put everything I say into your own actions . .

One of the first qualities needed to become an outstanding baseball player . . is to have an intense interest in the game . . Having an intense interest in the game . . gives you a solid reason to make a personal commitment . . to want to keep improving your skills . . The desire to keep improving will result in continuous training for keeping your body in top physical condition at all times . . Your trainers and coaches are the most important people on your team . . They will advise you but it is up to you to follow through . . From now on, you will exercise your body regularly . . and practice to keep your body strong and finely tuned . . so that your reflexes and coordination . . will always function perfectly . . By staying in top condition . . you will also avoid unnecessary injuries . . A part of that conditioning should include dancing . . or ballet lessons . . to improve your skills in spinning and making quick turns on the field . . Your desire to become an excellent baseball player will continue increasing . . and that will cause the subconscious levels of your mind to motivate you . . into doing the proper training needed . . to be an outstanding baseball player . .

A second quality of being an outstanding baseball player . . is to practice the skills of your position correctly . . Every sport requires that you have good speed . . good timing and coordination . . You need to have the necessary strength and energy . . and proper reflexes . . to enable you to make the right moves in the right way . . to handle your position perfectly . . Your trainers and coaches are there for your benefit . . Think of your trainers and coaches as being the most important members of your organization . . They will guide you . . but only you can create your success . . So from now on you will devote an increased amount of time . . to all of their requirements . . thus, improving on the requirements of your position . . including, making every move correctly . . So that when you participate in competition . . you will automatically make every play perfectly . .

You will watch outstanding professional baseball players . . who play the same position that you play . . You will observe everything they do to make every play correctly . . And talk with them whenever you have the opportunity . . The subconscious levels of your mind will remember . . everything they do, correctly . . and enable you, as well, to make every play correctly . . every time you are required to do so in competition . .

The most important thing you can do . . to help yourself improve . . on your talents, skills and abilities, as a baseball player . . is to take out an hour each day for meditation . . You will sit down or lie down in a quiet, comfortable place . . and visualize yourself performing all of the actions . . and all of the techniques required . . for the position you play on the team . . When you begin your meditation . . you will close your eyes and . . at first, clear away all of the noisy nonsense from your mind . . concentrate on the little light spots in front of your eyes and focus them down . . to only one white spot . . Then begin to see yourself on the playing field . . Visualize yourself in action . . doing everything perfectly . . Concentrate on every little move . . every slide . . every twist and turn . . See yourself jumping even higher than you have ever jumped before . . Reach for the ball from a different position than you are normally in . . and throw the ball with complete accuracy, every time . . Your visualizing time is equally as important as your actual practice time . .

You will do every maneuver correctly in your mind . . and that will enable you to do it correctly . . whenever you are participating in a game . .

Visualize yourself going over each play . . time and time again . . Always doing it perfectly . . in an easy, natural way . . Go over each play in slow motion . . in your mind . . so that you may understand and absorb . . exactly what is happening and when . . To better improve your timing as well . . As you are playing your position in actual games . . your mind will direct your body . . to perform the right moves and actions needed . . The subconscious levels of your mind will cause you to . . instinctively play your position correctly . . each time you are actually participating in a game of baseball . .

A third quality in becoming an excellent baseball player . . is to be calm and at ease, at all times . . regardless of the condition of the field you play on . . regardless of the weather and . . regardless of the attitudes of the fans . . Baseball is an outdoor sport . . and each field is different . . Weather conditions may be different each time you play a game . . The sun may be too bright or it may be raining . . You are now increasing your ability and your poise . . to adapt to any situation you may be required to play in . . with calmness and ease . . You will be calm and relaxed at all times . . whenever you are taking part in a baseball game . . You will play your position perfectly . . even if the crowd is quiet . . or noisy . . Even if airplanes are flying overhead . . Your concentration will be firm and perfect . . at all times and under all conditions . . whenever you are participating in a baseball game . .You are the expert . . the professional . . You are the master of your position . . and of your spiritual game . .

And you will also be an outstanding hitter . . Everything you do to keep improving your skills at your position . . you will also do, regarding your batting abilities . . Whenever you are up to bat . . you will be calm, relaxed and confident . . And confidence comes with practice . . Your vision will be perfect . . When the ball is pitched, you will see it clearly . . So clearly that you will know immediately . . what kind of pitch it is . . The ball will appear larger than normal . . and it will seem to come toward you . . slowly . . almost in slow-motion . . allowing you plenty of time to see it clearly . . and to hit it firmly . . every time it is in the strike zone . . When you are batting, you will always do what is best for the team . . for the situation you are in . . If you need to bunt the ball . . you will have practiced bunting . . so you can do it perfectly . . If you need to get a base hit . . you will have practiced at that . . so you will be able to do that perfectly, as well . . You will be capable of hitting the ball with strength . . with accuracy and with power . .

Continue breathing easily and freely now . . Keep moving into a more peaceful . . more calm and relaxed state . . as your mind continues to receive and absorb . . the suggestions I am giving you . .

The fourth quality and attitude you are developing . . is a desire to always play to the best of your ability . . and to maintain a strong desire to always win . . It is important to win . . However . . If you lose . . you will remain calm and you will recognize the skills of your competition . . And you will continue practicing and improving your own skills . . to a greater and greater extent . . You welcome competition . . You always do your best and you always . . recognize the abilities of your competition . . The tougher the competition . . the more your abilities keep improving . .

On the days when you are participating in actual competition . . against another team . . you will always have the ability to perform . . in an exceptionally outstanding way . . You will be at your very peak of ability . . mentally, physically, emotionally and spiritually . .

You know that by continuing to practice, both on the field and . . in your mind . . you will always continue to improve . . So, if at any time you make a mistake . . you will accept it . . learn from it . . and continue practicing . . so that you will be able to continue performing more perfectly . .

One hour a day of quiet meditation . . to visualize yourself . . performing all the necessary moves and maneuvers required . . to capitalize on your playing position . . will pay off greatly in the long run . . Visualizing time is as valuable a tool as actual practice time . . That is the main tool needed . . for you to become an exceptional player . .

One final point you will be sure to remember . . is that all outstanding athletes get the proper amount of sleep and rest . . When you go to bed, for the purpose of sleeping . . you will easily drift into a calm, peaceful state of sleep . . You will sleep comfortably until it is time . . for you to awaken . . When it is time for you to awaken . . you will feel well rested and refreshed . . You will continue having more strength and energy . . after relaxing so soundly as you sleep . . Each day, your self-confidence, self-reliance and self-acceptance will keep increasing . . and your skills as a baseball player will continue to improve . .

Remain resting comfortably for a few moments longer . . Give your subconscious mind the time . . to absorb and analyze . . everything we have talked about . . (pause)

In just a moment now . . I will be counting to FIVE . . for you to awaken from the hypnotic state . . You will awaken a little more with each number you hear . . When I reach the number FIVE . . you will open your eyes and you will be wide awake . . You will feel refreshed and wonderful . . And you will feel much better than you did . . before we started this session . .

I will begin the count . .

ONE . . Coming back to reality now . .

TWO . . Tingling sensations and any numbness is wearing off . .

THREE . . Your body wants to stir now . . Move your fingers, your leg muscles and your arms . .

FOUR . . Coming up fast now . . Feeling good about yourself . . and

FIVE . . Open your eyes now and breathe deeply . .

Let yourself continue to relax now . . so that you can really enjoy this pleasant experience . . to improve your fielding skills in (Baseball or Softball).

Keep your eyes closed and experience . . your confidence level increasing . . as you keep realizing more and more . . that you have the ability to be an outstanding (Baseball or Softball) player . .

The subconscious levels of your mind are so sensitive to what I am saying . . that your conscious mind can easily continue relaxing . . The suggestions and instructions I am giving you . . are making a deep and profound impression on your subconscious mind . . and that is what will cause you . . to put them into your own conscious actions . .

The subconscious levels of your mind are what cause you . . to react automatically . . The subconscious mind is what controls your muscles, your ligaments, your tendons and your breathing . . Of course, you help all of those parts of your body . . to continue responding more perfectly . . by exercising them regularly . . And it is also true that . . your automatic responses keep functioning more perfectly . . by practicing in your mind . . as well as on the field . .

So, I am going to give you suggestions and instructions now . . that will produce automatic improvements for you . . in your fielding skills . .

I want you to visualize yourself . . actually participating in a game now . . Imagine yourself at your position . . on the field . . and visualize the ball being hit . . It goes a little to the right of you . . And now, see yourself getting to the ball . . and fielding it perfectly . . and throwing the ball quickly and accurately . . to the position it needs to be thrown to . . Then see the ball being hit to your left . . Again, you field the ball perfectly . . and quickly throw it to the proper player . . to make the play perfectly . . Continue doing this . . over and over in your mind . . See yourself correctly fielding one ball after another . . after another . . Catch the ball and throw it to the proper places . . again and again . . (pause)

See and think of your reflexes . . and your coordination . . functioning perfectly . . See yourself moving smoothly . . Your entire body is functioning correctly . . You handle every fielding situation that comes to you . . perfectly and accurately, each time . .

When you are practicing on the field . . I want you to take an hour every day . . to practice the same moves, the same maneuvers . . over and over . . in your mind . . Just as you are doing now . .

Continue to relax a moment longer . . to give your subconscious mind the time to absorb everything we have talked about today . . In a moment, I will count to FIVE . . to awaken you from your hypnotic state . . Just relax a little longer now . . (Pause)

I am going to begin the count now . . and you will awaken a little bit more with each number that you hear . . When you hear the number FIVE . . you will open your eyes and be wide awake . . feeling refreshed and wonderful . . You will feel much better than you did before we started this session . .

I will begin the count now . .

ONE . . Coming back to the real world . . Feeling refreshed . . Feeling wonderful . .
TWO . . Tingling sensations are wearing off now . .
THREE . . Feeling rested . . Feeling good about yourself . .
FOUR . . Coming up fast now . . Very fast . . Your muscles want to stir . .
FIVE . . Open your eyes now and tell me how you feel . .

Let yourself continue relaxing now . . so that you can really enjoy this pleasant experience . .

I am going to give you suggestions and instructions . . that will help you to relax and it will help you to become . . the outstanding athlete that you know you are capable of being . .

Every part of your body . . every muscle, every nerve, every ligament and tendon . . is controlled by your subconscious mind . . And you are finding that your subconscious mind . . is causing you to respond to the suggestions and instructions I am giving you . . and is also automatically improving your athletic abilities . . Your athletic skills are what you provide after much practice . .

You already know that practice is important . . for the proper development of skills and talents . . Whether you want to play a musical instrument . . shoot a bow and arrow . . dance or improve yourself in football, golf, bowling or any other athletic skill . . Practice is imperative . . All outstanding athletes practice for hours each day . . to develop their skills and talents . .

We sometimes hear people talk about someone being born with natural athletic talent . . but even a person born with the capability of being a superstar must practice . . if he wants to be successful . .

Practice is necessary . . and you realize that practice is necessary . . but there are other things that you can do to improve yourself rapidly . .

First of all, you can learn a great deal by observing others . . who are already outstanding stars in your particular sport . . You can go to their games or see them on videos . . Talk with them personally, whenever you can . .

We continuously hear of records being broken in various sports . . One of the main reasons for new records being set . . is that each new generation of athletes . . learns from the experiences . . of those who have already developed their skills . . By observing other outstanding athletes . . your mind absorbs what they do . . And that, unconsciously . . improves your own athletic abilities . .

One of the greatest pleasures . . of being an athlete . . is to experience the joy of continuous improvement . . And that improvement comes from having the correct practice habits . .

Great athletes practice every move . . over and over . . so that it becomes automatic . . Then, when they are participating in a competitive way . . they can be relaxed and natural when different situations arise . . So, a second key to being successful as an athlete . . is to keep practicing on the best and most effective ways . . to improve your abilities . .

One of the most effective ways of doing that is with hypnosis . . Hypnosis enables you to remain calm . . and relaxed . . when you are participating in any athletic event . .

From now on, every time you look at water . . Any water . . That is your signal . . Seeing water will trigger your response . . to become more calm and relaxed . . and remain calm and relaxed for at least six hours . . You will be able to do everything . . in a calm and relaxed way . . And that will cause your reflexes and coordination . . to respond perfectly . . And will enable you to use your athletic abilities . . and skills . . correctly and consistently . . Remaining calm will improve your timing . . and your reflex action . . so you will consistently perform freely and smoothly . . Think of water . . That is the key to your inner strength . . your stability . . your calmness . . and . . your winning ways . .

You will be calm and relaxed at all times . . and the easy, natural, coordinated . . muscle movements you need . . will function automatically . . Your muscles, nerves, ligaments and tendons . . will function smoothly and perfectly . .

As you continue practicing . . your subconscious mind will become programmed . . and will automatically cause you to perform correctly . . in every situation . . Just as you do when you perform other activities . . such as brushing your teeth, walking . . or washing your face . . without consciously thinking . . about the movements and actions you go through . . to do those things . .

And third, I'm going to explain another technique . . for you to use . . to improve yourself . . To automatically become more perfect in your athletic performances . .

Your muscles, nerves, ligaments and tendons . . respond to commands from your subconscious mind . . And to build strength in your muscles . .

129

they need to be exercised . . But to train them . . you must train your mind . . which causes them to respond . .

I want you to take out one hour every day . . or in the evening before you go to sleep . . to visualize yourself participating in your sport activity . . Imagine yourself performing when you are at your best . . Make every move . . every twist and turn . . But do more than only what you do best in your sport . . I want you to see yourself running . . faster and faster . . And jumping . . higher than you have ever jumped before . . I want you to excel in every athletic event you can imagine yourself participating in . . Do all of the moves and maneuvers you are familiar with . . over and over . . in your mind . . But don't be satisfied until you perform as well as the greatest athletes perform . .

In your meditation time . . sit in a quiet, comfortable place . . Close your eyes and concentrate . . on the little flecks of light in front of your eyes . . Focus those light specks into one distant light . . until it gets very small . . Then, see yourself in action on the field . . It will become easier with practice . . Then begin to visualize yourself participating in actual competition . . See yourself performing perfectly every time . . Watch your moves closely . . in slow motion . . to fully understand exactly what is happening . . and how it happens . .

You can easily visualize yourself performing on the field . . right now, can't you ? . . I want you to practice on the field . . at the direction of your trainer or coach . . as often as they require you to . .

And I want you to take an hour, every day or evening . . to use your imagination and practice performing perfectly . . in your mind . . over and over again . . (pause)

When you need to calm yourself and relax . . think of water . . or find water to look at . . It will calm you and relax you for at least six hours . .

You will remember everything you have heard here today . . and you will find that your subconscious mind will cause you to keep performing better . . And you will automatically keep improving in actual competition . .

Continue relaxing for a little longer . . Then I will count to Five . . (Pause)

At the count of FIVE, you will awaken, feeling alert, invigorated and ready to take on your next challenge . . You will awaken a little more with each number you hear . . ONE, TWO, THREE, FOUR and FIVE.

Open your eyes now . .

Let yourself continue relaxing now . . so that you can really enjoy this pleasant experience . .

I am going to give you suggestions and instructions . . that will help you to relax and it will help you to become . . the outstanding athlete that you know you are capable of being . .

Every part of your body . . every muscle, every nerve, every ligament and tendon . . is controlled by your subconscious mind . . And you are finding that your subconscious mind . . is causing you to respond to the suggestions and instructions I am giving you . . And is also automatically improving your athletic abilities . . Your athletic skills are what you provide after much practice . .

You already know that practice is important . . for the proper development of skills and talents . . Whether you want to play a musical instrument . . shoot a bow and arrow . . dance or improve yourself in your athletic skills . . Practice is imperative . . All outstanding athletes practice for hours each day . . to develop their skills and talents . . They have the desire to be winners . .

But winning is not always the most important achievement . . with regards to being an outstanding athlete . . More important than winning is being a good athlete . . By that, I mean . . good in all areas of your life . . Being a good person . . Being a good loser . . Being a good winner . . Having good attitudes . . And feeling good about another person who has outstanding athletic abilities . .

Jessie Owens seemed like a certain winner in the long jump . . at the 1936 Olympics in Germany . . The year before, he had jumped 26 feet, 8 ¼ inches . . A record that stood for 25 years . .

As he was walking around, before jumping . . he noticed a tall, blue eyed, blond German . . taking practice jumps in the 26 foot range . . Owens felt nervous and was aware of the nazi's desire . . to prove their superiority . . especially over the 'lesser races' . .

On his first jump, Owens fouled . . stepping over the take-off board a couple inches . .

Being even more nervous now . . he fouled on his second attempt . . One more foul, he would be eliminated . .

At that point, the tall German introduced himself as . . Luz Long . . He said . . "The way you jump, you should qualify with your eyes closed", making reference to Owens' first two jumps . .

He talked with Jessie Owens a few more minutes, then made a suggestion . . He said, "Since the qualifying distance is only 23 feet, 5 ½ inches . . why don't you make your starting mark a few inches in front of the take-off board . . and jump from there . . Just to play it safe" . .

Owens followed his advise and . . qualified easily . . In the finals, he set an Olympic record . . and earned the second of four Gold Metals . . The first person to congratulate him was . . Luz Long . . in full view of Adolph Hitler . .

Luz Long later died in World War II . . and Jessie Owens never saw him again . . However, Jessie later remarked, "You could melt down all the metals and cups I have . . and they would never compare to the 24 carat friendship I felt . . for Luz Long" . .

And that is what I mean by . . the importance of having other qualities . . in addition to being an outstanding athlete . . Being a good sport . . and being a caring, loving person . . is far more important . . than winning . . Another important key . . with regards to being . . an outstanding athlete . . is to have the determination to always do your best . .

I heard about a runner . . who always entered every marathon . . And in most of the events . . he would finish in last place . . One day after running a couple of miles . . he was again in last place . . But as he was running, he thought to himself . . Twenty six miles is a long run . . If I can run just a little faster . . I think I can pass the guy in front of me . . So he picked up his speed, just a little . . and soon passed the runner in front of him . . He then decided the same thing . . about the next runner in front of him . . and continued doing this throughout the race . . Finally, when the race was completed . . to his amazement, he discovered . . he was the winner . . He kept passing each runner . . and without realizing it . . had passed all of the other runners in the race . .

We are always capable of doing 'just a little better' than we have been doing . . And the subconscious level of your mind is remembering . . that you too, are capable of running faster . . You are capable of continuing to improve . . in your running skills . .

From now on . . every time you are running . . you will be relaxed and calm . . Your pulse rate will be lower and your heart will beat slower . . Your lungs will expand and contract . . at the proper rate . . You will experience no debilitating pain in your organs or in your muscles . . Your coordination and reflexes will continue improving . . All of your muscles, ligaments and tendons . . will keep functioning more perfectly . . And your running time and skills . . will continue improving . . each time you run . .

You are continuing to feel more comfortable and more relaxed . . from the top of your head to the tips of your toes . . The subconscious level of your mind . . is hearing and absorbing the suggestions I am giving you . . and is causing you to put them . . into your own actions . . Your subconscious mind is very receptive . . to everything I am telling you . . and is accepting what I say . . Everything I tell you is true . . and is making a deep and lasting impression on your mind . . The subconscious level is causing you to be in charge . . of your automatic reactions . . The movements of your muscles, your nerves, your ligaments and tendons . . are responding to your conscious desire . . to be an outstanding runner . . Your natural running ability is continuing to improve . . (pause)

Now, I am going to give you a few suggestions . . that will improve your concentration . . I want you to imagine that you are out on the track, running . . In your mind, you are realizing that you are an outstanding runner . . You have developed perfect coordination of all your muscles . . your ligaments and your tendons . . Everything is working together perfectly . . You are a well coordinated, steady runner . . Being a good, steady runner means . . that you are capable of winning . . So, from now on . . whenever you are participating in any athletic running event . . you will have confidence that you . . are capable of winning . . regardless of the competition . . Your concentration will be perfect . . Your coordination will be perfect . . Your mind will be ready and your body will be ready . . You will keep practicing and exercising . . to keep your body in good condition . . And your stamina will improve tremendously . . Your self-confidence, your self-acceptance and your self-reliance . . will keep improving . .

Your successes in running will continue mounting up . . You will find that the subconscious level of your mind . . will cause just the right amount of adrenaline to flow through your body . . to cause you to run smoothly . . effortlessly . . calmly and easily . . You will be very pleased with all of the improvements you will notice in your running ability . .

Continue relaxing a moment longer, then I will count to FIVE . . You will wake a little more with each number that you hear . . When you hear the number FIVE, you will open your eyes and be wide awake . . and feeling wonderful . . (Pause)

I will begin the count now . . 1, 2, 3, 4 and 5 . . Open your eyes . .

ATHLETIC - SKILLS

(Follow Relax Induction)

Continue relaxing now as I give you suggestions and instructions . . that will help you to relax deeper . . and will help to improve your athletic skills . . Your subconscious mind is absorbing everything I am saying . . So you can continue to relax . . and go deeper into your hypnotic state . .

The power in your subconscious mind . . is the key to improve your athletic performance . . This has become widely recognized . . Your mind cannot give you the skills you need . . However, it can improve the abilities you already possess . . And we all have many abilities . . that we are not consciously aware of . .

The power of using your mind to visualize yourself in practice . . for developing your athletic skills . . is so great . . that many professional teams are using it in basketball . . football, track and field . . and baseball . . and in tennis . . And it is even being used by various Olympic teams . . such as the U.S. Olympic Judo Team . . It has effectively improved their skills, tremendously . .

The key to improving your athletic abilities . . through the power of your own mind . . is to rehearse the skills that you want to improve on . . over and over again . . in your mind . . And continue to rehearse the skills you already know . . in your mind . . When you rehearse these skills . . always imagine yourself performing perfectly . . By doing that, it reinforces the abilities correctly . . in the subconscious levels of your mind . . Your mind causes you to perform that skill correctly . . when you need to use it in competition . .

Select a time every day, for one hour, of meditation . . During the day, or the evening, just before you sleep . . Be consistent in your schedule . . Select a quiet, comfortable place for your meditation . . where you won't be disturbed by anything . . Simply focus your mind on seeing yourself in action . . Performing everything you do in your event . . And don't be afraid to excel . . Perform every move and maneuver . . Every twist and turn . . Run faster and jump higher than you think you can . . When you use your imagination to perform your skills . . always envision yourself doing it correctly . .

By doing it correctly in your mind . . you will soon be performing more perfectly . . whenever you participate in actual competition . .

As each move is made . . slow the action down to a slow-motion . . That way you can better see and understand . . exactly what is happening . . Why and how it is happening . . What you perform in your mind will quickly translate into reality . . You can do it . . if you, first, do it in your mind . . Visualization is the key to your future success . .

Another way to improve your athletic skills is by selecting . . a professional player . . who performs all of the skills correctly . . Observe that professional athlete as often as possible . . Memorize every move he makes . . Talk with him, if you have the opportunity . . Watch him on TV or on videos . . As you observe other outstanding athletes performing . . it makes an impression on the subconscious levels of your mind . . and you soon find yourself performing exactly the same way . . as the athletes you admire . .

When you are visualizing yourself performing . . in your mind . . see yourself dressed as you would be . . in actual competition . . See the environment and the people around you . . the weather conditions . . the way you expect it to be . . Imagine yourself performing your skills perfectly . . over and over again . . Do this as vividly as possible, each time . . See yourself and others, dressed appropriately . .

If others take part in the event . . see the others clearly . . The more you make this mental exercise as real as the actual competition . . the more powerful it will be . . for improving your capabilities . . in the real life event . .

Practice your visualization . . for one hour each day . . and again for a few minutes each night . . just before you go to sleep . . It will continue becoming more deeply reinforced in your mind . . And that will give it more power . . when you are actually participating . . in real competition . .

Your trainer and your coach . . are the most important people on your team . . They are there to advise you and to guide you . . to be successful . . by training you hard . .

And by urging you to practicing hard . . You will work hard under their guidance . . and you will live by the schedule they establish for you . . You will feel yourself becoming more talented . . and more skilled . . as you participate in your normal . . practice routines . . This prideful feeling you instill in yourself . . and your abilities to perform correctly . . will carry over into the time . . when you take part in real competition . . And you will notice your performance abilities . . continuing to improve . .

Your confidence . . derived from your successes . . will keep increasing . . and you will be more aware of your skills . . continuously improving . . day by day . .

I am going to give you a few more moments to continue relaxing . . to give your subconscious mind enough time . . to absorb everything we have talked about . . Everything I have told you is true . . And you will remember everything I have said to you . .

Contemplate on what you have heard, as you relax . . In a moment, I will begin my count . . to bring you out of your hypnotic state . . Just relax for a little longer . . (Pause)

I am going to begin my count now . . I will count up to five . . With each number you hear . . you will awaken a little more . . When you hear the number FIVE . . you will open your eyes and be wide awake . . Feeling good . . Feeling wonderful and feeling confident.

ONE . . Beginning to stir now . .

TWO . . Your fingers and toes want to move a little . .

THREE . . Becoming more aware of yourself and feeling good . .

FOUR . . Take in a deep breath now . . and . .

FIVE . . Open your eyes . .

We are going to conclude this session in a few minutes . . I will be counting from ONE to FIVE . . and you will awaken a little bit more . . with each number you hear . .

Each time I say a number . . your conscious mind will keep becoming more alert . . and when you hear the number FIVE . . your eyes will open easily . . and you will be back in a wide awake, fully alert state . .

You will feel wonderful when you open your eyes . . You will feel better . . both physically and mentally . . You will feel as though you have awakened from . . a very deep, peaceful and restful sleep . .

Each time I hypnotize you . . you can continue going into a deeper . . more peaceful . . more detached state . . Much more quickly . . And you'll continue gaining benefits from each session we have . .

Continue relaxing now for just a little longer . . Giving your subconscious mind opportunity . . to analyze and absorb everything we have talked about . . (Pause) Everything I have said to you is true . . and you will remember everything I have said to you . . I will begin my count now . .

ONE . . You are beginning to awaken . . a little at a time . . You will soon awaken . . and feel fully alert, confident and happy . .

TWO . . You are experiencing a wonderful, glowing feeling . . all through your body . . Each day you will feel more alive . . and more happy with yourself . . And you will continue to experience more improvements . . in all areas of your life . .

THREE . . All of the suggestions I have given you . . are now in the storehouse of your mind . . They will continue becoming more effective each day . . It is a cycle of progress that grows stronger as you progress . .

FOUR . . You are feeling rested and refreshed . . Your mind is alert . . And you will continue having more strength . . more energy and more vitality . . Breathe in deeply now and . .

FIVE . . Open your eyes, feeling healthy . . happy and confident . . You're back in a wide awake, fully alert state . . Tell me now , How do you feel ?

(NOTE :   If, after a minute or so, the client has not yet opened his or her eyes, say to them, "I am going to lift up your hand and arm.   You will awaken easily as I lift up your hand and arm". As you are lifting body parts, continue giving suggestions similar to those above.)

024 Prescript.   BACKACHE - ELIMINATING
(Follow Golden Glow Induction)

You are responding well to the suggestions I am giving you . . and you are beginning to experience some pleasant changes . . that will get rid of the aches and pains in your back . .

Permitting yourself to be hypnotized . . lets your subconscious mind know . . that you sincerely want your back . . to be healed . . You are dissatisfied with the feelings of discomfort you have been experiencing . . And you want to be rid of those . . aches and pains . . for now and forever . .

It is natural for your body to be healthy . . It is natural for all of the bones in your back . . to be in perfect alignment . . It is natural for the ligaments, tendons and nerves in your back . . to function perfectly . . It is natural for the muscles in your back . . to be strong and hold your spinal column . . in the proper alignment . . And it is natural for your subconscious mind . . to cause all of the activities of your body . . to function properly . . Keeping your back structure in perfect alignment . .

And you will be pleased . . that your mind is assessing everything I am saying to you . . And you will be pleasantly surprised at the rapid way . . in which your back is being healed . .

You have no reason to consciously remember . . what I am telling you . . because your subconscious mind will remember everything I am saying . . And your subconscious mind . . will cause all of the various parts of your body to work automatically . . and correctly . . And you will be happy to continue experiencing . . the comfortable way your back is healing . .

In the past, you may have had some doubts . . That is natural . . But now those doubts are leaving . . and you will really be happy to know . . those doubts will soon be gone completely . . Because they are being replaced with feelings of confidence and security . . When you were doubtful, you were probably wondering . . if your subconscious mind . . would cause your back to be completely realigned and healed . . this week . . Or will it take two weeks . . for your back to be completely realigned and healed . . Or will you be surprised to find . . your back perfectly realigned and healed . . by the time you awaken from this hypnotic state . .

One thing I have learned after hypnotizing many, many people . . is the fact that your subconscious mind . . can cause your healing processes to work rapidly . . and make the proper adjustments in your back, very quickly . . Another thing I have learned is that your subconscious mind . . knows exactly what needs to be done . . to work out the solution . . regardless of what it was . . that caused you to begin having a back problem . . Your subconscious mind knows how fast it can work . . in getting those improper understandings cleared up . . And you will be happy to find . . your body will make all the proper adjustments . . and heal your back completely . .

You are responding automatically to everything I say to you . . because you have decided . . that you want your back to be completely healed . . Right now you are experiencing the flow of golden energy . . still flowing through all of your systems . . You may notice the healing warmth of the energy . . penetrating throughout your body . . as well as in your back . . You are going through a very pleasant corrective experience . . right now . . without even realizing it . .

At this very moment . . your systems are making comfortable adjustments . . Proper alignments are taking place . . And although you are not sure of exactly what is happening . . you can sense that it is a good thing . . Just relax and . . let it continue . .

 It must be pleasing for you to know . . that it is your own mind . . that is causing those adjustment to take place . . In its own quiet way and . . for your benefit . . And for the healing of your body . . This experience of healing your back . . carries with it, a feeling of accomplishment . . And the feeling of knowing that it is being done . . carries with it . . a strong sense of satisfaction and contentment . .

So you can be proud of what you are accomplishing . . And proud to realize that your back is . . being perfectly realigned . . And to know that the muscles are strengthening . . to keep your back properly aligned and straight . .

Your subconscious mind understands the meaning . . of everything I am saying to you . . and is causing everything I tell you to work automatically . . And all of the changes are being accomplished . . in your own terms . .

And the pleasant feelings are with you . . as your subconscious mind silently works . . And you realize that it is all worthwhile . . and will be helpful to you . . in so many ways . .

You understand that what you are doing is very important . . and it will enable you to be an inspiration . . to many other people . . You will find pleasure and enjoyment . . in giving respect to the fact . . that your body is a temple of God . . And that you are having a healthy body . . So, too, will you be a perfect example of God's creation . . of beauty, health and strength . .

You are already feeling much better . . You are already feeling enthusiastic . . about what you are achieving . . And you will be very pleased to find . . that it will continue after you awaken . . from your hypnotic state . .

You are doing so well now . . I just want you to relax another moment or two . . and then I will begin my count to bring you back to the surface . .
(pause)

I am going to begin counting now . . from Five down to One . . When you hear me count out the number, One . . you will open your eyes, feeling good about yourself . . and good about your accomplishments today . .

Five – Your conscious mind is beginning to revive itself . . It is time to awaken . .
Four – Beginning to stir now . . Your body is in need of movement . . Let your arms and legs move a little . .
Three – Nearing the surface now . . Rising up higher . . and higher . .
Two – Almost there . . Almost there . . Inhale deeply now and . .
One – Open your eyes and adjust to your surroundings . .

Every cell in your body . . has a specific job to do . . And effortlessly . . performs functions . . that the world's most outstanding chemists, scientists and physicians . . have never been able to duplicate . . And all of the cells of your body . . do their work by receiving directions . . from your own subconscious mind . .

Your subconscious mind is directing . . the cells in your scalp . . to activate your molecular processes . . so they will renew, rejuvenate and restore . . the hair in your scalp follicles . .

When you were a tiny baby . . your mind knew what to do . . to cause the hair on your scalp to grow . . And your mind is now remembering what it needs to do . . to rejuvenate the growth processes of the hair in your scalp . .

Your subconscious mind is causing the sebaceous glands in your scalp . . to be stimulated . . and cause increased secretion . . and improve the condition of your scalp and hair . .

You will soon notice a new growth of hair in your scalp . . And you will be pleased . . as you become aware . . of a continuous improvement . . in the condition of your scalp . .

I heard of a farmer who found a sack of seeds . . that had been hidden for many years . . in the corner of a shed out near his barn . . He knew the seeds must be at least twenty years old . . because he hadn't cleaned out that shed for about twenty years . . Anyway, he decided to plant those seeds . . He waited patiently and, sure enough . . one day stalks of corn began coming up through the ground . . And the stalks continued growing taller and taller . . Finally, harvest time came . . and they produced a beautiful supply of corn . . And just as those seeds still had life in them . . after lying dormant for twenty years . . your scalp still has life in it, too . . And all of the cells, atoms and molecules in your scalp . . are being rejuvenated . . And are causing new hair to grow on your scalp . .

(Have client use imagination to envision his new hair growing as he desires it to be .)

Each night, before you go to sleep . . close your eyes and visualize your scalp . . full of hair . . the way you want it to be . . Keep reinforcing the image in your mind . . and your subconscious mind will cause it to happen . .

Your subconscious mind . . is causing your scalp to produce a continuous growth of hair . . You are developing your hair exactly . . the way you want it to be . . Your appearance keeps improving and your self-confidence . . continues increasing . .

All of these suggestions are already working . . and you will be very happy . . with the continuous improvement in your hair . .

EMERGE

One of the most helpful conditions of being . . in a hypnotic state of relaxation . . is that it enables your subconscious mind to examine . . review and explore . . the imprints, impressions, thoughts, ideas . . and other information . . in the storehouse of your mind . .

Your subconscious mind can review and examine . . all that information . . as it was understood when it went into your mind . . And can better understand it now . . from a different point of view . . A more adult . . more mature point of view . . Because you have had a lot of experience . . and have accumulated a much better understanding . . of your life circumstances . . since that time . .

You have numerous memories . . and many different kinds of understandings . . that can enrich and improve your life . . in scores of ways . . Physically, emotionally, mentally and spiritually . .

One day, a friend and I were walking through the woods . . We had walked for a long time . . and, finally, we came upon a huge tree . . that had fallen across the path . . We decided to sit down on the tree and rest for a while . . And I asked my friend to see if he could discover something new . . Something he had never noticed before . .

He looked around for a moment and then . . picked up a leaf from the tree . . Upon examining it closer, he discovered . . that it had hundreds of tiny veins . . Something he had never noticed before . . Then he looked around some more and realized . . that all the trees were leaning in the same direction . . and nearly all of them had moss growing on them . . but only on the north side . .

It's really easy to discover things for yourself . . when you take the time to do so . .

Of course, I don't know what you are doing right now . . You are merely reviewing . . and exploring . . for your own benefit . . You may be recalling things that happened when you were a tiny baby . . or it may be something from your early days at school . . Or perhaps, you may be recalling information from your Jr. High School days . . You are reaching understandings . . You are making new alignments of understandings . . Or even realignments of words . . and their actual meanings . . There is so much to explore . . And this is what you are doing . . You are exploring . .

Not knowing what is going to come up next . . It might be anything from somewhere in your past . .

I want to suggest a very comfortable examination . . An examination which will show you . . how your understandings have grown . . and changed . . You can . . make use of the imprints and impressions in your mind . . Imprints and impressions . . from various learning's and experiences . .

You continue breathing easily and freely . . And you hear the words I am saying . . without any kind of physical effort . . And all the time . . you are focusing on the inner experiences . . that are important to you . . And you can remember at any level you wish . . Many people can recall the day of their birth . . You can also do that . . Right now, you may be going through an emotionally corrective experience . . Recalling an understanding you thought was true . . but now you can see it differently.

At this very moment . . your system is synthesizing proteins . . And all of the various chemicals and substances in your body . . are beginning to function, harmoniously . . Rejuvenation is taking place, as it is needed . . I don't know exactly what is going on but . . you can sense something good is happening . . inside you . . So, let it continue . .

You will now enjoy the opportunity to broaden your horizons . . Your thinking will expand . . Your levels of knowledge will improve greatly . . And your creative talents will blossom . . You are becoming aware of a need for centering your life . . Bringing mind, body and spirit together . . Focusing on your life's direction and . . purpose for being . . And too . . this is a very creative time . . It must be pleasing for you to know . . your mind is doing all this . . in its own way . . for your own personal well being . . For your own benefit . . And for your own self-improvement . . You will now enjoy new ways of looking at things . . Your thinking will be more open to creativity . . Your yearnings for knowledge will improve . . And your creative abilities will shine through . . You are going to make many new discoveries . . These newly broadened thought patterns . . are opening up new horizons for you . . New discoveries are waiting . . And many new opportunities . . will be yours . .

When changes have begun . . and your subconscious mind knows that you will continue improving . . your mind will cause one of your fingers on your left hand to raise up . . (Wait for finger to raise up - then tell it to go down..)

Continue to relax for a little longer . . Giving a bit more time for your subconscious mind to accept and absorb . . all that we have talked about . . Relax and enjoy these peaceful moments . . (pause)

In a moment, I am going to count from One to Five . . You will awaken a little more with each number you hear . . When you hear the number FIVE . . you will open your eyes and be wide awake . . alert . . And you will feel wonderful . . For you truly are a wonderful person . . (Pause)

I will begin my count now . .

ONE . . You're coming up now . . slowly . . Soon you will awaken . .

TWO . . Your fingers and toes want to wiggle now . . Let them move a little.

THREE . . Feeling good . . Feeling refreshed and confident . .

FOUR . . You're nearly there . . Take in a deep breath now and . .

FIVE . . Open your eyes . . and tell me . . How do you feel ?

BED WETTING - ELIMINATE

Now as you continue to go deeper . . deeper relaxed . . I am going to give you . . some suggestions . . to assist you in keeping your bed dry at all times . . In fact, you realize that from this time on . . you are going to be able to keep that bed 100 % dry . . You are going to be able to keep your bed 100 % dry because . . now, you are in control . . You have full control over your spincter muscles . . Those are the little muscles that turn the urine off and on . .

As you sink deeper . . and deeper down . . you realize that from this time on . . you are going to be able to keep that bed 100 % dry . . 100 % dry because now you have the control . . Sufficient control over your spincter muscles . . Those are the muscles that shut off the urine . . You have control over those muscles . . so they will be able to hold up all night long . .

And I am also giving you a suggestion so that . . as your bladder fills up in the night . . if you do sleep for a long time . . and your bladder does become full . . your left hand will raise up and . . pinch your nose . . or tug on your ear . . and wake you up . . So that you keep the bed completely dry at all times . .

Because, before your bladder is completely full . . your left hand will pinch your nose and wake you up . . Which means, you will then get up and go to the bathroom . . Then go back to sleep . .

Now, you probably won't have to get up and go to the bathroom . . because your bladder probably won't be full during the night . . But if it is full . . and if it gets to the point where you might wet the bed . . if there is any chance of it at all . . then your left hand will reach up and touch your nose . . and wake you up . . And you'll get up and go to the bathroom . . And then go back to bed . . so you won't wet the bed . . ever again . . Isn't that wonderful ? . .

As a matter of fact . . you are through wetting the bed altogether . . And when you do go to the bathroom . . in order to strengthen the muscles that control urination . . every time that you urinate . . you will shut it on and off . . at least five times . . on-off, on-off, on-off, on-off, on-off . . And as you practice that . . you are actually working that muscle . . strengthening that muscle . . exercising that muscle . . Just like you would exercise and strengthen any other muscle . . And so, you will exercise and strengthen that muscle . .

every single time that you go to the bathroom . . shutting the stream on and off . . on and off . . on and off, at least five times . . And you will also do this if you are awakened in the middle of the night . .

And so, you are going to be able to keep the bed completely dry . . And it is going to be easy for you . . Especially now that your bladder muscles are becoming more and more developed . . The spincter muscle . . the one that controls the urination . . is becoming more and more strengthened . . more and more strong . . more and more developed . .

Now, as you sink deeper and deeper . . every one of these suggestions . . take complete and thorough effect upon you . .

First of all . . you keep the bed 100 % dry . . Second . . Your control of the spincter muscle . . the muscle that controls the urination . . is becoming greater and greater, every day that passes . . Third . . you strengthen this muscle by turning the urine stream on and off . . every time you go to the bathroom . . And, Fourth . . when you are sleeping at night . . if your bladder does fill up . . and before it gets to the point that you would urinate . . your left hand will raise up and pinch your nose . . and wake you . . so that you will immediately get out of bed and go to the bathroom . . Just like an alarm clock . . It wakes you up . . Only it wakes you up before you urinate in the bed . .

Now, all of these suggestions take complete and thorough effect upon you . . in mind, body and spirit . . Sealing themselves in, at the deepest part of your subconscious mind . . And you can be dry all the time . . At a friend's home or a relative's home . . Anywhere . . And this, of course, means that you are growing older . . and more mature . . that you are having better control over yourself . . and over your musculature . .

Now, you sink deeper and deeper relaxed . . as all of these suggestions take complete and thorough effect on you . . in mind . . in body and spirit . . And you sink further and further down . . Deeper and deeper . . relaxed . . Deeper and deeper . . relaxed . . Deeper and deeper . . relaxed . .

(pause)

148

All of the suggestions that I have given you . . are going to be reinforced in your mind . . ten times over . . making them very, very strong . . and keeping you 100 % dry . . All of the suggestions I am giving you . . are enforcing themselves . . over and over ten times . . keeping you 100 % dry . . All of the suggestions I am giving you are repeated and reinforced . . in your mind . . ten times over . . keeping you 100 % dry at all times . . Reinforced ten times over, and over again . . during the period of silence . . which begins now . . (pause)

EMERGE or go to Bed Wetting METAPHOR

(Follow Relaxation - Confidence)

Now as you continue to go deeper . . deeper relaxed . . And as you continue drifting into a deeper hypnotic state of relaxation . . you can feel yourself growing . . You will soon be a grown up person . . You do want to grow up, don't you ? . . (Pause - wait for answer)

Good . . I knew you wanted to grow up . . And that's one of the reasons you want to stop wetting the bed, isn't it . . You want to grow up and do things the way grown-ups do . .

You want to graduate from school . . You want to be able to drive a car . . And some day, you'll want to have your own home . . And you sure want to stop wetting the bed, don't you ? . . (Pause - wait for answer)

Good . . Since you want to quit wetting the bed . . I'm going to tell you something that will keep you from ever wetting the bed again . . How does that sound to you ? . . (pause for answer)

From now on, you will be able to sleep all night . . in a nice dry bed . . You are grown up enough now that you want to always sleep in a nice dry bed . . just like grown-ups do . .

You are old enough and smart enough that, from now on . . if you ever need to use the toilet during the night . . you will wake up . . and you will get out of your bed . . and go to the toilet . .

After you use the toilet . . you will go back to your bed . . and go beck to sleep . . And sleep in a nice dry bed for the rest of the night . .

Most of the time . . you will be able to sleep all night . . without needing to go to the toilet . . because you are growing up . . And you are learning to control yourself . . And you will never wet in the bed again . .

Just before you go to bed each night . . you will use the toilet . . and that will make it easy for you . . to go all night in a nice dry bed . . You will go to sleep in a nice dry bed . . and you will wake up each morning . . in a nice dry bed . .

You know, your bladder is made like a balloon . . so that it keeps stretching to hold fluid . . all night long . . And that enables you to sleep comfortably . . all night long in a nice dry bed . .

You will be very happy and proud of yourself . . because you realize that you are growing up . . And you keep having more and more confidence in yourself . .

You will be happier with your friends . . and you'll be able to have friends stay all night with you . . because your bed will always be nice and dry . . If you ever need to use the toilet during the night . . you will always wake up and go to the toilet . . And that way, you will always sleep in a nice dry bed . . that you will be proud to have your friends see . .

Now that you don't wet in your bed any more . . you will be more relaxed in school . . and you will find that your school grades keep improving . . more and more . .

You can really feel proud of yourself . . You know that your bladder will stretch enough . . for you to sleep in a nice dry bed all night . .

During the day . . if you need to use the toilet . . but can't get to a toilet right away . . you know how to control yourself until you can get to a toilet . .

During the night . . while you are sleeping . . your subconscious mind will cause you . . to automatically control yourself . . or to wake you up, if it gets to be too much . . And enable you to sleep comfortably in a nice dry bed . .

From now on . . if you are sleeping and need to use the toilet . . you will wake up and go to the toilet . . just like you do during the day, whenever you need to use the toilet . . But most of the time you will sleep comfortably . . all night long, in a nice dry bed . .

You are too grown up and too smart to wet the bed any more . . You feel good now, don't you ? . . You feel confident . . And you can really feel proud of yourself . . because you know . . you will always sleep comfortably, in a nice dry bed . .

EMERGE or go to **METAPHOR**

BED WETTING - METAPHOR
CHILD DISCOVERY

(Follow Bed Wetting)

(NOTE : Have client do something, such as, make one arm heavy and the other arm light, to demonstrate the ability of the mind to control body responses. Follow that by using finger response to get client released from imprints and impressions, that have been causing the bed-wetting problem.)

Your subconscious mind indicates . . that you are now released . . from everything that has been causing you . . to urinate in your bed when you are sleeping . . So you will find that you are getting rid of the habit . . of urinating in your bed . . your subconscious mind controls your body functions . . and is now getting rid of the bed-wetting habit . . completely and forever . .

From this moment on . . you will urinate only . . when you consciously make the decision . . to eliminate urine from your bladder . . into a toilet . . You will urinate only when you make a conscious decision . . to cleanse urine out of your bladder . . unless there is an emergency . . an illness . . or some other reason . . that would make your conscious consent impossible . .

You are continuing to drift into a deeper hypnotic state . . and your subconscious mind is accepting . . the suggestions, guidance and instructions . . I am giving you . .

Once upon a time . . there was a poor little girl who lived alone with her mother . . When they had nothing left to eat . . the little girl went out into the forest . . where she met a woman . . who already knew she was hungry . . So, the woman gave the little girl a small pot . . and instructed her to say, "Little pot. Cook!" . . and the little pot would make a good, sweet porridge . . Then, to make it stop cooking . . the little girl was to say . . "Little pot. Stop!" and it would stop cooking . .

The girl took the pot home to her mother and put an end to their hunger . . From then on, they had porridge as often as they wanted it . .

One day, the little girl had gone out . . And while she was away, her mother said . . "Little pot. Cook", and it began cooking . . After she had eaten her fill, she wanted the little pot to stop cooking . . but she had forgotten the right words . . and the little pot kept on cooking . . And the porridge ran over the rim and filled the kitchen . . And then, filed the whole house . . And then, the house next door . .

152

And out into the street . . And the little pot kept cooking and cooking . . as though it wanted to feed the entire world . . And nobody knew what to do . . Finally, the little girl came home and merely said . . "Little pot. Stop!" . . And it stopped cooking . . And for a long time after that . . any people who wanted to go into that town . . had to eat their way from one street to the next . .

And, just as easily . . you have now stopped wetting the bed . .

From this moment on . . you are in control of your urinary elimination processes . . and you have decided that you will never . . ever again . . urinate in your bed . . Just think of . . "Little pot. Stop!"

As you continue relaxing . . all embarrassments you have experienced . . from wetting in your bed . . are fading away from your memory . . and are being replaced by strong, proud feelings of achievement . . and confidence . . You are proud to have stopped wetting in your bed . . And you realize that . . your decision to end bed-wetting is a great accomplishment . . that lets you know you are capable . . of making other choices and decisions . . that will improve your life . . You will be more calm and relaxed during the day . . and you will sleep more comfortably . . at night . . in a nice dry bed . .

Your decision to stop wetting your bed . . is causing you to feel more at ease . . more confident and . . more secure . . Your self-confidence will continue increasing more each day . . And you will have the confidence you need . . to conquer any other problems . . that ever come up in your life . . You will be more successful in all the other goals you ever want to achieve . .

What I want you to do is to accept yourself . . for who you are . . Realize that you are the one . . who must choose your place in life . . Know that while you can control yourself now . . you can also control your destiny . . You have a number of goals you want to achieve . . So, you want to focus your efforts . . You want your mind to review, explore and examine . . all misunderstandings . . and get them straightened out . .

It is a wonderful thing for your mind to review . . to explore . . to discover . . And there are so many discoveries you will make . . Some are personal . . and will belong only to you . . Some, you will want to share with others . . One of the nice things about it is . . you don't know what you are going to discover . . But you're going to have an enjoyable time . . when you discover it . .

And you can find out everything you want to know . . because you have the background of understanding . . And it has to be your background . . to understand it . . You can draw from your background to do your own self – exploration . .

Many people question what their goals in life really are . . They learn their goals in the process of getting there . . You may not know exactly what your goals are . . but you're going to enjoy discovering them . . And when you are through . . you will know exactly what they are . .

Life isn't something you give an answer to . . You enjoy the process of waiting . . The process of discovery . . The process of becoming . . who you are . .

Upon graduating from college . . George Washington Carver prayed and asked God, "How do you want me to help you to run the universe?" He received no answer . . He, then, asked God, "How do you want me to help you to run the world?" Again, he received no answer . . Then he asked God . . "What DO you want me to do ?"

Finally, from a state of meditation, he decided to work as a chemist with what was considered, the lowly peanut . . And he developed many food and industrial uses for the peanut . . And later, for the sweet potato . . He revolutionized the agricultural industries and changed economic history . . all because he took the time to explore his mind . . and make the discoveries for his life to be complete . .

And that is what you are going to do . . Explore, Examine and Discover . .

In a moment, I am going to count from One to Five . . You will wake up a little more with each number you hear . . When you hear the number Five . . you will open your eyes and feel wonderful . . Because you certainly are a wonderful person . . You will remember everything you have heard today and know that everything I have told you is true . . I will begin the count now . .

One . . etc.

You are realizing more and more . . that your subconscious mind controls all of the activities . . and processes of your body . . So, your conscious mind can continue relaxing now . . because there is nothing it needs to do at this time . . Your subconscious mind is receiving everything I tell you . . and is causing everything I tell you . . to begin working immediately . .

In just a moment . . when I tell you to begin . . I want you to count from TEN . . down to ONE . . slowly . . in your mind . . And notice what is happening to your RIGHT hand . . as your LEFT hand becomes completely numb . .

Start counting now from ten down to one . . and notice what is happening to your RIGHT hand . . Start from ten and when you reach the count of one . . lift your RIGHT hand up to let me know . .

(Note : After the client lifts the RIGHT hand up, pinch the LEFT hand with your finger nails, and ask, "What does it feel like I am doing" . . The LEFT hand should feel numb. If the response is good, then pick up the LEFT hand with your finger nails, pinching it tightly. Then have the client open his or her eyes and look at the finger nail marks . . Then pinch the RIGHT hand to show that it is not numb and pinch the LEFT arm, to show that it is not numb.) Now, you realize that your subconscious mind . . can cause changes in your body automatically . .

So in just a moment, I want you to count backwards again . . from TEN down to ONE . . slowly in your mind . . And notice the normal feeling . . coming back into your LEFT hand . . as your blood pressure is stabilizing at around 120 over 70 . . When you reach the count of ONE, lift up your LEFT hand . . to let me know the normal feeling is back . . (pause)

You are responding perfectly to everything I say to you . . Your subconscious mind is causing your entire organism . . your body . . to cooperate with everything I tell you . . And you will be pleased to have that continue . . even after you awaken from the hypnotic state . .

You are beginning to feel a sense of confidence and a sense of competence and sureness . . And the feeling of calmness you are experiencing will continue . . as you go about the activities of your daily life . .

Before I had you get the numbness in your hand . . you may not have realized . . that your subconscious mind controls your physical body . . and you may still have some doubts in your mind . . But those doubts will soon be leaving you . . Those doubts are being replaced . . with a strong sense of confidence and sureness . . And before this session is completed . . you will be sure that the problem you have been experiencing . . will be completely healed . .

(Use Magnetic Hand demonstration. Show how the mind controls the body.)

Now you are realizing even more . . that your subconscious mind . . controls every part of your body . . without any conscious effort by you . .

You understand that if someone came into the room . . and said something to embarrass you . . your face would turn red . . The blood would rush to your face . . and cause your face to become red all over . . And realizing that your subconscious mind . . controls the flow of blood to your face . . And, too, you understand that your subconscious mind also . . controls the flow of blood . . in all of the other parts of your body . .

Your subconscious mind and your body . . have had a lot of experience . . You know that if you decide to wiggle your finger . . immediately your finger will begin to wiggle . . And it is your subconscious mind that is causing . . all of those ligaments, tendons and bones . . to move . . You know that if you decide to have a bite of food . . it is your subconscious mind that causes you to chew the food . . and swallow it . . And it is your subconscious mind that causes the food . . to digest . . And it is your subconscious mind that causes you . . to have bowel movements . . to get the digested food out of your body . . through the normal, natural processes of your elimination system . .

Your subconscious mind and your body . . have had a lot of experience . . And that lets us know . . that it is capable of controlling . . the capillary flow of blood . . Just like your subconscious mind can control your salivary glands . . as you look at food or see someone eating a lemon . .

You can say something sad to someone . . and produce tears . . Tears require an alteration of the flow of blood . . in the tear ducts . . Even though you don't know how those tear ducts are supplied with blood . . So, you are realizing that your subconscious mind has a tremendous amount of information . . of which you are totally unaware . . And your mind is using that information . . to work out a solution to the problem you are having . . and heal your body completely . . and perfectly . .

So, I want you to use your imagination now . . and imagine how it would feel to be relaxing comfortably . . at some place you enjoy very much . . Perhaps at the beach . . feeling the sand under your back . . and a pleasant breeze blowing across your body . . And you are continuing to become more calm . . and more relaxed . . You watch the seagulls drifting in the wind and . . you can see a fishing fleet . . far out on the horizon . . And smell the salty, sea air . . So peaceful . . (pause)

You understand that your inner mind is controlling . . your breathing . . Notice how easily and calmly . . you are breathing now . . without any conscious effort by you . . Your subconscious mind is also controlling your pulse . . your blood pressure . . the blood in your arteries and veins . . In fact, your inner mind knows exactly how to control your bleeding . . completely and perfectly . . and it is healing you even now . . as you are relaxing in this comfortable position . .

Notice how relaxed and comfortable you are now . . as you are allowing your subconscious mind . . to help you . . Your mind is reviewing what caused that problem . . and is working out the solution . . Your inner mind is causing you . . to experience pleasant changes . . that are healing your body perfectly . . Even after you awaken . . from the hypnotic state . . and come back to a wide awake, fully alert state . . Your subconscious mind will cause the healing processes of your body . . to continue working . . Healing every part of your body . . in a gentle, pleasant way . .

Continue relaxing now, for a few more minutes . . to give your subconscious mind the time . . to accept and absorb . . everything we have talked about today . . We have covered a lot of things, haven't we . . So continue to relax . . (Pause)

In a moment, I will count to FIVE . . and you will awaken feeling refreshed and wonderful . . You will awaken a little more with each number you hear . . You will remember everything I have told you and . . everything that I have said to you is true . . I will begin my count now . .

ONE . . etc.

You are responding well to everything I tell you . . and you are ready now for your subconscious mind . . to begin making changes in your body . . that will bring your blood pressure down . . to its normal level . . about 120 over 80 . . And keep it down at that level . .

It is natural for your body to be healthy . . It is natural for your heart . . to pump blood . . through your circulatory system perfectly . . It is natural for your blood pressure . . to be 120 over 70 or 80 . . And it is natural for your subconscious mind . . to cause all of the activities of your body . . to function normally . .

These are some of the reasons . . your subconscious mind . . is receiving everything I am telling you . . And it is understanding . . that everything I am telling you is natural for your body . . to keep it functioning properly . . And you will be quite happy with your ability . . to achieve everything I am telling you . .

As I am talking to you . . your subconscious mind is working out . . the best way to bring your blood pressure down . . to its normal level of 120 over 80 . . And you will be pleased to find . . that your blood pressure will stay down . . at its normal level of 120 over 80 . .

Your subconscious mind does many things during the day . . and even at night while you are sleeping . . although you are not consciously aware of what is happening . .

Your subconscious mind keeps your digestive system . . actively functioning . . whether you are awake or asleep . . It causes you to continue breathing . . 24 hours a day . . When you decide to talk . . it causes your tongue to move to the right position in your mouth . . and causes your mouth to form in the right position . . And it causes the right amount of air and oxygen . . to move through your vocal cords so you can make the sounds . . of each word you want to say . .

And your subconscious mind knows how . . to keep all the activities of your body functioning correctly . . including . . keeping your heart pumping the blood . . through your circulatory system properly . . and keeping your blood pressure at 120 over 80 . . without any help from your conscious mind . .

So, it is perfectly natural for your subconscious mind . . to bring your blood pressure down . . to 120 over 80 . . And keep the activities of your body functioning properly . . And keep your blood pressure down . . at its correct level . .

You are realizing more and more . . that your subconscious mind controls all of the activities . . and processes of your body . . So, your conscious mind can continue relaxing now . . because there is nothing it needs to do at this moment . . Your subconscious mind is receiving everything I tell you . . and is causing everything I tell you . . to begin working immediately . .

In just a moment . . when I tell you to begin . . I want you to count from TEN . . down to ONE . . slowly . . in your mind . . And notice what is happening to your RIGHT hand . . as your LEFT hand becomes completely numb . . Start counting from TEN down to ONE, now . . and notice what is happening to your RIGHT hand . . When you reach the count of ONE . . lift your RIGHT hand up to let me know . .

(Note : After the client lifts the RIGHT hand up, pinch the LEFT hand with your finger nails, and ask, "What does it feel like I am doing ?" The LEFT hand should feel numb. If the response is good, then pick up the LEFT hand with your finger nails, pinching it tightly. Then have the client open his or her eyes and look at the finger nail marks. Then pinch the RIGHT hand to show that it is not numb and pinch the LEFT arm, to show that it is not numb.)

Now, you realize that your subconscious mind . . can cause changes in your body automatically . .

So, in just a moment . . I want you to count backwards again . . from TEN down to ONE . . slowly in your mind . . and notice the normal feeling . . coming back into your LEFT hand . . as your blood pressure is stabilizing at 120 over 80 . . When you reach the count of ONE . . lift up your LEFT hand . . to let me know the normal feeling is back . . (pause)

You are responding perfectly to everything I say to you . . Your subconscious mind is causing your entire organism . . your body . . to cooperate with everything I tell you . . And you will be pleased to have that continue . . even after you awaken from the hypnotic state . .

You are beginning to feel a sense of confidence . . and a sense of competence and sureness . . And the feeling of calmness will continue . . as you go about the activities of your daily life . .

You do not consciously understand . . what caused your blood pressure to go up . . but that doesn't make any difference . . Whatever caused it, is past now . . and your subconscious mind . . is getting those incorrect understandings cleared up . . and your blood pressure will remain . . at its normal level . . of about 120 over 80 . . You will be pleased to know that . . this will cause all other parts of your body . . to keep becoming healthier . . and continue functioning more perfectly . .

By accepting everything I say to you . . and putting it into your own actions . . you will find that it will benefit you in many ways . . And everything you achieve . . will be of your own accomplishment . .

Having your blood pressure down . . at a normal level . . will give you a feeling of satisfaction . . You are already beginning to feel happy about it . . And you will be pleased to find that this will continue . . long after you are back in a wide awake . . fully alert state . .

Continue relaxing now for a few more minutes . . to give your subconscious mind the time . . to accept and absorb . . everything we have talked about today . . We have covered a lot of things, haven't we . . So continue to relax . . (Pause)

In a moment, I will count to FIVE . . and you will awaken feeling refreshed and wonderful . . You will awaken a little more with each number you hear . . You will remember everything I have told you and . . everything I have told you is true . .

I will begin my count now . .

ONE . . You are coming up now . . Soon you will awaken . .

TWO . . Your fingers and toes want to move now . . Let them move a little.

THREE . . Feeling good now . . Feeling refreshed and wonderful . .

FOUR . . You're almost there . . Take a deep breath now . . and . .

FIVE . . Open your eyes . .

You are deeply relaxed now . . and I want you to continue to relax . . while I give you suggestions . . that will cause you to be more calm and relaxed . . as you go about your daily routines . .

Your subconscious mind has amazing capabilities . . for sorting out information and understanding it . . even if it is received in parables . . or symbolic terms . . The subconscious level of the mind . . seems to deal in symbols . . much more than does the conscious mind . . That may be the reason why so many dreams are revealed in symbols . .

As the result of many years of research with hypnosis . . it has been found that your mind . . can often work out the solution to a problem quite rapidly . . when it is explained in parables or in symbolic terms . . And that's one of the reasons I want to tell you . . about a little clock that was in the bedroom . . of a very pretty little house, for many years . .

Year after year, the little clock kept faithfully ticking, on and on . . sitting on the night stand by the bed . . All day and all night . . for 365 days of every year . . As long as the clock was wound properly . . it continued ticking . . and always keeping accurate time for its owner . .

One day, the owner of the clock was in a hurry . . She grabbed the clock quickly . . winding it rapidly . . And she seemed tense . . Perhaps because she felt she just had too much to do . . And after winding the clock . . she set it down on the bedside table . . But then she noticed that it had stopped ticking . .

She picked it up hurriedly . . and shook it a few times . . and put it back down on the table . . But it still was not working . . She looked at it angrily, said a few words under her breath . . and left the room, muttering . . "I don't have time to mess with you now . . I have too many things to do" . .

That evening, she came into the room again . . looked at the clock and said, "That no-good clock is still not ticking" . . And she picked it up, shook it a few more times . . and hit it with her hand . . But all of her shaking, hitting and angry words . . did not cause the clock to start ticking again . .

The next day, she did the same thing again . . and when it would not begin ticking . . she angrily threw it into the waste basket . . Then carried it out and dumped the basket into the trash bin . .

The little clock lay in the trash bin for several days . . Finally, the collectors came and took away the trash . . They drove it to the dump, and there . . the little clock lay . . with all of the other discarded junk . . And the little clock thought, "Oh, I feel terrible . . This must be the end for me" . .

One bright morning, several days later . . a little boy, walking by the dump, noticed the little clock, laying all by itself . . As he picked it up, he said, "This is really a pretty clock . . I wonder what's wrong with it ?". .

He shook it gently and tried to wind it, carefully . . but soon, had to admit that it just would not start ticking . . Yet, it was so pretty that he decided to take it home with him . . And when he got home, he set it beside his bed . . and sat down beside it, just to look at it . . And he wondered what he might do . . to get it to start ticking again . .

Then he remembered that only a few blocks down the street . . was a clock repair shop . . He picked up the little clock . . and he ran all the way to the clock repair shop . . Inside the shop, he saw a man behind the counter, sitting with his back to the door . . The boy looked around and didn't see anyone else in the shop to wait on him . . so he finally said . . "Mister. Can you make this clock tick for me?"

The clock repair man got up from his seat . . Took the clock in his hand, and said . . "Let me see what you have here" . .

As the repair man examined the clock, the young boy looked around the shop . . There seemed to be hundreds of clocks all around him . . ticking, chiming . . and some were even cuckoo clocks . .

"I sure hope you can fix my pretty little clock, Mister" . . The boy said as he looked up at the clock repair man . .

The repair man lifted the back off the little clock and said, "Someone has wound it too tightly . . I will see what I can do . . but I can't promise anything . . You come back in two days and I will let you know if anything can be done for it" . .

The boy turned and ran out of the clock shop . . His heart was beating fast as he thought anxiously . . "I do hope he can fix my pretty little clock . . so it can tell time again" . .

After he got back home . . he went into his room and was making all kinds of promises to himself . . in his mind . .

'If the clock can run', he thought . . 'and tell the time again . . I'll make my bed every morning . . I'll brush my teeth every day . . I'll keep my clothes picked up off the floor . . and I'll go to bed on time every night . . I'll really be good, I promise . . If only the clock will be able to tick . . and tell the time again' . .

He could hardly wait for the two days to pass . . so he could go back to the clock repair shop . . and see if the clock could be fixed . . Those two days seemed like two weeks to the little boy . .

Finally, the two days had passed . . and the little boy hurried down to the repair shop . . and he opened the door . . He was almost afraid to go in . . He felt so fearful . . of hearing the repair man say, "The clock . . could not be fixed" . . But he straightened up his shoulders and walked right up to the counter . . He stood there for a moment, waiting . . But the clock repair man didn't turn around . .

Finally, the boy coughed, and asked . . "Mister . . Were you able to get my clock fixed ?" . .

The repair man turned around and asked, "What clock are you talking about?" . .

The little boy's heart sank . . "Oh, Sir, You must remember . . It's been here for two whole days . . It's a pretty little clock . . You said you would see if you could fix it . . Remember ? You said someone had wound it too tight . . Don't you remember ?" . .

The repair man got up slowly and, with a smile, said, "Let me take a look." . . He walked over to a cupboard . . and pulled out the pretty little clock . . Then, he asked, "Is this the one"? . .

The little boy jumped up and down, and said, "Yes, Sir . . That's the one"! The repair man held it up and said, "Well, here it is, my boy . . Ticking away" . .

"Oh, Thank you, Sir . . Thank you very much . . How much does it cost?" . .

"I'll tell you what I'll do, Son" . . said the happy repair man . . "You come into my shop . . every once in a while . . and tell me how your little clock is doing . . and I won't charge you anything" . .

The little boy hugged the clock . . and said once more, as he turned to leave the shop . . "Thank you again for fixing my clock, Mister" . .

And the boy ran all the way home, as fast as he could . . so he could put his little clock on the bedside table . . And the little clock kept perfect time for him . . for many, many years after . .

All that was needed to repair the clock was . . to loosen the tension from the main spring . . that had been wound too tightly . . by the woman with . . so much on her mind . .

Just as it was easy for the repair man to loosen that spring . . it is even easier for you . . to be relaxed . . and calm . . and peaceful . . through your own ability to listen to the suggestions . . and guidance . . I am giving you . .

Your subconscious mind is cooperating by . . causing you to be calm, relaxed . . and peaceful . . as you go about your daily activities . .

Continue to relax a few moments longer . . Then . . I will begin my count . . from one to five . . (Pause briefly.)

When you hear the number FIVE . . you will be wide awake, feeling refreshed and relaxed . . And ready for new challenges . .

ONE - You will remember everything you have experienced today . . You are feeling good now . . Relaxed . . In control . .

TWO - Coming up now . . Move your fingers and your toes a little . . Let the body awaken . .

THREE - Move your arms and legs a bit now . . Feeling good . . Feeling wonderful . . For you are, truly, a wonderful person . .

FOUR - We're nearly there now . . Take a deep breath and . .

FIVE - Open your eyes. Focus on your surroundings . . And tell me . . How do you feel ?

You are deeply relaxed now . . and I want you to continue to relax . . while I give you suggestions . . that will cause you to become even more calm and relaxed . . As you continue listening to the soothing sounds in the background . . I want you to use your imagination . . And feel yourself moving into . . the situation I am describing . . where you find yourself sitting beside . . a gently flowing stream . . in the woods . . on a beautiful summer day . . You may hear the sounds of birds . . off in the distance . . And you are aware of the sun shining . . through the trees . . You can smell the soft scent of pine needles . . And hear a gentle breeze . . rustling through the branches of the trees . . As well as the rippling sounds of the nearby stream . . It is very peaceful . . As you sit there quietly . . a squirrel gathers nuts for winter . . and a rabbit hops near the stream . . In this beautiful place of leisure . . you are just relaxing . . and having an enjoyable time . .

Feel your body absorbing the stillness and beauty of this harmonious place . . Without noticing it you are continuing to sink deeper . . into relaxation . . Becoming more relaxed . . more peaceful . . and at ease . .

Hold onto those peaceful, happy feelings . . as you visualize yourself going forward into the future . . Moving forward in time . . And you will soon find yourself, four weeks ahead . . Four weeks ahead of now . . And you are trying to remember exactly where those bone spurs used to be . .

They have faded away so naturally and easily . . it is now difficult to remember . . exactly where they once were . .

You are now looking back . . at the time when you used to have those troublesome bone spurs . . It is now only a memory in your mind . . And your bones and skin are becoming healthier . . and more perfect each day . . Notice how comfortable and relaxed you are . . Each day, you are able to do your daily activities . . more easily . . more comfortably . .

And you are looking forward to the other things . . you will be doing . . as you go about your normal daily activities . .

Now, let that image fade from your mind . . as you continue to feel relaxed and at ease . . Feel the blood flowing through your entire system . . which is being pushed along by your pulse . . Carrying with it . . all the nutrients and chemicals needed . . to provide the proper healing energy . . which will dissolve those bone spurs . . and cleanse them out of your body completely . . Through the natural processes of your elimination system . .

You are experiencing perfect peace of mind . . relaxing comfortably . . And all the while . . your subconscious mind is resolving that bone spur problem . . in its own easy . . and natural way . .

You are becoming more aware of the flow of healthy blood . . flowing through your circulatory system . . Eliminating any unwanted objects in its natural function . . of cleansing the body . .

In a few moments . . you will be returning to a fully alert state of consciousness . . Feeling healthy and confident . . that the subconscious level of your mind . . is resolving that problem in a way that is pleasing to you . .

I am now beginning my count, from ONE to FIVE . . When you hear the count of FIVE, you will open your eyes . . feeling wide awake and alert . . rested and relaxed . . You will become more fully awake . . with each number that I say . .

ONE, TWO, THREE, FOUR, FIVE . .

As you go deeper and deeper into relaxation . . all of the sounds fade away into the background . . Going deeper and deeper . . Relax and hear only the sound of my voice . . Relax . . Relax completely . .

Now, allow yourself to go even deeper . . Deeper relaxed . . completely relaxed . . Every muscle and every fiber of your being . . completely relaxed . . Just let it all go . . Relax . . Just relax . .

Before reaching maturity . . you had no breast development . . Then, you began to mature . . And your hormones and other body processes began to make changes in you . . And your breasts began enlarging . . However, that process stopped . . all too soon . . It stopped before your breasts became a full, well developed, satisfactory size . . in proportion with the rest of your body . .

I am speaking now, directly with your subconscious mind . . Allowing it to hear and to understand this situation . . Your subconscious mind is understanding that now . . and is directing your body processes . . to reactivate the growth activities in your breasts . . And cause your breasts to begin enlarging once more . . And become perfectly proportioned to the rest of your body . .

Beginning right now . . the processes in your body . . which are responsible for the growth of your breasts . . are functioning to increase the size of your breasts . . And this enlargement process will continue . . until your breasts are full, firm, smooth and round . . Exactly the way you want them to be . . The process will stop . . when you want it to stop . .

I want you to take a little time now . . to visualize the flow of energy . . coming down from the top of your head . . flowing into your body . . The energy is pulsing through your circulatory system . . penetrating your diaphragm . . And it is permeating your breasts . . I want you to flow with this energy now . . Go with it . . inside your body . . You can see all of the tiny capillaries and larger veins . . inside your breasts . . The incidental flow of blood carries with it all of the nutrients . . the nourishments . . and the pure energy needed . . to begin the stimulation . . for your breasts to grow larger . . from the inside, out . .

167

The circulation of your blood is now improving . . in the areas of your breasts . . and your blood stream carries with it . . increased nourishment's to the delicate tissues on the inside . . and outside . . of your breasts . . You will notice that the flowing energy . . permeating your body . . is a soft blue color . . But as it begins filling your breasts . . the colors change to a softer pink . . spreading into . . and around your breasts . .

Take this opportunity . . to examine your breasts carefully . . inside . . for any kind of spots . . or blemishes . . no matter how small . . Also, examine higher up . . under your arms . .

There may be times, in the future . . when you feel a pleasant warmth and perhaps . . small muscle spasms . . or mild tingling sensations . . in your breasts . . That is perfectly normal . . You will merely be experiencing the pleasant increase in the size of your breasts . .

These suggestions and instructions . . are going into the storehouse of your subconscious mind . . And your mind is causing the processes of your body . . to continue functioning properly . . to increase the size of your breasts . .

It is perfectly normal and natural for you to have . . fully developed, firm, smooth, round breasts . . And your body processes are functioning perfectly . . to provide the nourishments needed in your breasts . . Enabling them to grow more fully . . and more perfectly . . until they are exactly the way you want them to be . .

If you had seeds for flowers hidden away in a closet . . they could lay there for years and never grow . . But, if you finally found those seeds and planted them . . and nourished them properly . . they would grow into a beautiful bouquet of flowers . . Your breasts are comparable to those seeds, that had been hidden away . . For some reason, your breasts did not receive the proper nourishment to blossom . . when you began maturing . . But now, your hormones and other body processes are functioning properly . . And your breasts will continue growing . . until they become firm and full . . and very beautiful . . the way you want them to be . .

(Have client do an imagination demonstration such as, "Magnetic Hands" or "Hand clasp" and then, continue as follows:)

Now, you have a better understanding of the power . . . of your subconscious mind . .

I want you to use your visualizing powers again . . only this time . . I want you to see your body . . as being beautiful . . perfectly shaped . . and with your breasts full, firm, smooth and round . . and perfectly developed . . Just the way you want to see them . . Think of your body now, as you are standing naked . . in front of a full length mirror . . Seeing your body . . including your breasts, perfectly developed . .

Visualize your feet, your legs and your thighs . . as beautiful . . and perfectly developed . . Now, see your abdomen and stomach, flat and tight . . Your waist is slim and trim with well proportioned hips . .

And now, look . . and feel, your breasts . . Firm and full . . smooth, round and perfectly shaped . . Just as you want to see them . . And see your shoulders and arms . . long and trim and slender . .

Keep that image in your mind clearly . . It is becoming deeply implanted . . in the storehouse of your mind . . And your mind is causing it to happen . . You are experiencing some very pleasant changes taking place within you . . as your breasts continue enlarging . . Until they are exactly the way you want them to be . .

Each night, just before you go to sleep . . I want you to close your eyes for a few minutes . . and visualize yourself . . exactly the way you want your breasts . . and your body . . to be . . It will keep becoming more clear . . and more real . . each night . . As you continue visualizing this way . . each night . . your subconscious mind . . and all other levels of your mind . . will continue to cause all of your body processes to function perfectly . . just as they are doing now . . And your breasts will continue to become more full and firm . . Exactly as you want them to be . .

Every cell, every atom and every molecule of your body . . is continuing to function more perfectly . . Your skin keeps becoming more flawless, more smooth and clear . . taking on a youthful appearance . . And you continue developing a more perfect . . a more beautiful body . .

You will be quite happy and pleased with yourself . . as you notice how your body is reshaping itself . . to accept the new development of your breasts . . as they become more full and mature . .

Your self-confidence and self-acceptance will keep increasing . . And you will be more successful in all other areas of your life . .

These suggestions and instructions are now in your subconscious mind, permanently . . And they will keep becoming more effective each day . .

Every time you inhale, deeply . . you will experience the tissues in your breasts being nourished . . rejuvenated and stimulated to grow . . until they are fully and completely developed . .

You will enjoy a wonderful feeling of well being . . throughout your entire body . . And you will continue feeling more alive and more happy with yourself . .

You will enjoy experiencing this continuous cycle of progress . . that keeps growing stronger each day . . And you will be proud of your continuous improvements . . in all areas of your world . . Physically, Mentally, Emotionally and Spiritually . .

You are going to build yourself up . . more and more . . with every breath you take . . as you go deeper and deeper . . Deeply relaxed . . Deeper and deeper as you relax . . You are going to remember . . everything you have experienced in this session . . And all of the suggestions you have received . . will be reinforced in your mind . . again and again . . every single day . .

I want you to relax more now . . Go deeper and just relax . . as your subconscious mind takes over . . absorbing . . ratifying . . and instilling within itself . . everything you need . . to help you to be the person . . you are to become . . And may God be with you . .

I will give you another moment of silence . . (pause)

I am now counting to five . . And at the count of five . . you will feel wide awake, alert and refreshed . . You'll be completely relaxed and invigorated . . with the knowledge of your accomplishments . .

One . . You are coming up now . . You feel the energy and the vigor flowing through your body . . From head to foot, you are feeling refreshed.

Two . . Rising up now . . Coming to the surface . .

Three . . Feeling wonderful . . For you are . . a wonderful person . .

Four . . Now, more alert . . You feel vigorous . . energetic . . Relaxed.

Five . . Open your eyes now . . Refreshed and awake . .

BREAST ENLARGEMENT - 2
BODY IMPROVEMENT

Begin with Relaxation

As you go deeper and deeper into relaxation . . all of the sounds fade away into the background . . Deeper and deeper . . Relax and hear only the sound of my voice . . Relax . . Relax completely . . Now, allow yourself to go even deeper . . Deeper relaxed . . Completely relaxed . . Every muscle and every fiber of your being . . Completely relaxed . . Just let it all go . . Relax . . Just relax . .

Now that you have learned how to relax . . you are going to be able to use that ability . . to enlarge your breasts . . And improve yourself . . in many other ways . . You can automatically be more relaxed and more at ease in your daily life . . And that will allow all of the processes of your body . . to function properly . . And every part of your body will reshape itself . . Exactly the way you want your body to be . .

(Use technique of having the client develop heaviness in left arm and lightness in right arm, by using imagination.)

You are responding well to everything I tell you . . and now you have a better understanding of the power of your subconscious mind . . You realize that when you imagine something in your conscious mind . . the subconscious mind causes your physical body to respond to your thoughts . . Now, you can use that principle to cause your breasts to enlarge, gradually . . And to develop every part of your body . . to be just the way you want your body to be . .

I want you to use your imagination again now . . This time, I want you to visualize yourself with a perfect body . . Exactly the way you want your body to be . . Envision yourself . . standing naked . . looking into a full length mirror . . Look at yourself deeply now . . See yourself having a slender waist . . and with your stomach and abdomen flat, smooth and firm . . Imagine your hips and buttocks, smooth and perfectly developed . .

Look now, at your thighs and legs . . slim and trim . . Now, look at your arms . . long and slender . . And your face and neck . . smooth and graceful . . Your skin is clear, beautiful and youthful looking . . And all of your muscles, firm and perfectly developed . . And now, look closely at your breasts . . Feel them . . So full and round . . Both breasts, exactly the same size . . firm and perfectly developed . .

Carefully inspect your whole body . . so beautiful and so perfect . . with full, firm, perfectly developed breasts . .

That image of your body is becoming implanted . . in the storehouse of your subconscious mind . . And your mind is causing all of your body processes . . to keep functioning more perfectly . . to shape your body . . to be just the way you want it to be . .

Each night, just before you go to sleep . . you will close your eyes for a couple of minutes and visualize your body . . Just as you are doing now . . As you continue to envision yourself this way . . your mind will cause you to develop a more beautiful, perfect body . . The body you have always wanted . .

Everything I am telling you is true . . and is already happening . . And your subconscious mind is continuing to help you . . to develop a more perfect body . . With perfectly shaped . . breasts . .

Your appearance is continuing to improve more each day . . And you will be happy to find . . your self-confidence and self-acceptance . . is also increasing . . more each day . .

Your mind knows the foods you need to eat . . to enable you to develop a slender body . . with full, round, smooth, firm breasts . . And your mind is controlling your appetite . . causing you to eat only the right foods . . and the right amounts of foods that your body needs . . to be slender . . healthy and strong . . with full, firm, round, smooth breasts . . Your eating habits change . . to continue meeting the needs of your body . . You eat only when your body needs food . . And you eat only the foods needed by your body . . to provide the proper proteins, vitamins and minerals . . fiber and potassium and other nutrients needed . . to keep your body healthy and strong . . As soon as you begin to eat . . you will start feeling content and satisfied . .

And the moment you have eaten the amount needed by your body . . at that time . . you will feel perfectly content and satisfied . . From now on . . you eat only when your body needs food . . And you will eat only the small amount needed by your body . . at that time . .

The growth processes in your breasts are re-learning to function perfectly . . and they are continuing to enlarge your breasts . . until they are full and firm . . And your circulatory system is carrying the proper amounts of nourishments to your breasts . . Causing the size of your breasts to keep increasing . . until they are exactly the way you want them to be . .

You will be very proud and pleased . . as you notice how your breasts are gradually enlarging . . And you will feel overjoyed with pleasure . . by your accomplishments . .

I want you to relax even more now . . Go deeper and just relax . . as your subconscious mind takes over . . Absorbing . . ratifying . . and instilling within itself . . everything you need . . to help you to be the person . . you are to become . . And may God be with you . .

I will give you another moment of silence . . (pause)

I am now going to count to five . . And at the count of five . . you will feel wide awake . . alert and refreshed . . You'll be completely relaxed and invigorated . . with the full knowledge of your accomplishments . . For you will recall everything you have experienced . . during this session . .

One . . You are coming up now . . You feel the energy and the vigor flowing through your body . . From head to toe, you are feeling refreshed . . physically, mentally and spiritually . .

Two . . Rising up now . . Coming to the surface . .

Three . . Feeling wonderful . . wonderful . . For you truly are . . a wonderful person . .

Four . . Now you are more alert . . More and more aware . . You feel vigorous . . energetic . . and relaxed . .

Five . . Open your eyes now . . Refreshed and awake . .

As you go deeper and deeper into relaxation . . all of the sounds fade into the background . . Deeper and deeper . . Relax and hear only the sound of my voice . . Relax . . Relax completely . .

Now, allow yourself to go even deeper . . deeper relaxed . . Completely relaxed . . Every muscle and every fiber of your being . . Completely relaxed . . Just let it all go . . relax . . You are relaxing deeply now . . And I am going to give you suggestions . . that will help you with your situation . .

You are here because you want to reduce the size of your breasts . . The subconscious level of your mind . . and all levels of your mind, are cooperating . . to reduce your breasts to a size . . that is comfortable and pleasing to you . . consciously . .

Before reaching maturity . . you had no breast development . . Then, you began to mature . . and your hormones and other body processes began to make changes in you . . And during those changes . . your breasts began enlarging . . However, that process continued . . perhaps, longer than necessary . . Your breasts quickly became full but also . . overly developed . . in proportion to the rest of your body . .

I am now speaking directly with your subconscious mind . . Allowing it to hear and to understand this situation . . Your subconscious mind is understanding now . . Is responding . . and is directing your body processes . . to counter the growth activities in your breasts . . And is causing your breasts to begin lessening in size . . so they may become perfectly proportioned to the rest of your body . .

Beginning right now . . the processes in your body . . responsible for the growth of your breasts . . are functioning to decrease the size of your breasts . . And this . . down-sizing process . . will continue . . until your breasts are smaller . . yet full, firm, smooth and round . . Exactly the way you want them to be . . The process will stop . . when you want it to stop . .

I want you to take a little time now . . to envision the flow of energy . . coming down from the top of your head . . flowing into your body . . The energy is pulsing through your circulatory system . . Penetrating your diaphragm . . And it is permeating your breasts . . I want you to flow with this energy now . . Travel with it . . You can

174

see all of the tiny capillaries and larger veins inside your breasts . . The incidental flow of blood carries with it all of the nutrients . . the nourishment's . . and the pure energy needed . . to begin the necessary stimulation . . for your breasts to remain healthy . . but also to become smaller . . from the inside, out . . The circulation of your blood is now improving . . in the areas of your breasts . . And your blood stream carries with it . . increased nourishment's . . for the delicate tissues on the inside . . and outside . . of your breasts . .

You will notice that the flowing energy . . permeating your body . . is a soft blue color . . But as it begins filling your breasts . . the colors change to a softer pink . . spreading into and around your breasts . . This soft pink color allows you to see more clearly, any blemishes which may be present . . Take this opportunity to examine your breasts, carefully . . inside . . for any kind of spots or blemishes . . no matter how small . . Also, examine higher up . . under your arms . .

There may be times when you feel a pleasant warmth and perhaps . . small muscle spasms . . or mild tingling sensations . . in your breasts . . That is perfectly normal . . You will merely be experiencing the pleasant changes taking place in reducing the size of your breasts . .

These suggestions and instructions . . are going into the storehouse of your subconscious mind . . And your mind is causing the processes of your body . . to continue functioning properly . . to diminish the size of your breasts . . causing them to be smaller . . and lighter . . You will enjoy the pleasant changes taking place in your body . .

It is perfectly normal and natural for you to have . . fully developed, firm, smooth, round breasts . . And your body processes are functioning perfectly . . to provide the nourishments needed in your breasts . . enabling them to flourish while reducing in size . . They will remain full . . and perfectly shaped . . while their size becomes, gradually, smaller . . until they are exactly the size you want them . .

As you were growing and becoming a mature woman . . your breasts continued enlarging . . until they became larger than you desired them to be . . And so . . now you want them to reduce in size . . You want your breasts to become smaller . . You want them to reduce down to a size . . that is pleasing and comfortable for you . . consciously . .

Since you became fully developed . . your breasts have grown larger . . They have enlarged to such a point that they have become . . troublesome for you . . And you want them to become smaller . . and more in proportion to the rest of your body . .

You know that women's breasts . . are really a wonderful and beautiful part . . of their bodies . . And I want you to think of your breasts now . . the way you want them to be . . First of all . . think about your hands . . The human hands are a very important part of the body . . They enable you to do the work that you want to do . . They enable you to pick up dishes and children . . They enable you to write . . They enable you to wash your face and comb your hair . . and do many other things you desire to do . . You respect your hands and you are happy that you have your hands . . The same is true of your breasts . . You respect your breasts and you are very happy that you have them . . And you are continuing to have a much better attitude about your breasts . . Even so . . you are, now, giving your breasts the opportunity to reduce to a smaller size . . They are reducing to a size that is pleasing to you . . And you will be even happier . . when your breasts are perfectly proportioned to the rest of your body . .

Each time you look at your breasts in the mirror . . you will see them becoming more perfectly proportioned and more beautiful . . Your beasts will soon be the size you want them to be . .

While you are continuing to become more relaxed and at ease . . the subconscious levels of your mind are working on the very best way to reduce your breasts to a smaller size . . And as you are becoming drowsier . . and sleepier . . perhaps you would like to shift in your chair . . or shift your hands . . or feet . . I want you to be completely comfortable . .

And while that is taking place . . your mind is continuing to cause your breasts . . to become smaller . . And when the subconscious levels of your mind . . know the changes have started . . to cause your breasts to reduce . . to the size you consciously desire them to be . . one of the fingers on your left hand will lift up . . toward the ceiling . . And your finger will remain up . . until I tell it to go back down . . (Wait for finger to lift.)

You are doing very well . . You will remember everything I have said to you today . .

And you will greatly benefit from everything I have told you . . Continue now, to relax, for just a little longer . . (Pause)

In just a moment we will be concluding this session . . I will be counting to FIVE for you to awaken . . You will come up to a wide-awake, fully alert state, when I say the number FIVE . .

I will begin now . .

ONE - Feeling so good . . feeling wonderful . . all over . .

TWO - your hands are tingling and your legs are feeling a bit numb yet . . Get the feelings back into your body . .

THREE - Coming up now . . More alert . . More aware . . Stirring into conscious awareness . .

FOUR - Gently inhale now . . Breathe out . . and . .

FIVE - Open your eyes and focus on your surroundings . .

(Follow Stress Reduction - 1st Session)

You are deeply relaxed now . . and I want you to continue to relax
. . while I give you some information and suggestions . . concerning
your problem . .

You have come to realize that mouthwashes . . only cover up the
odor . . caused by bad breath . . And that they do nothing . . to
correct the cause of the problem . . The origin of bad breath could
possibly be . . from a number of sources . .

One possibility is that it might be caused from decaying matter inside
of decaying teeth . . Which can be eliminated . . with proper
treatment from a dentist . . who can eliminate the odor . . as well as
preserve the teeth . .

Occasionally, bad breath can be a result of congestion . . or infection
in the nasal cavity . . Or the sinuses . . Or it might also originate
. . from the respiratory or alimentary tract . . which sometimes draws
bile odors from the liver . . or related organs . .

By virtue of your agreement to allow me to hypnotize you . . to get
to the root of this ailment . . it also lets your subconscious mind
know . . that you are determined to correct this problem . . Now that
your subconscious mind is aware of your determination . . it will
review and examine . . what has been causing the problem . .

Bad breath has controlled your life long enough . . and you are
determined that you are going to overcome this problem . . for now and
forever . .

I am going to give you some suggestions now . . that will be of
great benefit . . to increase the process . . of the complete healing of
all of your body's systems . .

I want you to visualize a radiant, blue light . . coming down onto the
top of your head . . This radiant, blue light is pure energy . . from
the astral realm . . It is shining directly onto your head . . pouring
energy onto your brain . . You can see your brain glowing now . .
vibrating with the energy . . A soft, blue, glowing aura . . softly
radiating around your brain . . (pause)

You can see how it is emanating from your cranial mass, into your nervous system and . . blood system . . Starting at the top of your spine . . and filtering its way downward . . through your spinal column . . You can watch the blue glowing energy . . permeating, all throughout your entire body . . From the top of your head . . all the way down to your toes . . The energy flows . . wrapping itself around your rib cage . . entering every gland and organ in your body . . It has entered your blood stream . . reinforcing the production of white corpuscles . . Bringing up their numbers to their proper count . . Your immune system may have been weak in certain organs and glands of your body . . But the astral flow of the blue energy will prime your system . . And rejuvenate any shortfalls you may have had in the past . . Your immune system is gaining the power . . and the strength . . to replace any dysfunctional cells . . Wherever they are needed . . throughout your body . .

I want you to travel now . . on a tour . . throughout your body . . Anywhere you want to go . . Simply follow the blue glowing light . . as it travels through your blood veins . . your glands . . your various organs . . Follow the flow of energy . . and be sure it saturates everywhere it is needed . . If there are any organs or glands that your subconscious mind is aware of . . that need specific attention . . go there and concentrate the blue light . . to be sure every point is permeated with the energy . . For this energy is powerful . . It is the healing power given directly from God . . And it cannot fail . . Because failure is impossible . . at the astral level of the soul . . (pause)

Now, I want you to use your imagination . . Imagine your body as being healthy, strong . . and in perfect physical condition . . Imagine your immunity system . . functioning perfectly . . Think of your skin as healthy, smooth and youthful looking . . Think of your circulatory system . . functioning properly . . Producing a sufficient amount of white blood cells to keep your immunity system healthy . . And know that the bad odors from within you have disappeared . . completely . . Get all of these ideas of a healthy, glowing body, in your mind . . (pause) Your mind is now accepting these images . . and is causing you to experience the changes needed . . to heal your body, perfectly . .

In the past you have had some doubts . . but those doubts are fading rapidly . . All doubts are being replaced with a strong feeling of confidence and sureness . . that the healing processes in your body are already taking place . . It may take a week to even three weeks for your entire body to be completely healed . . and functioning perfectly . . But you will be noticing yourself improving . . more each day . .

You may not understand the processes your subconscious mind is using . . to cause your body's systems to be healed and to function properly . . But that's okay . . You can be pleasantly surprised . . as you become more aware . . of the progress you continue to achieve . .

At this very moment . . all systems are making comfortable adjustments . . Your systems are now synthesizing proteins, nutrients and other chemicals and substances . . And they are traveling . . all throughout your body . . Rejuvenation is now taking place . .

Your expectations are, naturally, increasing . . And you will be sensing the pleasant changes taking place within you . . You can feel pleased and proud of what you are accomplishing . . The feeling of knowing it is happening . . gives you a strong sense of satisfaction . .

When your subconscious mind knows the changes have started . . and the healing processes have begun . . your subconscious mind . . will cause one of the fingers . . on your left hand to raise up . . toward the ceiling . . And it will remain there . . until I tell it to go back down . .
(After getting response, tell finger to go back down.)

You are responding very well to these suggestions . . to eliminate the bad odors from within you . . that you have experienced . . And to eliminate any other bad areas that your immune system might detect . . Now, I want you to rest a few moments . . while your subconscious mind continues to absorb . . all that we have talked about . . (Pause)

I am now going to begin my count from ONE, up to FIVE . . When you hear the count of FIVE . . you will be wide awake and alert . . and you'll feel refreshed and wonderful . . You will remember everything we have talked about today . .

ONE - Beginning to emerge now . . Move your fingers and toes a little . .
TWO - Waking more now . . Coming up . .
THREE - Your arms and legs may still be asleep . . Let them move now . .
FOUR - Take a deep breath now and . .
FIVE - Open your eyes . . feeling good . . feeling wonderful . .

038 Prescript. BURNED CLIENT - HYPNOSIS (1st Session)

The acutely burned patient (client) arrives in the emergency room in a state of frightened anxiety and is already in a state that makes him or her extremely susceptible to both good or bad suggestions. The inflammation is mediated through the central nervous system by release of a Bradykinin-like substance, which is released during the first two hours after the burn stimulus. However, this enzyme is kept in abeyance by icing the wound. The damaging inflammatory reaction can be blocked by early hypnosis, permitting healing to occur rapidly, thus, eliminating the need for skin grafts or plastic surgery. When proper hypnotic techniques are applied very quickly, after the initial burn, it can even prevent scarring of any kind.

When a newly burned patient arrives in the emergency room, his mind is focused, causing hypnosis to be easily induced. Since he is most likely a stranger to the hypnotherapist, the first communication is an introduction and a suggestion.

HELLO, I'M _____, AND I'M HERE TO HELP TAKE CARE OF YOU . . DO YOU KNOW HOW THEY TREAT THIS KIND OF BURN ?

Patient : NO (This is the standard reply. Rarely, a nurse or physician may be the patient.)

THEN YOU MAY NOT KNOW THAT YOUR OWN MIND CAN HELP SPEED UP THE HEALING PROCESSES . . ACTUALLY, YOU'VE ALREADY DONE THE MOST IMPORTANT THING, IN GETTING TO THE HOSPITAL QUICKLY . . YOU ARE SAFE NOW, AND IF YOU WILL RECEIVE WHAT I TELL YOU . . YOU WILL BE ABLE TO REST COMFORTABLY, WHILE YOUR BODY IS HEALING RAPIDLY . . JUST RELAX . .

THE FIRST THING I WANT YOU TO DO IS TO REALIZE THAT THE STAFF HERE IS VERY WELL-TRAINED AND WILL BE GIVING YOU THE BEST OF CARE . . AND THE SECOND THING IS FOR YOU TO REALIZE THAT, WHATEVER YOU THINK . . WILL MAKE A BIG DIFFERENCE IN THE HEALING OF YOUR SKIN . . HAVE YOU EVER SEEN A PERSON BLUSH . . OR TURN WHITE WITH FEAR ? . .

Patient : YES

WELL, YOU KNOW THEN THAT WHAT HAPPENED TO THEM CAME FROM A MERE THOUGHT OR IDEA . . AND ALL OF THE LITTLE BLOOD VESSELS IN THE FACE EITHER OPENED UP AND TURNED RED . . OR CLAMPED DOWN AND TURNED WHITE . . WHATEVER YOU THINK AFFECTS THE BLOOD SUPPLY TO YOUR SKIN . . AND THIS IS WHAT AFFECTS THE HEALING . . AND WE CAN BEGIN THAT HEALING, RIGHT NOW . .

REMEMBER WHAT BRIA'R RABBIT SAID ? . . HE SAID, EVERYBODY'S GOT A LAUGHING PLACE . . AND NOW, I WANT YOU TO GO TO YOUR LAUGHING PLACE . . BY THIS, I MEAN, I WANT YOU TO CLOSE YOUR EYES AND IMAGINE THAT YOU ARE IN A SAFE, PEACEFUL PLACE, ENJOYING YOURSELF . . YOU'RE TOTALLY FREE OF ANY RESPONSIBILITY,

JUST TAKING IT EASY . . THE PLACE WHERE YOU GO . . IN YOUR MIND . . MAY BE A BEAUTIFUL BEACH OR IT MAY BE HIGH UP IN THE MOUNTAINS . . MAYBE YOU JUST WANT TO RELAX AND WATCH A LITTLE TV . . OR MAYBE YOU ARE OUT ON THE GREENS . . PLAYING A ROUND OF GOLF . . (To a young child) OR PERHAPS YOU ARE DOING NEEDLEPOINT, OR PLAYING WITH TOY SOLDIERS OR DOLLS . . WHEREVER YOU DECIDE TO GO, I WANT YOU TO CONTINUE TO RELAX . . THERE IS NOTHING TO CONCERN YOURSELF ABOUT . . JUST BREATH EASILY . . AND RELAX . .

FROM NOW ON, EVERY TIME YOU ARE TOLD TO GO TO YOUR LAUGHING PLACE . . YOU WILL CLOSE YOUR EYES (IF POSSIBLE) AND IMMEDIATELY GO TO THIS PLACE . . OR, ANY TIME YOU WANT TO RELAX AND FEEL EVEN MORE COMFORTABLE . . YOU WILL CLOSE YOUR EYES AND THINK OF THAT PLACE . . AND YOU WILL AUTOMATICALLY BE . . AT YOUR LAUGHING PLACE . . SO, THINK OF YOUR LAUGHING PLACE NOW . . FEEL YOURSELF THERE . . REALLY ENJOYING YOURSELF . . GET EVEN MORE COMFORTABLE NOW . . BY HAVING YOUR EYES CLOSED . . AND ROLL YOUR EYEBALLS UP . . AS THOUGH YOU ARE LOOKING AT THE TOP OF YOUR FOREHEAD . . AND TAKE A VERY DEEP BREATH . . AS YOU INHALE . . FEEL THE MUSCLES IN YOUR EYES . . BEGINNING TO RELAX . . AS YOU EXHALE . . FEEL YOUR EYELIDS . . AND ALL THE MUSCLES AROUND YOUR EYES . . RELAXING EVEN MORE . . FEEL THAT RELAXATION CIRCULATING . . THROUGHOUT YOUR ENTIRE BODY . . YOUR MIND IS TAKING YOU OFF NOW . . TO YOUR LAUGHING PLACE . .

I READ AN ARTICLE THE OTHER DAY ABOUT SNOWFLAKES . . THAT WAS QUITE INTERESTING . . IT TOLD ABOUT RESEARCH THAT WAS CONDUCTED . . BY A SCIENTIST . . WHO DEVOTED HIS LIFE TO THE STUDY OF SNOWFLAKES . . HE FOUND THAT EVERY SINGLE SNOWFLAKE . . HAS SIX SIDES . . AND EVERY SNOWFLAKE IS HEXAGONAL IN SHAPE . . YET, NO TWO SNOWFLAKES ARE EXACTLY ALIKE . . DURING HIS RESEARCH, HE PHOTOGRAPHED MORE THAN 10,000 SNOWFLAKES . . HE CLAIMED THAT THE ENTIRE COUNTRYSIDE . . FROM MAINE TO CALIFORNIA . . COULD BE COVERED IN SNOW A FOOT DEEP . . AND YET, NO TWO FLAKES WOULD EVER BE FOUND TO BE EXACTLY THE SAME . .

WHILE YOU ARE CONTINUING TO ENJOY YOURSELF . . AT YOUR LAUGHING PLACE . . WITHOUT EVEN NOTICING IT . . YOUR BODY IS CONTINUING TO FEEL COOL . . AND MORE COMFORTABLE . . AND WHEN YOUR BODY ACHIEVES A VERY PLEASANT STATE . . OF COMFORT AND COOLNESS . . YOUR SUBCONSCIOUS MIND WILL LET ME KNOW . . BY CAUSING ONE OF THE FINGERS . . ON YOUR RIGHT HAND . . TO RISE UP TOWARD THE CEILING . . THAT WILL BE THE SIGNAL . . THAT ALL AREAS OF YOUR BODY . . ARE FEELING COOL . . AND COMFORTABLE . .

(Wait for finger to raise, then continue with :)

AND NOW, PERMIT YOUR INNER MIND TO BECOME TOTALLY AWARE . . OF THE SENSATION . . OF BEING COOL AND COMFORTABLE . . AND IT WILL KEEP YOU THAT WAY . . UNTIL YOUR BODY HAS HEALED COMPLETELY . .

Note : In burns under 20%, one session of hypnosis is usually sufficient. For larger burns, it has been found helpful to have repeated sessions to help control pain, anorexia or other problems.

CANCER CONTROL

Sometimes, when people experience a physical problem . . they immediately become worried . . Often, they run directly to a physician to describe what they are experiencing . . And have him make a diagnosis to give them a prescription . . or do surgery . . What people forget to remember . . is that there is an intelligence within us . . that can, and does, change things . .

Someone once made a wise statement when he said . . "Go first, direct to God, and then to man, if God directs" . .

When we experience any kind of physical illness . . disease or handicap . . we make a wise decision if we peacefully and calmly . . go to a quiet place . . Breath deeply and exhale slowly . . four or five times . . and let our body become relaxed . . In that state of relaxation . . we can reflect on what would be the best thing to do . . And then, follow the intuitive feelings that guide us . . to make the right decision . . with regards to the wisest thing to do . . to overcome the problem . .

In reality . . you are the master of your own body . . Keep this truth foremost in your mind . . Let the healing energies and powers within you . . freely work in your body . . the way they normally do . . to heal your skin, if it is cut or bruised . . or to heal your bone, if it is broken . .

As you continue listening to the soothing sounds of the air conditioner . . and to my voice . . you are becoming more and more aware of that part of your mind and body . . where you have an inner harmony . . and an inner calm . . A place of inner healing powers and life giving energies . .

You are remembering that . . from the beginning . . when you first came into existence . . your mind and body have always known . . how to heal themselves . . Your body knows how to heal scrapes, wounds, cuts, bruises and injuries . . Your body knows how to generate new cells and new tissues, whenever needed . . And your body knows how to regulate and rejuvenate itself to function properly . . It knows how to keep you breathing . . even when you are sleeping . . It knows how to keep your body temperature stabilized . . It knows how to maintain its own healthy blood chemistry . . It knows how to maintain the necessary hormonal and chemical components . . for a healthy, functioning, body and mind . .

And it is normal and natural for your subconscious mind . . to keep your immune system functioning . . perfectly . . Automatically eliminating any organisms that your body does not need . . Your immune system knows how to function perfectly, at all times . . The white blood cells do their job perfectly . . overcoming any invading bacteria . . or viruses . . trying to come into your body . . And cleansing them out of your body . . in an easy, natural way . . through the normal processes of your elimination system . .

And your body knows how to regulate the metabolism . . and stabilize your body at a normal, moderate, healthy level . . In every way, your mind and body are doing their job perfectly well . . healing your body . . keeping it functioning properly . .

Now, I want you to repeat the following statements . . in your mind . . and let them become deeply embedded . . in your subconscious . . And know that they are beginning to work immediately . . through your subconscious mind . .

(1) I am calm and at ease . . (2) I know that the tremendous power of my mind can help me . . both mentally and physically . . (3) I have a built-in immune system . . My immune system can eliminate all cancerous cells from my body . . (4) My immune system is powerful . . My immune system is doing what needs to be done, to heal my body perfectly . . (5) I am becoming healthy . . I am being healed . . I am getting well . . I am rejuvenating perfectly and completely . . (6) I am living my life in harmony and love . . (7) I am spiritually whole and complete . .

EMERGE

CANCER HEAL - 1

You are calm and relaxed . . Resting peacefully in a quiet hypnotic state . . I want you to go a little deeper now . . Deeper . . Submerge yourself in this relaxing, peaceful feeling . . Deeper, now Deeper . . and relax . .

The fact that you are having these sessions . . and have permitted yourself to be hypnotized . . reveals your determination . . to be rid of the cancer from every part of your body . . And to have your whole body restored and rejuvenated . . to a healthy, strong body . .

Being in a hypnotic state causes your body to completely relax . . And that enables the processes of your body to function more perfectly . . Which, in turn, causes . . the Healing Energies of your body to function properly . . with a curative power to heal many ailments . . including cancer . .

Your conscious mind is continuing to relax now . . And you are not thinking of anything in particular . . Your subconscious mind is hearing and absorbing everything I say . . and is causing your body processes to respond . . to everything I tell you . .

You will be very pleased that you decided to allow yourself to be hypnotized . . because it makes it much easier for the activities of your body to function properly . . And it allows the healing energies to flow . . into every cell and molecule of your body more readily . .

It isn't necessary for you to consciously remember . . what I am saying to you . . while you are hypnotized . . Because your subconscious mind will remember . . and will cause everything I tell you . . to begin working immediately . . And you will be happy to notice a continual improvement in your health . .

One of the things I have learned, from hypnotizing people . . is that your subconscious mind knows how . . to work out solutions to the problems you are experiencing . . And I have witnessed many, many people . . who have been healed . . from nearly every kind of illness . . including cancer . . And I know you can be healed completely . .

Your subconscious mind has the ability to recall . . Everything you have seen, heard and experienced . . since your soul came into existence . . And your mind knows how to assess that information . . and clear out information that has been misunderstood . . and resolve the problem completely . .

Your subconscious mind can begin reviewing and examining the information . . in the storehouse of your mind . . that has caused the cancer . . And your mind will realize there is no reason . . for it to continue with the misinformation . . which has been the cause of your problems . . Then your subconscious mind . . can automatically work out the solution . . and cleanse the cancer out of your body . . And the healing energies of your body can do their work . . Healing your body completely . .

Continue relaxing now . . keeping your eyes closed as you rest . . Think about what is happening in your body now . . You are beginning to experience wonderful feelings and sensations, all throughout your body . . You can begin noticing a very pleasant sensation of warm, healing energy . . flowing, throughout your bodily systems . . Your blood system . . your nervous system . . your oxygen intake . . All bodily systems are being nourished with revitalizing energy . . Just relax and enjoy the pleasant healing energies . . flowing all through your body . .

You are already beginning to experience some pleasant changes . . that will bring you much greater happiness and joy . . And you will be pleased with your inner ability . . to make true . . everything I am saying . .

It may take a little time . . for your subconscious mind to review and examine . . all the information in your mind . . that has caused the cancer to develop in your body . . and work out the solution to the problem . . But your subconscious mind is working on the solution right now . .

Getting rid of the cancer may not happen all at once . . Instead . . you will probably get rid of some of the cancer today . . and tomorrow, you'll get rid of a little more of the cancer . . The following day, a little more will be gone . . The healing and cleansing processes will go on . . until all of the cancer is cleansed out from your body completely . . You may not, consciously, understand what originally caused the cancer to develop . . But whatever caused it, is past now . . Your subconscious mind is understanding that there is no reason you need it anymore . . And you are enjoying the pleasure of discovering . . that your body is being healed . . completely and permanently . .

Doing it this way is giving you a tremendous feeling of accomplishment . . By permitting your subconscious mind to do it for you . . you can experience a continual process of healing . . And therefore, you can become stronger and healthier . . throughout your entire body . .

It is natural for your body to be strong . . It is natural for all of your organs, glands, and the cells of your body, to function properly and to keep your body healthy . . Everything I am telling you is natural for your body . . so it is natural for your subconscious mind . . to receive what I am telling you . . and to cause the processes of your body to function properly . . and restore your body to its natural, perfectly healthy, strong condition . .

Your body needs proteins to keep you strong . . So you will eat the proper amounts of lean meats and fish . . to supply your body with the proteins it needs . . You will also enjoy eating good, fresh vegetables, fruits and other body-strengthening foods . . that provide your body with a proper balance of vitamins, minerals and fibers . .

Your subconscious mind will cause your tastes . . to correspond to the real needs of your body . . And you will desire those foods, needed by your body, each day . . to keep improving your health . . The cells of your body are alive . . and they know how to perform their tasks . . of keeping your bones healthy . . causing your hair to continue growing . . providing the proper nourishment to keep your fingernails and toenails growing . . And those cells in your body also know . . how to provide the proper nourishment, strength and energy . . to all other parts of your body . . in a perfect and natural way . .

All of the cells in your body know how to cooperate with each other . . and they know how to perform their functions properly . . And they work in unison . . and in harmony . . to restore and rejuvenate your body perfectly . . Your subconscious mind is directing the minds of every cell you have . . to work in harmony with all other cells . . and to heal your body completely . .

Each day, you learn to be more relaxed and steady . . And you continue developing more strength . . more energy . . and more vitality . .

Right now, you can notice something good happening in your body . . Your circulatory system is carrying nourishment, oxygen and healthful energy, to every part of your body . .

Your system is synthesizing proteins . . And all of the chemicals and healing energies in your body . . are functioning harmoniously . . Rejuvenation and regeneration are taking place now . . And will continue . . even after you awaken from your hypnotic state . .

You don't know exactly what is happening in your body right now . . but you can sense that it is good . . So, let it continue . .

It must be pleasing for you, to know that your mind is doing this, in your own best interest . . And in the best way . . for the improvement of your health . . And for your overall well being . .

When your subconscious mind knows . . that the improving changes have begun . . and that your health will continue to improve . . one of the fingers on your right hand will lift up towards the ceiling . . And will remain there . . until I tell it to go back down . .

(Pause for about 30 seconds. Then, if finger has lifted, conclude the session. If finger has NOT lifted, continue with suggestions from, 'Self - Confidence' Prescription.)

All right now . . Rest and relax for a few moments . . You have done very well . . I am going to count forward now . . from One to Five . . When you hear the number Five, you will be back in the present . . And you will remember every thing you have experienced . . You'll feel very relaxed and refreshed . . and you'll be able to do whatever you had planned for the rest of the day or evening . . You will feel very positive about what you have experienced here today . . And very motivated about your confidence and your inner abilities . . Play this tape again . . to re-experience your higher self . .

Now, I will begin my count . .

ONE   - You are very, very deep . . You are gradually coming towards consciousness . .
TWO   - You're getting a little lighter now . . Feeling better . . Feeling good about yourself . .
THREE - You're much, much lighter . . Let your fingers and toes move a little now . .
FOUR   - Coming up now . . Very, very light . .
FIVE   - Awaken . . Wide awake and refreshed . .

(Follow Relaxation)

You are calm and relaxed . . Resting peacefully in a quiet hypnotic state . . I want you to go a little deeper now . . Deeper . . Submerge yourself in this relaxing, peaceful feeling . . Deeper, now Deeper . . and relax . .

The suggestions and instructions that I am giving you . . are being received and absorbed by your subconscious mind . . and they will help you to be completely cured from cancer . .

Every tissue and organ in your body . . is controlled by a complex interaction among your natural chemicals . . circulating in your bloodstream . . And they are interacting with the hormones . . secreted by your endocrine glands . .

This mixture is controlled by your Pituitary Gland . . which is your 'master' gland . . located in the middle of your head . . just below your brain . . The output of pituitary hormones . . in turn, is controlled by both chemical secretions and nerve impulses . . from a neighboring part of your brain, called, the Hypothalamus . . That tiny region regulates most of the body's unconscious maintenance processes . . such as your heartbeat . . your breathing . . your temperature . . your digestive system . . your blood pressure . . and all of the other activities of your body . . And all of those processes function by . . receiving directions from your subconscious mind . . Thus, the more positive your subconscious mind is programmed . . the healthier your body becomes . . That is one of the reasons it is so important for you . . to develop a positive, loving attitude towards others . . But more importantly . . about yourself . . So that, each day . . your self - confidence . . your self-acceptance and your self-esteem . . will keep increasing . . And you will continue realizing, more and more . . your own self-worth . .

William James, a well known psychologist, wrote, "The greatest discovery of my generation is that human beings, by changing the inner attitudes of their minds, can change the outer aspects of their lives" . .

Years of working to help people overcome physical problems, through hypnosis . . have taught me that cancer, diabetes, asthma and all other illnesses . . are caused by the mind . . And by changing the ideas of the mind . . the mind can cause the processes of your body . . to function properly . . and heal the cancer . . and all other illnesses . .

The simple truth is . . happy people are usually healthy people . . Your attitude towards yourself . . is the single most important factor . . in overcoming the cancer and maintaining a healthy body . .

There is a sound scientific reason why Norman Cousins was completely cured from a deadly disease . . Laughter . . From getting comedy films and watching them for several hours each day . .

Laughter produces complete, relaxed action of the diaphragm . . It exercises the lungs . . increases the blood's oxygen level . . and gently tones the entire cardiovascular system . .

Laughter also increases . . the production of a class of brain chemicals called, catecholamines . . which activates a different part of the immune system . . and increases the production of . . endorphins . . The body's natural opiates . .

You may not consciously know what caused the cancer . . But you are realizing that, whatever caused it, is past now . . And, you are developing a happier attitude . . a greater self-confidence . . along with the understanding that whatever your mind caused . . it can also cure . .

Beginning now, your subconscious mind is reviewing . . and examining . . the information stored away in your mind . . You have tremendous amounts of information in your mind . . that has been accumulating there . . since your soul came into existence . . The information is there . . It is about you and it belongs to you . . It is there for you to use for your own self-improvement . . And it will help you to overcome your cancer, completely . .

I want you to use your imagination now . . I want you to go deep inside your own body . . You are going inside your body now . . Your body is still the same size . . but you have become like a tiny, snoopy little cell . . and you are exploring, deep inside your own body . .

Now, take your time and look around, carefully . . Travel wherever necessary until you have located the (cancerous cells / tumor) . . (pause) Tell me when you have it located . . (pause)

Now, in this cancerous area . . I want you to look at your white blood cells . . or corpuscles . . They are the healers of your body . . There are thousands of them . . Look at them carefully . . And tell me what you find . . (pause)

You may see those white blood cells as nurses . . Or, maybe as friendly, white animals . . Or, perhaps, you may see them as soldiers . . Whatever image your mind gives them . . so they can help clear the cancer out of your body . . is just fine . . Nod your head when you have given them an image . . (pause)

Now, send a command to those white healers . . to eliminate all the cancerous cells . . from your body . . And see them as they surround the cancer cells . . And escort each one of them out of your body . . in an easy, natural way . .

And, you can see, there are thousands more of the white blood cells remaining in that area . . to protect your body and keep improving your health . .

Now, send a second command to your red blood cells . . to carry nourishment . . which will give you strength, energy and vitality . . in every part of your being . . Wherever it is needed . . to keep your body healthy and strong . . (pause)

When you see your white and red blood cells . . doing their work properly . . and know that changes have started . . and your body is being healed . . one of the fingers on your left hand will lift up towards the ceiling . . and will remain up until I tell it to go back down . .

Rest and relax a few moments now . . You have done very well . . (Pause)

I am going to count forward now . . from One to Five . . When you hear the number Five, you will open your eyes . . feeling awake, alert and very refreshed . .

One - Feeling good now . . feeling wonderful . . You will remember everything . .

Two - Get the feelings back into your body . . Let your hands and legs stir.

Three - Coming up now . . More alert . . More aware . .

Four - Gently inhale now . . Breathe out . . and . .

Five - Open your eyes and focus on your surroundings . .

You are very relaxed now . . Relaxing deeper . . and deeper . . Enjoy this relaxation . . as we begin to talk about . . your body . .

The fact that you are having these sessions . . and permitting yourself to be hypnotized . . reveals that you sincerely want to be healthy . . And it also reveals that you are willing to accept my guidance and suggestions . . And that means your subconscious mind . . will cause your body to heal in an easy, natural way . . You will overcome this situation . . by directions from your mind . .

I want you to use your imagination now . . I want you to imagine a very bright, white light . . coming down from above you . . and entering the top of your head . . permeating your entire body . . You can see it . . and feel it . . And it becomes reality . . It fills your entire body with a positive, protective, God given energy . . Causing you to be safe from any harm . .

Now, imagine an Aura of pure white light . . emanating from your heart region . . This pure white Aura . . is surrounding your entire body . . protecting you . . You can see it . . and feel it . . and it becomes reality . .

Now, only your higher self, masters and guides . . and highly evolved, loving entities . . who mean you well . . will be able to influence you . . during this, or any other hypnotic session . . You are totally protected by your Aura of pure white light . . And it will surround you with love and protection . . each time you are hypnotized . .

In a few moments, I am going to count from One to Twenty . . And as I do so . . you will feel yourself . . rising up, to the superconscious mind level, where you will receive information . . from your higher self . . and from your masters and guides . . You will also be able to overview . . all of your past, present and future . .

Go deeper now . . DEEPER . . and relax . . and just allow yourself to flow with me . . as I begin the count . . with Number 1 . . Rising up . . Rising up . . 2, 3, 4 . . Rising higher now . . gently rising higher . . 5, 6, 7 . . Letting information flow . . as you are rising higher . . 8, Letting information flow freely . . 9, 10 . . You are halfway there . . 11, 12, 13 . . Feeling yourself rising even higher . . higher . . 14, 15, 16 . . Almost there now . . 17, 18, 19 and . . number 20 . . You have arrived . . Take a moment and orient yourself . . to the superconscious mind level . .

You are now in a very deep, DEEP, hypnotic trance . . And in this superconscious mind level . . there exists a complete understanding and resolution . . to the cancer problem . .

Your problem . . may have derived from a condition . . or situation . . in your past or present . . or even from your future . . I want you to discover . . in your own way . . how this problem developed . . You are in complete control . . and are able to access this information . . by tapping into this limitless power . . of your superconscious mind . . I want you to be open to anything . . and everything . . And to flow with this experience . . You are always protected by the Aura of white light . .

At this time . . I want you to ask your higher self to explore the origin . . of your health problem . . Trust your higher self . . and your own ability . . to allow any thoughts, imprints or impressions to come into your subconscious mind, concerning this goal . . Do this now . .
(Pause several minutes)

Now, I want you to remain coupled with your superconscious mind . . but for a few moments, I would like you to let go of this situation . . regardless of how simple or complicated it may seem . . At this time, I want you to visualize yourself . . in your current life and consciousness . . Free of this issue . . Imagine yourself being at your ideal level of good health . . See a friend or mate . . sharing in your joy and happiness with you . . He or she, is amazed at your excellent recovery and perfect health . .

You are doing very well . . Now, I want you to further open up the channels of communication . . by removing any obstacles . . and allowing yourself to receive information and experiences . . that will directly apply to . . and help better . . your present life situation . . Allow yourself to receive more advanced . . more specific information . . from your higher self and masters and guides . . to raise your frequency and improve your physical health . . Do this now . . .
(Pause a few minutes)

It is your God given birthright to have a healthy body . . Everything about the body reveals that it was created to be healthy . . If your skin gets cut, it heals . . If you get a bruise on your body, it heals . . If you experience a broken bone, it heals . . Your intestines . . glands . . organs . . are all interconnected . . And they heal, as well . . And it isn't medicine that does the healing . . Your body heals itself . . through the power of your superconscious mind . .

From that level, you are transferring the vital information that will heal you . . into your subconscious mind . . By opening up the channels of communication . . And by removing any obstacles that may hinder you . . from receiving or transmitting from your experiences . .

The subconscious part of the mind controls every bodily function . . Negative thoughts or ideas can go into the mind . . and can cause the body to develop illness or disease . . But, as positive thoughts or ideas enter the mind . . they will cause the body processes to function correctly and properly . . And they will heal any kind of illness or disease . . Positive thoughts HEAL . .

In the Bible, it says, "You can be transformed by the renewing of your mind" . . Hypnosis provides the means of renewing your mind, with positive thoughts and ideas . . that cause your body processes to function properly . . And that is what causes your health to keep improving . . more and more each day . .

Now, visualize yourself, having a perfectly healed body . . Hold that image . . and that thought . . in your mind . . For that is, as you will soon be . . Hold onto that positive image . . in agreement with your higher self . . And mentally, tell yourself that you are thankful . . to be healed . .

NOTE : ENCOURAGE CLIENT TO VERBALIZE EXPERIENCES TO STRENGTHEN MEMORIES LATER ON.

All right . . Rest and relax a few moments . . You have done very well . (Pause a moment)

I am going to count forward now . . from One to Five . . When you hear the number Five, you will be back in the present . . And you will remember every thing you have experienced . . You will open your eyes and feel very relaxed and refreshed . . And you'll be able to do whatever you had planned for the rest of the day or evening . . You will feel very positive about what you have experienced today . . And be very motivated about your confidence and inner abilities . . Play this tape again . . to re-experience your higher self . . Now, I will begin my count . . EMERG

(Induction included)

Before beginning, advise client to wash hands as a symbolic gesture of bodily purification, and to dry them well.   Then, drink a glass of water to symbolize the desire for purity on the inner plane.   Advise, "The more your actions and thoughts express your humility and respect toward the cosmic, the more you combine within yourself, the ideal conditions for conscious attunement with the Celestial Sanctum ."

Now, I would like you to close your eyes and . . begin breathing deeply . . and slowly . . But before you let go completely and slip into a deep hypnotic state . . just let yourself listen to everything I say to you . .

If you are ready to proceed, I would like you to repeat the following invocation after me . . "May the Divine Essence . . of the Cosmic . . infuse my being . . and cleanse me . . of all impurities . . of mind and body . . that I may enter . . the Celestial Sanctum . . and attune myself . . in pureness . . and worthiness . . So Mote It Be !"

Very good . . Now, I must ask that you prepare, in your mind, the reason for your desire to go to the Celestial Sanctum . . Not because I am curious but because . . it is a very long journey and not one to make too hastily . . When you are asked the reason for your being there, you should know the reason . . Perhaps it is for medical reasons . . or perhaps you need enlightenment about something . . You may want to inquire about a dearly departed loved one . . Whatever the reason, get it firmly in your mind now . . Let me know when you are ready . . (pause)

And now we will begin . . There is nothing to be concerned about . . Whatever is going to happen will happen automatically . . so you don't need to think about that now . . and you will have no conscious control over what happens . .

The muscles in and around your eyes will relax all by themselves . . as you continue breathing deeply . . easily and freely . . Breathe deeply now . . through your nose . . and slowly exhale . . Do that three or four times . . and notice the cosmic energy coming into your mind and your body . . A relaxing energy . . filling your lungs with life . .

Without thinking about it . . you will soon enter a deep, peaceful, hypnotic trance . . without any effort . . There is nothing important for your conscious mind to do . . There is nothing really important except the activities of your subconscious mind . . and that is where

196

all events will take place . . but you will notice many events taking place . . on your conscious plane . . after this event has passed . .

You are responding very well, without even noticing it . . You have already altered your rate of breathing . . You are breathing much more easily and freely . . and you are revealing signs that indicate you are beginning to drift . . into a very restful state of being . .

You can enjoy relaxing more and more now . . and your subconscious mind will listen to each word I say . . and will guide you through the steps of your journey . . so it becomes less and less important for you to consciously listen to my voice . .

Simply relax . . Relax . .

I want to take you . . first, to a restful . . quiet place deep in the forest . . where you will find peace and relaxing comfort . . in a totally relaxing world of your own . . We will only stay for a little while . . You're going to take a short journey . . up a mountain trail . . where tall trees nestle high up . . in the rain clouds . . The clouds bump and mesh together . . swirling . . in shades of pink and soft azure blue . . Occasional drops of rain settle softly . . on your face . . But you smile because . . the rain drops make you feel excited and . . happy inside . .

It is time now to let go . . Let yourself be free to slowly drift up . . up . . to the tops of the trees . . high above the trees . . where you are free to sail on the wind . . Look away and you will see the far mountain ranges . . covered in white snow caps . . many miles away . . You can see them clearly in the distance . . Beautiful patches of white snow . . against the blue and green background . . of the Earth . . But you are not going there now . . Perhaps, another time . .

Let yourself slowly drift through the branches of the elm trees . . and the oak trees . . Tall and majestic . . You are settling down into the top of . . the great elm tree with its mighty . . spreading branches . . Where birds flutter past in darting flashes . . Chipmunks and squirrels . . find food to store for the winter. And there . . far below . . you hear and see where a gurgling brook trickles . . with singing waters . . winding through the forest grasses . . far below . .
You are drifting now . . Slowly rocking on the winds . . like the leaves . . Drifting slowly, to the left . . then to the right . . Back

197

and forth, as you slowly, gently, sail down . . down . . Deep . . deeper . . toward the green grasses of the forest . . far below . . Slowly turning . . circling . . through the huge branches of the trees . . Drifting in high circles . . Swaying to the right . . Sailing upward with the leafs in the wind . . Then to the left . . Circling . . circling . . among the drifting leafs . . The winds carry you gently in a downward motion . . Drifting and circling . . Down . . down . . Deep . . Very Deep . . Until at last . . your feet touch the soft, green grasses . . covering the earth . . Here, you will find peace . . tranquility . . complete relaxation . . Here, you are as one . . with all that God . . has created . . for your absolute tranquility . .

Here, there are no sounds . . besides my voice . . and the noise of rushing waters in the distant brook . . flowing through the forest . . Any other sounds you may hear will only support you . . in your relaxed and comfortable state . . Your mind and body are open . . to complete trust . . Trust in the power of your mind . . to benefit you on your journey . . Your mind is very relaxed now and . . open to receive the beneficial suggestions . . I will soon give you . . But for now we will stay here . . in this beautiful meadow . . For here . . there is much to experience . . and to learn . .

Enjoy this time . . here in this beautiful garden . . where birds chatter happily in the trees . . The animals roam freely . . without fear . . with nothing to disturb their natural way of life . . The swaying grasses in the meadow are filled with colorful flowers . . blown by the soft winds of springtime . . The high alpine peaks glisten on the distant horizon . . and love is in your heart . . You are not alone . . Love is everywhere . . Rest now for a moment before we continue . . (pause)

I want you to look upward now . . through the branches of the trees above you . . I want you to lift yourself up now . . up . . up . . into the branches . . Keep going up . . until you are at the tops of the trees . . Look all around you . . You can see for many miles in all directions . .

Such a beautiful country . . You will continue rising up now . . Rising higher . . and higher . . Into the blue sky above you . . The town is in the distance . . as you rise up, even higher . . The town gets smaller now . . fading from view while you go higher . . and higher . . There, at the horizon of the Earth . . is the ocean . . A darker blue . . with the setting sun far to your left now . . You can see almost the entire country . . And the Earth is outlined before you . . Rising higher now . . higher . . Beneath you, the Earth looks like a large beach ball as you continue traveling upward . . and away from the big blue marble . . And it gets smaller and smaller . . in the far distance . . Now . . it seems to be only a small . . revolving sphere in the corners of your memory . . Continue your journey beyond . .

AT THIS TIME, CLIENT MAY ENCOUNTER MANY "EYES" WATCHING. ASSURE HIM / HER THEY ARE GUARDIANS OF THE CELESTIAL SANTUM.

Now, you may turn your gaze toward the infinite Cosmic . . Continue your spiritual ascent . . until you perceive the Celestial Sanctum . . just as you have visualized it to be . . See it the same as you have imagined it . . It may take the form of a cathedral . . a mosque . . synagogue . . temple or a landscape . . The fact that you now see it, rising in the cosmic . . and bathed in celestial light . . fills your spirit and soul with an indescribable inner joy . .

ENCOURAGE CLIENT TO RESPOND TO QUESTIONS.

You are arriving on a plane just above the Celestial Sanctum . . and you can see how very beautiful and large it is . . Q. What does it appear to be made of ? Are there many people here ? Can you describe the buildings to me ? Are they like palaces with stained glass windows ? I am told . . you can hear beautiful music everywhere . . and smell the odor of incense . . The visual beauty must be fantastic . . Tell me what you can as you look at it from the outside . . Would you like to go in now ?

You are walking up the stone stairway to a huge entryway . . leading into the inner sanctum . . where many people are mingling . . You may speak to anyone here . . for they are all welcome . . just as you are welcome . . Each of them is God's child . . Each with a purpose . . You may freely walk through the crowds and notice the people here . . Perhaps there is someone you know . . from now, or from the past . . Someone is noticing you now . . there, to your right . . as though you are familiar to them . . Why don't you stop and communicate for a moment . . We have time . .

Now that you have arrived in the Celestial Sanctum . . let yourself become totally immersed in the sacred, inspiring and comfortable feelings which pervade it . . With your body and soul bathing in this harmonious atmosphere . . the time has arrived for you . . to express to the God of your heart . . the reason for your coming to this place . . of high spirituality . . It may be a health problem . . or you may wish to be enlightened . . concerning some family, social or professional problem . . Simply refer to it mentally . . as though you were informing the most conceivable, pure Cosmic Intelligence about it . . for that IS what you are doing, isn't it . . Your presence in the Celestial Sanctum is highly valued . . You have made a great effort to be here . . and it is greatly appreciated . . So, if your goal is simply to pray . . or meditate upon some philosophical subject . . do it in this harmonious setting . . and proceed according to your feelings and beliefs . . (pause)

You are no longer alone, are you ? . . You are now in the company of friends . . An angel and your earthly guide . . Later on, perhaps you will tell me about them . . Be sure to ask them, What are their names ? . . (pause)

The time has now come for you . . to present the reason . . that has caused you to ascend to this most sacred place . . the Celestial Sanctum . . Do this now . . in the presence of these holy beings . . Take whatever time you need . . to interact with them . . When you have finished . . you will raise your hand as a signal to tell me you are ready to continue . . (Pause. It may take some time)

You have presented your reason for ascension to the Celestial Sanctum . . and perhaps you have received an immediate answer . . However . . do not think about it any more . . but remain immersed in this characteristic harmony . . and . . this is very important . .

Place yourself, now . . in a state of total receptivity . . At the exact moment you reach this state . . you will receive a Cosmic Influx that will cure you . . inspire you . . or bring you the answer you are seeking . . This does not mean that you will be immediately conscious of receiving this influx . . because it is situated at a psychic level . . which cannot be perceived, objectively . . However . . as the hours or days go by . . you will begin to notice the full impact . . that this cosmic communion will have on you . . Such a spiritual contact always has beneficial results . . It is impossible to fail when experiencing the Celestial Sanctum . . because failure is impossible at the level of the soul . .

(Offer an option) Q. Do you feel you have accomplished everything you can at this time ? Is there a reason you wish to stay longer or . . would you like to return home now ? If you wish to go home . . we will do that now . . Take one last look around you . . notice everything you can and . . remember everything that you will . . You may never again have opportunity to return to this sacred place . . in this lifetime . . It has been, truly, a wonderful experience, hasn't it . .

Make your way now to the main entryway leading to the outer chambers . . and out beyond . . into the courtyard . . This is where we were when we first arrived and . . it is now familiar, isn't it . . And so, we will depart from here, as well . . Lift yourself gently upward . . up . . up . . above the Celestial Sanctum . . for one last look . . You will always remember this vision . . As you will remember everything . . you have experienced . . on this celestial journey . .

Turn slightly to the left now and you will see a small, blue dot . . far off in the distance . . near our sun . . Watch it closely as it becomes larger and larger . . We are speeding very quickly through time and space . . Getting nearer now . . closer . . It is appearing like a big, blue marble . . notice the streaks of clouds . . wrapping around it . . It is getting larger now . . as we draw nearer and nearer . . Soaring gently and silently . . above the North American Continent . . You can see the Rocky Mountains . . and the great American Desert . . stretching from Canada to Mexico . . Coming in swiftly now . . Now, slowing a bit, as we turn . . gliding in, silently, toward home . . There . . you can see the lights of the city now . . We are nearly there . . Yes, we are touching down now . . Safely home at last . . Your wonderful journey has happily ended . .

I will count from five down to one . . and you will open your eyes . . feeling refreshed . . feeling wonderful . . for you are . . truly . . a wonderful person . .

FIVE - Feeling good . . feeling wonderful . . all over . .

FOUR - your hands are tingling . . Get the feelings back into your body.

THREE - Coming up now . . Stirring into conscious awareness . .

TWO - Gently inhale now . . Breathe out . . and . .

ONE - Open your eyes now and focus with your mind . . because it is imperative that you repeat this invocation after me . .

"May the God of my Heart - Sanctify this Attunement of Self . . with the Celestial Sanctum ! So Mote It Be !" Bless you.

CEREBRAL PALSY

START WITH GOLDEN GLOW INDUCTION. USE FINGER RESPONSE OR
OTHER TECHNIQUE TO FIND CAUSE OF PROBLEM. ENSURE CLIENT IS
RELEASED FROM UNDERLYING CAUSE BEFORE PROCEEDING FURTHER.

Your subconscious mind agrees that you are released . . from the
imprints and impressions in your mind . . that had been causing you
to experience Cerebral Palsy . . That means that it is now okay . .
for your body processes to function properly . . and heal your body in a
perfect way . .

You are calm and relaxed now . . And you can continue slipping into
a deeper, more peaceful hypnotic state . . Your subconscious mind is
accepting the suggestions and instructions . . that I am telling you now . .

The suggestions and instructions I give you will go into the
storehouse of your mind . . And they will begin working immediately in
your body . . And will keep becoming more effective each day . .

Even after you awaken from the hypnotic state . . the healing
energies in your body will continue working . . And you will be
noticing the improvements . . no matter how slight they may seem to
be . . Each day the improvements will become more apparent . .

All of your body processes will now continue working in perfect
harmony . . repairing cells, nourishing tissues, strengthening muscles
and ligaments . . correcting deficiencies in your nervous system . .
and cleansing impurities out of your body . . through the natural
processes of your elimination system . . Every feature of your body is
working in smooth, perfect harmony . . Your body possesses all of
the chemicals and minerals it needs . . to heal your body in a
perfect way . .

Each cell of your body effortlessly performs amazing functions . . that
the world's most outstanding chemists, medical doctors and scientists
. . have not been able to duplicate . . And all of those natural
healing energies are activated . . simply by means of receiving
positive directions from your subconscious mind . .

By thinking positive thoughts . . your subconscious mind responds by
activating the natural healing energies within your body . . and causes
them to function properly . . thereby, producing your perfect health . .

As you continue to think only positive thoughts . . about every part of your body, being healthy . . those thoughts and impressions move into your subconscious mind . . causing the processes of your body to renew and rejuvenate every cell . . every atom and every molecule in your anatomy . .

Every day you will continue to experience improvements in your physical movements . . And your physical movements will continue becoming more perfectly coordinated . . And you will easily move your arms and legs in perfect harmony and coordination . . Your whole body is becoming more perfectly coordinated . .

Now concentrate on all of the muscles, nerves, ligaments and tendons in your face, head, neck and spine . . And visualize them as they continue to improve . . and function more perfectly . . (pause)

Envision your head and neck . . becoming more perfectly coordinated with your torso . . Your arms and hands, functioning in more perfect harmony . . Your arms and legs, along with all other parts of your body . . continue to function in more perfect harmony and coordination . . Submerge these positive thoughts, of your body . . into your subconscious mind . . and allow the natural healing processes to take control . . (Pause)

During your daily life, you will be more calm and relaxed . . More stable and more settled . . as your health continues its improvement . . As your health continues improving . . your confidence will keep growing stronger . . And you will achieve greater accomplishments . . in all areas of your life . . These healing processes are already working in your body . . because you want them to work . .

Your subconscious mind is eagerly obeying your desires and directions . . for your body to be healed and strong . . To be completely healthy . . and perfectly coordinated . . in all of its physical senses . .

You are doing very well . . And now, I want you to rest and relax for a few moments . . Giving your subconscious mind a little time to absorb all that we have talked about today . . Just relax a little longer . . and focus your mind on the healing processes, as they repair and realign . . (pause)

I am going to count from 1 to 5 now . . And on the count of 5, you will open your eyes to an alert waking state . . feeling clear of mind . . relaxed . . and wonderful . . I will begin . .

One - You will remember everything you have experienced today . . with understanding and clarity . .

TWO - You are now connected to your inner strength and higher power . . supporting your good . . You will carry that inner strength with you throughout your day . .

Three - Everything I have told you is true and is already happening . . and you are already successful in manifesting the positive suggestions that I have given you . . into your daily life and consciousness . .

Four - You are beginning to be more aware of your body as it fully awakens and wants to stir . .

Five - As you open your eyes now, you are feeling clear, rested and wonderful. For you are a wonderful person . .

THESE SUGGESTIONS ARE TO BE REPEATED WHILE THE CHILD IS SLEEPING.   A PARENT SHOULD READ THE SUGGESTIONS, JUST AS THEY ARE.   THE SUGGESTIONS HAVE BEEN CAREFULLY DESIGNED FOR MAXIMUM EFFECTIVENESS.   READER SHOULD SPEAK IN A WHISPER, LOUDLY ENOUGH TO BE HEARD BUT SOFTLY, SO THE CHILD CONTINUES SLEEPING.   SUGGESTIONS CAN BE GIVEN EVERY NIGHT, IF DESIRED, THEN ONCE OR TWICE A WEEK, WHENEVER NEEDED.

YOU ARE A WONDERFUL PERSON.
I (WE) LOVE YOU, VERY, VERY MUCH.
YOU ARE LOVED AND RESPECTED.
YOU CONTINUE TO FEEL MORE AND MORE SELF CONFIDENT EVERY DAY.
YOU ARE A VERY GOOD FRIEND.

YOU MAKE FRIENDS EASILY BECAUSE PEOPLE NATURALLY LIKE YOU.

YOU ARE HEALTHY AND HAPPY.
YOU ARE VERY INTELLIGENT.
YOU ARE VERY LOVING AND KIND, TO YOURSELF AND TO OTHERS.
IT IS EASY FOR PEOPLE TO LIKE YOU.

YOU LEARN SCHOOL SUBJECTS VERY EASILY AND YOU ENJOY LEARNING WHAT YOUR TEACHER TEACHES YOU.

YOU ENJOY SCHOOL MORE AND MORE EACH DAY.

YOU FEEL VERY SELF-CONFIDENT.
YOU LOVE YOURSELF AND RESPECT YOURSELF AND YOU TAKE GOOD CARE OF YOURSELF.
I (WE) LOVE YOU MORE AND MORE EACH DAY.
YOU ARE WONDERFUL.
YOU ARE A WONDERFUL AND LOVING PERSON.
IT IS EASY FOR YOU TO LEARN AND REMEMBER GOOD THINGS.
YOU ARE HEALTHY AND HAPPY.

YOU HAVE PLEASANT, ENJOYABLE DREAMS EACH NIGHT.

You can keep your eyes open now and . . look up at the ceiling . . Right up over your head . .

You don't need to look at anything special . . Just whatever you find interesting . . But keep looking up over your head . .

I'm going to count from TEN down to ONE, and I want you to close your eyes, a little more, with each number I say . . I want you to have them stuck shut by the time I reach the count of ONE . . You can test your eyes after I reach the number ONE, to be sure you have them stuck shut . .

TEN . . NINE . . Feel your eyes closing shut . . EIGHT . . SEVEN . . Your eyelids are closing tighter . . SIX . . FIVE . . They feel like they are growing together now . . FOUR . . They feel like they are glued tightly shut . . THREE . . TWO . . After I say the next number, you can test your eyelids to be sure they are stuck shut . . ONE . . Okay, test your eyelids now and be sure you have them stuck shut . .

Now, let all the little muscles around your eyes completely relax . . And keep them closed until I tell you to open them . .

You are following my suggestions real good . . Now, just relax your body, all over . . And you may begin to feel like you are drifting into something that feels very much like sleep . . And that's okay . . You'll still be able to hear what I say, so . . just relax . . Relax . .

I want you to pretend that you are going to play near a swimming pool . . Or a lake . . Or right by the ocean . . It's a nice warm day . . If you are by the ocean, just imagine that you are digging in the sand . . As you keep digging down . . deeper and deeper . . the sand feels cooler, doesn't it . .

The air smells nice and fresh . . You are feeling so good and so happy . . and you are really enjoying yourself . .

Some of your friends are coming to play with you now . . You can have fun, splashing and playing in the water . . You are feeling so good that you want to tell your friends just how good you feel . . It feels so good to be alive . . And it's really good to be you . . You are really enjoying yourself . . running on the beach and playing hard . .

As you run in the sand and play in the water . . you can meet other friends and enjoy talking with them . . Notice how good the warm sand feels on your feet . . You have really been enjoying yourself . . And now, you feel like you want to find a shady place to lie down and rest a while . .

Now, you are lying down . . Just take a deep breath and feel yourself really relaxing . .

And now, you are holding a very special flashlight . . That flashlight can shine any place you can imagine . . Imagine that light, shining inside of you now . . It's shining all around the inside of you . . making sure that every part of your body is healthy . . You can see all through the inside of your body . . so you can see that it is in a good, healthy condition . . That flashlight shows that your body is getting healthier and stronger each day . .

And now, the flashlight is shining inside of your head . . Showing that you are very intelligent . . And it shows that you have a good mind and that you learn very fast . . It also shows that your grades in school will keep improving more and more . .

And now, shine that flashlight all over your whole body . . That light is helping you to continue growing happier and stronger . . Enabling you to keep enjoying life, more and more, every day . .

You are feeling happiness and joy all around you now . . And you are feeling thankful aren't you . .

Just say to yourself, "I am thankful" . . Because being thankful helps you to feel good . . And feeling good enables you to sleep better at night . . And you wake up each morning feeling strong and healthy and happy . .

Every day you keep having more confidence in yourself . . and you continue improving in all areas of your life . . You realize that you are safe and you are loved . . Because you're such a wonderful person . . And your happiness just keeps increasing more every day . .

Now, I want you to count to yourself . . 5, 4, 3, 2, 1 . . And when you say ONE, you can open your eyes . . Okay ? I'll count with you . . 5, 4, 3, 2 and ONE . . You can open your eyes now . .

Jim was a boy I knew when I was in school . . And Jim always wanted to be special . . He was in the third grade . . The same grade I was in . . His best friend was a big, strong, tall boy named Charley . . He admired Charley because . . Charley could throw a football real far . . And when he played baseball, he could really hit the ball a long way . .

Maybe you've wondered at times about being taller, like someone you know . . Or bigger or stronger . . like someone else . .

A lot of times, when Jim was in class . . he would think of how he would like to be as smart as Billy . . because every time the teacher asked a question, Billy always seemed to know the answer . . Many times, Jim would know the answer too, but he was afraid to raise his hand like Billy did . .

And as you are sitting there . . you may be thinking of what it's like for you . . when the teacher asks a question . .

When Jim was on the playground at recess . . he always noticed how really fast Patty could run . . She was the fastest runner in the class, and Jim wished he could run as fast as Patty . .

And Jane was very small . . She was the smallest girl in the room . . And she had lots of friends . . Everyone seemed to be very kind and gentle with her because she was so small . . And every once in a while Jim found himself wishing he could be small, like Jane . . so everyone would be kind and gentle with him too . .

But Jim felt like he was just an ordinary guy . . He was always wishing he could be different and be able to do something very special . . Anything . . So he was surprised one day, to hear the teacher say that everyone is special in some way . . And then she said, "You need to take some time to stop and think of how you are special". But then she handed out report cards . . And Jim looked at his and noticed that he still had average grades . . Nothing very high . . and nothing low . .

The third grade class was getting ready to do a spring concert . . And Jim noticed that tiny Jane was put in front of the class . . And Mike, who had a good speaking voice, was given a speaking part . .

And his friend, Charley, who was big and tall, was going to carry a flag . . because everyone would be able to see him . . And Stacy and Brett were going to sing a duet because they had nice singing voices and sang real good together . .

But Jim ? . . Well, he was just going to be a part of the group . . He wasn't given anything special to do . . As he was standing there, he was thinking about all the special things the others were given to do . . And he thought how wonderful it would be . . if he could do something special too . .

Then something happened . . After school that evening, he began reading a book his uncle had given him called, "The Phantom Tollbooth" . . And as he was reading the story about a young boy named Mylo, who received a magical Tollbooth as a gift, he noticed that whenever Mylo would go through the magic tollbooth . . he would find himself in the land beyond . . And throughout his travels in this great land . . he was always joined by 'Humbug' and a watchdog named, 'Toc' . . And in one of the chapters, Mylo began thinking that he must be lost . . And as he wandered around the countryside with Humbug and Toc . . they came to a small house . .

There were many doors going into the small house . . and on one of the doors was a sign the read, "The Giant" . . Mylo said, "Wow, A giant! I wonder if that giant can tell us if we're lost?" . .

So they knocked on the door . . and a man opened the door . . But he wasn't a giant . . He was sort of an ordinary sized man . . Mylo asked, "Are you the Giant?" The man answered, "Yes. I'm the smallest giant in the world." Then, Mylo asked, "Are we lost?" The giant replied, "I think you should go next door and ask the midget" . .

So Mylo went to the next door and knocked . . A man came to the door and he looked very much like the giant looked . . In fact, he looked to be the same man . . They looked enough alike to be twins . . And Mylo asked, "Are you the midget?". . The man answered, "Yes. I'm the tallest midget in the world" . . So Mylo continued, "Are we lost?" . . The big midget scratched his head and replied . . I don't know the answer to that question . . Why don't you ask the fat man next door" . . So they went next door and knocked again . . and the same man answered the door . .

Mylo asked, "Are you the fat man? . . "Yes", the man answered. "I'm the thinnest fat man in the world" . . "Are we lost?" Mylo asked again . . "I don't know." said the fat man . . "If you go to the back of the house and knock on the door marked, 'Thin Man', he may know the answer" . .

And, guess what ? When the door opened, it was the same man . . But Mylo politely asked, "Are you the thin man?" . . The man answered, "Yes . . I'm the fattest thin man in the world" . .

Mylo wisely replied, "I think you are all the same man" . .

The man responded, "Well, I always thought of myself as just an ordinary man . . but I like to feel special . . So I can be the fattest thin man or the thinnest fat man . . or the tallest midget or the shortest giant . . I can be whatever I think I am . . All I have to do is imagine what I want to be . . and I become whatever I imagine myself to be . . Pretty neat, huh . . ?"

After Jim read the story, he thought about it and, somehow, the idea remained in his mind . . On the night of the spring concert . . when everyone was running around in costumes and stacy and Brett were practicing for their duet and Jane was getting prepared to be the smallest person in the concert . . Jim calmly walked down the hallway . . Then, as he passed a doorway, he heard someone inside crying . . He stopped and peeked into the room and noticed . . it was Charley who he had always wanted to be like and . . And so, he asked, "What's wrong, Charley?" . .

You've probably seen someone crying and wondered what you could do to help, haven't you? . .

And that's just what happened to Jim . . Charley was crying and he said, "I know I'm the tallest, biggest and strongest kid in the class . . but I sure wish I wasn't . . I wish I could be like you, Jim. I wish I could just be your size . . Sometimes it's really hard to be the biggest boy in class" . .

Jim looked at his friend, Charley, and said, "Hey, Charley, Maybe you can be the tallest short boy in the class" . . Charley smiled . . Jim said, "Come on . . You've got to get that flag" . .

Charley replied, "Yeah, you're right, Jim. You're a pretty special friend, ya' know?" . .

They went to the stage door together, to be in the spring concert . . And after that, Jim did think of himself as someone very special . . He said to himself, "I can be very special . . In fact, I can be whatever I want to be" . .

EMERGE

210

The experience of having a baby . . is one of the greatest accomplishments . . a human being has the privilege of achieving . .

By having this baby, you are creating an opportunity . . for a soul to come into an environment of love and happiness . .

The baby is already conceived within you . . and is now developing, growing and preparing for its entry into the world . . And you are giving it the opportunity to enter . .

After its birth . . you will then have the opportunity to provide it with guidance . . love and affection . . that will enable your child to develop and grow . . into a happy, successful adult . .

God created the human body so that it is always capable of functioning perfectly . . Every cell and every organ in your body possesses life, wisdom and power . .

There is constantly a new, fresh, vitalizing force of energy . . flowing through your body . . And those forces in your body are now in the process . . of producing a new life . . a new child . .

You are looking forward to the time when your child will be born . . Your subconscious mind is causing all of your body activities to function perfectly . . And the birth will be an easy, normal event . . You are feeling happy about it . . Recognizing it as a truly great opportunity to be a co-creator with God . .

Your body is made so that it is able to handle . . the growth and development of the child within you . . in an easy, natural way . .

Having a baby is such a joyful experience . . It is a perfectly natural experience . . Because your body is made so that it will adjust easily and naturally . . as the child is developing within you . .

When it becomes time for the baby to enter the world . . your body will make all the proper adjustments, easily . . The long muscles of your womb will contract . . to expel the baby from your body . . And the round muscles . . which have been holding the baby safely in your body . . will relax . .

It is all normal, natural and easy . . and will be accomplished calmly and perfectly . . in a very comfortable way . .

You are feeling more peaceful about giving birth to your baby . . And you are looking forward, with great joy and expectation, to the time it will be born . .

There will be a continuous improvement in your health . . And you will be pleased about having the privilege . . of bringing a new baby into the world . .

Having these sessions with hypnosis . . enables you to learn how to remain relaxed and calm . . in your daily activities . . So, the birth of your baby will be accomplished in a comfortable way . .

When you walk, your baby will adjust . . and you will maintain a good posture . . And when you sit down, it will be easy for you to adjust your body . . into a comfortable position . .

Your subconscious mind is causing you to desire foods . . which will provide the best nourishment for you and for your baby . . And the processes of your body will function perfectly . . so your food will digest easily . .

When the time comes for your baby to be born . . the natural processes of moving your baby out of your womb . .and out of your body . . will be just as easy as eating, breathing, digesting food . . or any other natural process of your body . .

You will give birth to a healthy baby, easily . . because the process is natural and automatic . .

You will feel calm and relaxed . . and will have the baby just as easily and naturally as you achieve the other functions of your body . .

Your muscles will respond with perfect coordination . . When the long muscles contract to move the baby out of your body . . the round muscles will relax . . The more the long muscles contract . . the more your round muscles will relax . . The muscles in your body will work together in perfect harmony . . And the rest of your body will remain calm and relaxed . .

When it is time for your baby to be born . . you will be aware of the different feelings and sensations . . in your body . .

When you begin to feel some pressure of the contractions . . you will recognize it and quickly realize the time has come for the baby to be born . .

During the first few contractions . . you will be aware that you are merely feeling pressure . . You will be relaxed . . and will experience a wonderful feeling of satisfaction and relief . . You will go to the hospital with a feeling of joy and anticipation . .

At the hospital, when the baby begins passing out of the womb and through the birth canal . . you will experience a great sense of satisfaction . . You will feel relaxed, calm and happy . . And you will be very peaceful and serene . . You'll remain comfortable and at ease as you deliver the baby . .

You are one with God . . God is in command . . and you feel confident and capable . . You have peace of mind and self assurance . . This is a beautiful world . . And you are a beautiful person . .

You are having a wonderful experience and . . all is well . .

Your inner mind is causing you . . to experience pleasant changes . . that are preparing your body perfectly . . Even after you awaken . . from the hypnotic state . . and come back to a wide awake, fully alert state . . Your subconscious mind will cause the processes of your body . . to continue working . . Adjusting every part of your body . . in a gentle, pleasant way . .

Continue relaxing now, for a few more minutes . . to give your subconscious mind the time . . to accept and absorb . . everything we have talked about today . . So continue to relax . . (Pause)

In a moment, I will count to FIVE . . and you will awaken feeling refreshed and wonderful . . You will awaken a little more with each number you hear . . You will remember everything I have told you and . . everything that I have said to you is true . . I will begin my count now . .

ONE . . You are coming up now . . Soon you will awaken . .
TWO . . Your fingers and toes want to wiggle now . . Let them move a little
THREE . . Feeling refreshed and wonderful . . for you are, truly, a wonderful person . .
FOUR . . You're almost there . . Take a deep breath now . . and . .
FIVE . . Open your eyes . . and let me see a big smile . .

It's interesting to be aware . . of how we sometimes deceive ourselves . . Some people tell themselves, they can't stop smoking . . It is too hard . . Some people tell themselves . . they can't stop taking Cocaine . . It is too hard . . When they feel the urge to take Cocaine . . stopping the urge may, very briefly, seem too hard . . But, what makes it too hard? . . I want you to use your imagination now . . and you will demonstrate to yourself . . one of the things that makes it seem to be so hard . .

I want you to hold your left arm straight out in front of you . . and clench your left fist . . And make your left arm rigid and stiff . . Make it even stiffer now . . Make it so stiff and rigid that it feels like it will not bend . . Notice how it keeps getting stiffer and more rigid . . with each number that I say, as I count from ONE to TEN . .

ONE . . Notice the power and strength in your left arm as you keep making it stiffer . . TWO . . THREE . . You are making it so stiff and rigid, it will resist your efforts to bend it . . FOUR . . Making it even stiffer now . . FIVE . . SIX . . Notice that it is very stiff and rigid now . . SEVEN . . It feels as rigid as a bar of steel . . EIGHT . . It is already so stiff that if you tried to bend it, it would keep getting stiffer . . NINE . . When I say the next number, you will try to bend it . . so you can notice how stiff and rigid it remains . . The more you try to bend it, the stiffer it becomes . . TEN . . It is so stiff and rigid now that it will resist any effort you make to bend it . . Try to bend it now . . so you can notice that it keeps becoming stiffer and more rigid . .

If client is unable to bend arm, say, "Now you are aware of the power . . of your subconscious mind . . When it accepts an idea, it controls you, even when you consciously try to resist".

If client does bend arm, say, "Now you realize that you are in control . . and can overcome thoughts and ideas in your subconscious mind . . And you are realizing that you will also have the power to overcome the Cocaine habit" . .

Your left arm feels rigid and stiff because you are telling yourself it feels 'rigid and stiff' . .

I put the suggestion into your mind and your mind accepted it . . and became convinced that your left arm was stiff and rigid . . The only thing that makes it so, is your mind, irrationally, telling you that it is so . . While, in fact . . it is so . .

Now, I am going to touch your left hand . . and you will notice, immediately, that you can open your fist . . and bend your left arm easily . . (Touch left hand) Now you notice that you can easily bend your left arm . .

Think about that now . . A moment ago, you couldn't bend your left arm . . Now you can . . What made the difference? . . (Wait for response) Occasionally, when something seems to be very difficult . . some people say to themselves . . I can't do it, or, I'll never be able to do that . . They give up before they even try . . They deceive themselves . . Of course, they can do it . . Just like YOU can do it . . With self-determination, you can and will accomplish your goals . .

When a person becomes determined to stop smoking . . or stop drinking . . or rid themselves of the Cocaine habit . . They discover that the subconscious part of their mind . . is more than willing to cooperate . . enabling them to overcome the problem easily . . There is no logical reason why life should always be difficult . . When we choose to accomplish something that seems to be difficult . . we discover that we become stronger . . We progress as a person . . and we feel good about ourselves . . Remember that you can and will go on living without (Cocaine-cigarettes-alcohol) The solution is to simply take on the determination . . to accomplish your goal . . by using your mind . .

When you feel a momentary urge to take Cocaine again . . tell yourself you are FREE FROM IT . .

You have decided to treat your body well . . You need your body to live in . . and to transport your mind and your spirit from place to place . . And you want to live, for the rest of your life, in a healthy body . . You have chosen to be free from (cocaine - cigarettes - alcohol) . .

If you are around other people who are using _____ . . you will remain calm and relaxed . . And you will be thankful that you are no longer a user . . If you see other people taking _____ . . you will be even more thankful that you have stopped taking it . .

Your health will keep improving more each day . . and you will notice how much better you feel . . mentally and physically and spiritually . .

(USE OTHER 'STOP - SMOKING' PRESCRIPTIONS AS FURTHER SESSIONS ARE NEEDED.)

I want you to continue relaxing for another moment or two . . in silence . . to allow your subconscious mind to absorb . . and resolve . . everything we have talked about today . . (pause)

You are now very comfortable, relaxed and totally at ease . . You are experiencing perfect peace of mind . . And in the future . . you can enjoy this same perfect calmness and respite . . any time you want it . . All you will need to do is to sit or lie down in a comfortable position . . Close your eyes and imagine yourself in this . . comfortable state of mind . . Then count backward in your mind from TEN down to ONE . . By the time you reach number ONE . . you will be completely relaxed . . calm and at ease . . And you will know peace with the world . . And you can remain in that state for as long as you desire . . When you are ready to return to a wide-awake and alert state of mind . . you'll only need to open your eyes . . Whenever you do this . . you will always feel rested and refreshed . . full of energy, strength and vitality . . after relaxing this way, for only a few minutes . .

You will remember everything I have said to you today . . and you will greatly benefit from everything I have told you . . Continue now, to relax, for just a little longer . . (Pause)

In just a moment we will be concluding this session . . I will be counting to FIVE for you to awaken . . You will come up to a wide-awake, fully alert state, when I say the number FIVE . .

ONE - Feeling so good . . Feeling wonderful . . all over . .

TWO - your hands are tingling and your legs are feeling a bit numb yet . . Get the feelings back into your body . .

THREE - Coming up now . . More alert . . More aware . . Stirring into conscious awareness . .

FOUR - Gently inhale now . . Breathe out . . and . .

FIVE - Open your eyes now and focus on your surroundings . .

So, as you continue to relax . . I want you to be made aware . . that you have been doing a very harmful thing to yourself . . I want you to realize . . that you have been placing certain labels on yourself . . Labels which are harmful to you . . You have been sticking labels on yourself . . just like you would put labels on a bottle . . One of the labels that you have placed on yourself is called . . inadequate . . And every time you think the word, inadequate, of yourself . . you increase your own belief that you are, in fact, inadequate . . For you see, the difficulty is that people tend to believe or, act out, what they say, or feel, about themselves . . In other words, you are, basically, what you believe yourself to be . .

This is a very simple concept . . Just as you believe that, as an American, you should act like an American . . because you believe yourself to be an American . . And if you really thought of yourself as belonging to another nationality, then you would act like that . . Basically, we are all what we believe ourselves to be . . Those of us who believe ourselves to be doctors . . will act like doctors . . And those who believe themselves to be inadequate . . will act and feel . . inadequate . .

There are many people who place labels on themselves . . just as you have done in the past . . Then they say to themselves, "I'm just inadequate" . . after giving themselves that label . . But then, they feel the need to live up to that label . . or live down to it, as the case may be . . For you realize that all of their actions carry them, always, toward the image that they hold of themselves . .

Unfortunately, there are many negative labels that people place upon themselves . . Another such label you have accepted in the past is that of a lack of self-confidence . . And you may have said to yourself, "I just have no self-confidence" . . for whatever the reason was . .

Now, I'm telling you this because . . this is serious . . And it is serious because it doesn't take long for you to believe it, once you have placed these thoughts into motion . . Once you have given yourself the suggestion that your self-confidence is slipping . . it's just a step away from thinking, "I'm not worthy of anything really good happening to me" . .

There have probably been times in the past when you have kept yourself from being chosen by others for certain honors . . because you have said to yourself, "I can't accept their confidence because I'm too unworthy" . . "I'm too unworthy to be chosen by them because I'm undeserving", or

"I don't deserve any better breaks than have already come my way because of my present conduct . . or my past conduct . . or my present or past thoughts . . I don't deserve this because of what happened in my past" . . Well, you know more about your past than anybody . . but . . should that determine your future ? . .

You have been allowing your conscious mind to play tricks on you . . Playing tricks on you by letting you feel that your problems are too difficult to be resolved . . You have said things to yourself like, "I'm stuck in the mud and I'll probably be stuck there forever" . . "I'm inadequate . . I don't have enough self-confidence to accomplish what I want . . I'm unworthy - undeserving" . .

Now listen to me carefully . . All these things are simply labels . . They are all just little labels . . And, NO, they are certainly not you . . And why are they not you ? . . Perhaps I can explain it best by giving you some examples . .

Let us suppose you have a bottle of penicillin . . Oh, yes, it's a good bottle of penicillin . . And the bottle of penicillin could be used to fight infection by a doctor, if properly used . . But suppose you wrote out the label for it . . and you stuck that label on the bottle of penicillin . . and on that label, you had written, in big bold letters . . the word, POISON, on it . . You put the poison label on the bottle of penicillin, even though the bottle . . contained perfectly good penicillin . .

Now, with a label like 'POISON' on the bottle, neither you nor anybody else would dare take that penicillin and use it, now would they . . That penicillin might have saved a life . . but it is ruined now . . All because of a bad label . .

But, how much more important are people than bottles ? . . So, if you disregard this extremely important aspect of labeling yourself . . then, horrible mistakes can be made . . in your life . . And so, of all the people you are labeling . . what person is more important to you than yourself ? . .

Just think about it . . How did you come to label yourself, "inadequate"? Where did you get the idea that you had a lack of confidence? . . And, if you ever placed a label of 'unworthy' on yourself, why did you do that ? . . And, if you're so undeserving . . who, then, is 'deserving' ? . .

Maybe you applied still other labels to yourself . . Labels like, "I have a bad memory . . I have a bad temper . . I'm too aggressive . . I'm easily depressed . . I'm confused . . I'm this . . I'm that . .

Whatever it happens to be, you keep sticking labels on yourself . . And every time you do, you keep giving yourself negative suggestions . . But I want you to realize that it is not the label that counts . . It is the contents . . When a wrong label is glued onto a bottle of poison . . tragedy occurs . . And, likewise, when the wrong label is glued onto you . . tragedy occurs . . Just as it does when a drug is mislabeled . .

Now, there are a lot of reasons why a person might label themselves as, inadequate . . And one of the reasons why this might occur is . . because of their identification with someone else . . For example, If a person says to himself . . "I'm really just like my Father, and he is really inadequate . . Therefore, I must be inadequate" . . or, "I'm really just like my Mother . . She is inadequate, therefore, I must be inadequate" . . Now, if your parents were inadequate, do you have to be inadequate, too? . . Well, that doesn't make any sense at all . . If that were true, every person with inadequate parents would also be inadequate . . And it wouldn't be long before every person on earth were inadequate . . The truth of the matter is . . inadequate people may come from very inadequate parents but . . by the same token, inadequate parents may also produce a genius . .

Actually, most of the great geniuses of all time, came from very humble beginnings . . Many of our great men have been in some sort of trouble . . emotionally and, sometimes, politically . . Most of them, in fact, had difficulties . . But they overcame their troubles . . Just as you can learn to overcome your difficulties, too . . The truth is, most people, who are inadequate, are that way because they have labeled themselves as 'inadequate' . . Consequently, they are merely acting out the label that they themselves have placed upon themselves . . Yes, that's correct . . They are merely acting out the label that they have placed on themselves . .

The point I am making is this . . Inadequacy, carries a very strong meaning . . It is a very powerful, but negative, label . . And it is the wrong label for you . . And right now, you are going to delete that negative label you have imposed on yourself . . Delete it from your thinking . . From your conscious awareness . . You are not to use that label on yourself, ever again . .

Right now, you will allow yourself to accept the suggestion that you will be whatever you are capable of being . . Accept the suggestion that you will become what you believe yourself to be . . And you will do what you believe yourself capable of doing . . And you are going to rip off that label of inadequacy, that you have been placing on yourself from time to time . .

So, in your mind's eye, right now, as I speak . . I want you to let that label be seen . . in your imagination . .

I want you to imagine seeing yourself, with that label, inadequate, on you . . And I want you to reach up and grab that label, with your hand, and rip it off from you . . Right now ! Pull it off . .

You don't need it . . It never helped you at all . . You have used that label to hide behind, for a long time now . . But you don't need it any more . . And I don't care why you put it on . . Whether it was because you identify with your Mother or your Father or with somebody else who is inadequate . . It doesn't matter . . You no longer need to identify with that part of that person . . Remember that you are not that person in any way . . You are who YOU are . . And there is only one of you . .

Now, Lack of Confidence . . Is that one of the labels you have placed on yourself ? If it is, RIP IT OFF! See it in your mind's eye and see yourself ripping that label off ! Right now ! Because, from this moment on, you are going to allow yourself to be labeled, CONFIDENT . . Now, in your mind's eye, put that label on you . . In big, bold letters . . And wear it proudly . . Even if you feel completely empty of any confidence, right now . . label yourself, CONFIDENT anyway . . And you will begin filling yourself with confidence . . by using this powerful suggestion . . Of course, you understand . . that confidence is not achieved quickly . . It must be earned gradually . . It is the BI-product of talent, training, repetition and dedication . . But confidence . . translates into power, in any walk of life . . Because it makes you become absolutely certain of your position and your ability . . It is a powerful force that definitely influences your inner strength . . your charisma . . and your character . .

You needn't be an empty bottle any longer . . Every day in every way, you will allow yourself to become more self-confident . . You are what you believe yourself to be . . And what we think, in secret, comes to pass . . And since your picture of yourself determines your behavior . . you must have confidence in your ability to set goals for yourself . . and to go after those goals . . And if you don't go after them, you realize that you will fall prey to petty worries and petty fears . . Petty troubles and self pity . . All of which are self-destructive . .

Now, I want you to fully understand this . . Your vision is the promise . . of what you shall one day be . . That's right . . The vision you have of yourself is what you will one day become . . Now, accept that as absolute truth . . These are not simply nice sounding words that I speak . . Nor are they mere platitudes or cliches I am giving you . . They are facts! Believe it! Repeat it over to yourself . . Say to yourself, "My vision is the promise of what I shall one day become" . . And as you repeat these words, periodically, realize that you must continually re-appraise yourself . . almost daily . . So, make the adjustments . . Make changes for the better . . Make improvements . . I want you to repeat these words to yourself . . and never forget this important key to your future . .

"My vision is the promise of what I shall one day become" . .

Anyone who is overconfident has good reason to feel that way . . But, keep in mind that all great men and women . . constantly re-examine their actions, their thoughts and their goals . . They re- examine them to keep themselves on course . . Just like launching a rocket to the moon . . The goal, of course, is to get to the moon . . but getting there does not occur in a straight line . . Adjustments must be made, continually, to keep it on course . .

That is what you are going to allow yourself to do now . . You are going to allow yourself to set goals . . And you are going to remind yourself to re-examine those goals, periodically . . Re- examine them so that you can confirm your motives . . And so that you can understand more clearly what your actions ought to be . .

And more firmly grip onto your values . . And not let go of them . . Sense your goals so you can allow yourself to become . . what you really want yourself to be . .

In just a moment, I will give you a period of silence . . And during that silence . . I want you to contemplate . . all of the labels . . which you have placed on yourself . . The ones that really should not be there . . You know what they are . . During this moment of silence, you are going to see all of those labels on your body . . And you are going to rip them right off, without question . . Without hesitation . .

You are going to replace those old labels with all new ones . . Good, positive labels that you will place on yourself . . Labels of confidence . . Labels of self-assurance . . Labels of self-reliance and labels of love . . Labels of kindness and generosity . . And labels of skillful and artistic ability . . You're going to let all those harmful labels be gone . . All of the harmful identifications are now gone from your life . .

221

You are going to put good labels all over yourself . . because you are intelligent . . You are capable . . You are effective . . You are self-confident . . You are self-reliant . . You are self- assured . . You have the ability to completely relax . . You have the ability to be comfortable and CONFIDENT in any situation . . And you are going to allow all of this to happen . . Easily happen . . As you tear off those negative labels and replace them with all positive labels . . during this moment of silence, which begins . . now . . (Pause one minute)

Regardless of what comes up in your life . . you will be in control of your emotions and feelings . . That is what will cause success to be yours . . And soon you will have all that you want in your life . . Now, I am going to count from 1 to 5 . . And on the count of 5 . . you will open your eyes . . to an alert, waking state . . feeling clear of mind, relaxed and confident . . Very confident . . I will begin . .

One.   You will remember everything with complete understanding . .
Two.   You are now connected to your spiritual, inner supporting strength.
Three. Everything I have told you is true . . and is already happening . .
Four.   Becoming more aware of your body as it awakens and wants to stir.
Five.   Open your eyes now, feeling clear, rested and wonderful . .

CONSTIPATION

You are now in a pleasant, hypnotic state of relaxation . . And you will continue experiencing wonderful, peaceful sensations and feelings, that your relaxation brings . . You are letting yourself go completely . .

Your subconscious mind is hearing and receiving the suggestions and instructions I am telling you . . And your mind is ready to receive an explanation . . that will cause your elimination system to function properly . . So that you will eliminate all waste materials and waste products . . out of your body . . easily and regularly . . through the normal processes of your elimination system . .

Your entire gastrointestinal system is a muscular tube . . which is coiled around inside your body . . Various parts of that tube have different purposes . . and can be compared to specialized departments in a factory . .

For example; Your mouth is like the receiving department going into the factory . . You receive the food into your mouth . . And as you chew the food . . it mixes with saliva, provided by the glands in your mouth . . This is an immediate beginning of the digestive process . . By chewing your food thoroughly . . it prepares itself to be swallowed . .

Your throat is comparable to a conveyor system . . When you swallow, it moves the food through the conveyor canal and down into your stomach . . And the digestive process continues as it is moving down your throat . .

Your stomach does the processing of the food . . The food is received into your stomach and is prepared for your body to distribute it . . to all of the places where it is needed . . to keep your body healthy and strong . . It processes and distributes . . all of the nutrients, the energy, the strength and vitality that you experience . . through your blood stream and on . . to every part of your body, where it is needed . . And all of the waste products from the food is separated and cleansed out of your body . . through the natural processes of your elimination system . .

That whole system, inside your body, continues working twenty four hours a day . . in a way that is comparable to a conveyor system in a factory . .

The tubes . . which make up the conveyor system . . are composed of rings of muscles . . Those rings of muscles contract and relax . . contract and relax . . Continuing to push the food material along through the body just like an assembly line in a factory . .

Learning to relax enables your entire system to function properly . . The relaxation and contraction of the proper muscles will work perfectly . . From the receiving part of your body . . right on through to the disposal part of your body . . Notice how relaxed you are feeling now . . It's just as easy to have that relaxation in your mouth, throat, and on down through your entire digestive system . . And on into the tubes which eliminate the waste materials from your body . .

From now on, every time you look at food . . your subconscious mind will automatically cause you to become calm, relaxed and peaceful . . throughout your entire body . . And your intestinal tract will be relaxed . . And that will allow the natural contractions and muscle reactions . . to push waste materials through the colon . . and to the rectum . . in an easy, natural way . .

Your rectum can be compared to a waste basket . . And you know, you don't run to empty a waste basket every time you put a scrap of paper in it . . You wait until it's almost full and then you empty it . . That's the way your body functions also . .

The normal processes of your body cause waste materials to be carried through the colon and into the rectum, where it is stored . . As the rectum becomes full . . an automatic signal is sent out by your subconscious mind . . to your conscious mind . . Letting you know you are ready to have a bowl movement . . to cleanse the waste materials out from your body . . When you receive that signal . . that feeling . . you will go to the toilet . . And from now on . . as soon as you sit down on the toilet seat, that will be a signal to the round muscles which keep the waste valve closed . . to relax . . Sitting down, on the toilet seat will be a signal . . and will cause the round muscles to relax and become soft and flexible . . so they will stretch easily and comfortably . . That will be followed by waves of muscular contractions in the colon and rectum . . which will move the waste materials out of your body, in an easy, natural process . . When you feel the urge to have a bowl movement . . you will go to the toilet, sit down and wait . .

As you do that, it will be a signal to your subconscious mind to cause your rectum to empty itself, easily and comfortably . .

When you look at food, you will become relaxed . . And when you eat food, that will be a signal, which will cause your digestive system and elimination processes to function properly . . And your body will dispose of its waste materials in an easy, natural manner . .

All foods you eat will digest perfectly . . After you chew it thoroughly, it will easily pass down your throat and into your stomach . . That easy, natural movement will continue on through your intestines . . And at the proper time, you will know when you need to use the toilet . . The urge will be normal and natural for your body . . And you will respond to the urge by going to the toilet, eliminating the waste materials from your body . . Keeping your body clean and healthy . .

When you sit down on the toilet, that will be a signal for the round muscles to open the waste valve . . The muscular contractions in your colon and rectum will then cause the waste materials . . to move out of your body, easily . . Without any conscious effort by you . .

The whole process will work in a natural way . . When you eat, the relaxation starts . . Then at intervals, which are normal for your body, you will experience the urge to go to the toilet . . When you sit down on the toilet, that will be a signal for your anus to relax and become flexible . . So it will stretch easily as it needs to . . And your rectum will empty itself in a comfortable way . .

The only thing you need to do, consciously, is to . . go to the toilet when you feel the urge . . Your subconscious mind will cause your body processes to continue functioning properly . . Cleansing the waste materials out of your body in an easy, natural manner . . And you will always have an easy, natural bowl movement . . Whenever your body needs that normal cleansing out . .

When you have the urge to go to the toilet, you will go . . And your subconscious mind will take care of the part of causing you to have a bowl movement . . easily and naturally . .

The processes of your body will continue to function normally . . and regularly . . And that will cause your health to continue improving . . You will have more strength, more energy and more vitality . .

EMERGE

You will continue drifting into a deeper, DEEPER . . more peaceful, hypnotic state . . of relaxation . . as I give you suggestions and instructions . . that will cause you to experience continuous improvements . . in your life . . physically . . mentally . . and spiritually . .

As you submerge yourself, going deeper . . and DEEPER . . You can notice how you are becoming . . even more relaxed and settled . . Concentrate on that pleasant feeling of relaxation . . Your mind and body are relaxing, more and more . . All tension is leaving your body . . And all stresses and strains are moving out of your systems . . as though they are being drawn out of your body . . by a powerful magnetic energy . . You are learning to be relaxed and calm . . and will continue using these principles of relaxation . . during your daily life . . By learning to relax . . as you are doing now . . you will experience a happier, healthier, more enjoyable life . . And a more creative life . . than ever before . .

You will soon notice a feeling of energy and vitality . . flowing through your entire body . . Cleansing . . healing . . purifying and rejuvenating your body . . gradually and perfectly . .

The important thing for you to realize now is . . that you have a tremendous power within you . . that can renew old ideas, restore and rejuvenate old thoughts . . completely and perfectly . . And all of those revitalizing energies, that make this all possible . . are all directed . . by your own mind . .

You are continuing to have more confidence in your ability to concentrate . . The fact that you have been able to concentrate . . well enough to achieve a hypnotic state of relaxation . . indicates that you also have the ability to concentrate . . when you are reading, listening or studying . .

Concentration is imperative for creative thinking to occur . . You must know your subject well . . Analyze it . . Dissect it . . Probe it and test it . . Understand all of its best qualities . . and be aware of its hidden faults . . Ask yourself, "What improvements can I make . . that are more practical or desirable . . as well as, more . . cost effective" . . Before proceeding with any changes, you must, first, be thoroughly familiar with your subject, product or new concept . .

I am going to give you some suggestions and instructions now . . that will improve your ability to concentrate . . And improve your learning skills . . So much that your memory will keep improving more . . each day . .

From now on . . when you want to read or study . . or listen to a lecture or a speech . . you will get your materials ready . . such as, books or writing materials . . Then when you are ready to begin concentrating . . you will breath deeply and exhale slowly, three times . . And then, think of the numbers, 3, 2 and 1 . . As soon as you breath deeply and exhale slowly, three times . . And think the numbers, 3, 2, 1 . . you will become calm and relaxed . . the way you are now . .

Breathing deeply and exhaling slowly, three times and thinking the numbers 3, 2 and 1 . . will be a signal . . Your subconscious mind will respond to that signal . . and will cause you to become calm and relaxed . . just as you are now . . And your awareness will narrow down . . to absorb the reading . . studying or listening you want to do . . You will be less sensitive to surrounding noises or distractions . . while you are studying . . Your total involvement will be devoted . . to what you are concentrating on . . As you read, study or listen . . in that state of calmness and relaxation . . your close attention will increase to perfection . . and will remain that way for, at least, one hour . .

Your concentration will be perfect for at least one hour . . each time you use the signal . . of breathing deeply and exhaling slowly, three times . . while thinking of the numbers 3 , 2 and 1 . .

Your subconscious mind has capabilities . . far beyond what you have been aware of . . And your mind is remembering everything it needs to remember . . to cause the creative energies to function properly . . To instill thoughts or ideas . . or innovative insights . . into your conscious thinking . .

All limitations are being lifted . . And you are being revitalized with increased energy and inner strength . . Your body, mind and soul are continuing to function . . in a more harmonious way . .

Self-realizations and understandings are opening up within you . . A feeling of peace is moving through every part of your being . . Instilling greater awareness of the powers of God within you . .

You are realizing that you have the ability . . to remember and to recall . . everything you ever learn . . Your mind is comparable to a computer . . It records everything you see, hear and experience . . You are capable of recalling everything you learn . . And ever improving on concepts or ideas . . Some of the material you learn may not seem to be immediately important enough . . to remain in the conscious level of your mind . . So it goes into the storehouse of your mind . . But the information is always there . . And it is available when you need to recall it . . All you need to do is to let the subconscious level of your mind know . . you need to recall something . . And it will permit the information to come into the conscious level of your mind . . whenever you need it . .

Now you understand what real concentration is . . and that will cause your attentiveness to continue improving . . Your ability to recall . . will improve more each day . . Memories will stay in your conscious mind much longer . . And your ability to bring information out . . from the storehouse of your mind, more quickly . . will also improve dramatically . . You will become a memory giant . . And your future career . . will depend on it . .

You will also find your self-confidence and self-acceptance . . growing stronger . . And you will continue improving in all areas of your life . . physically, mentally, emotionally and spiritually . .

You will have the knowledge to solve every problem that comes up in your life . . You will look forward to each day of your life with anticipation . . And you'll find that each day will bring you greater happiness and joy . . You will arise each morning, feeling rested and refreshed . . And you'll continue having more energy, more strength . . and more vitality . . (pause)

The suggestions and instructions I have given you . . are now in the storehouse of your mind . . And they are already working to keep improving . . your way of life . . They are intended to influence your thoughts, feelings and actions . . in a positive, helpful way . . You will notice some very positive improvements . . And you will be very pleased . . with your continuous progress . .

I am going to give you a period of silence now . . as all of these suggestions seal themselves . . into the deepest part of your subconscious mind . . And they will reinforce themselves, over and over again in your mind . .

Your subconscious mind is absorbing everything I am saying . . And so, as you continue to relax deeper . . this period of silence will begin now . . (2 to 3 minutes of silence.)

In a moment, you will be, once again, in a normal state of mind . . Now, I am going to count from ONE to FIVE . . and when you hear the number, FIVE . . you will open your eyes and be wide awake . . feeling refreshed and wonderful . . For you are . . a wonderful person . .

ONE - Coming up now . . Feeling rested and refreshed . . You will remember everything with clear understanding . .
TWO - Coming up a little higher now . . You are connected to your inner strength . . Supporting your best interest . .
THREE - Everything I have told you is true . . And is happening now . . You will benefit greatly from this experience . .
FOUR - Becoming more aware of your body . . Move your hands and feet . . Let them stir a little . .
FIVE - You may open your eyes now . . Inhale and stretch a bit . . Tell me, "How do you feel ?"

As you continue to relax more peacefully and calmly . . the suggestions and instructions I give you . . are being completely understood by your subconscious mind . . And your mind will cause them to begin working immediately . . And they will keep becoming more effective each day . .

Your conscious awareness is narrowing down . . There may be times when I am talking . . but you may not be conscious of my voice . . And that is okay because your subconscious mind hears everything I say . . and will cause you to put everything into your own actions . .

Your subconscious mind learns rapidly . . and knows that you are an intelligent person . . You have great knowledge and ability . . that has developed . . as a result of your years of experience and education . .

From the very beginning of time . . when you first came into existence . . you have been absorbing countless impressions . . Learning many facts . . Storing ideas and all kinds of information . . in your mind . . So, you actually have great amounts and varieties of knowledge and wisdom . . Far beyond what your conscious mind has been aware of . .

You feel, growing within you, a realization . . that you have the ability to face any situation . . that ever arises in your life . . But, at the same time, you are feeling a hesitation . . of making important decisions . . Decisions that impact, not only your life but . . the lives of those around you . .

A friend of mine went through a similar experience recently . . that increased his wisdom on a number of levels . . He had wanted to get a new job . . One that paid more than his present job and would increase his prestige . . He applied for that job but found that it would require him to move to a distant city . . He really wanted that job . . but felt uncertain about whether he was willing to move to get the job . . So, he asked the company for a week to think the offer over . . They felt that was only fair . . so they extended the offer for another week . .

That whole week, his mind went back and forth . . trying to consider it from every angle . .

When they called him, after the week was up . . he asked if he could have three more days to make his decision . . They called him, three days later . . and he asked for "just one more day" . . They politely gave him one more day, to decide . . When they called him early the next day, he said he would call them later that afternoon . . And that was when they told him they had already given the job to someone else . . Someone more decisive and enthusiastic about the opportunity . . He was quite upset because he really wanted the job . . But he had been afraid of making the wrong decision . .

Rather than accept the job, a much better job, even though it had its down side . . he was unable to make any decision, until it was too late . . There are times in life when you simply must make decisions . . and profess confidence in those decisions, when you do . .

Many people miss out on wonderful opportunities . . Not because of a lack of skills . . but simply due to a fear . . of making decisions . .

When decisions are to be made . . instead of becoming overwhelmed with thoughts of negative things that could possibly result . . consider what will be gained by making a positive decision . .

You can make decisions . . with confidence . . You make each decision based on your present knowledge . . And once you make a decision . . you are confident, realizing that, if you attain new knowledge, you'll have the ability to make new decisions . . So, you have the confidence in yourself . . and confidence in the decisions you make . . because you know they are right . .

Your self-confidence is increasing daily . . And you have complete confidence in your own good judgment . . your own opinions and your own points of view . . You will continue to be more successful in everything you do . . You will remember that life is not a cup . . to be drained . . but is . . instead, a cup to be filled . . You will be successful in filling the cup of your life . . with joy, happiness and prosperity . .

When I was learning to drive a car . . a friend told me to put the car in reverse and back it up . . But he said it this way . . "Go ahead . . Back up" . . The moment he made that statement, I saw the humor in it and began to laugh . . He asked me why I was laughing and I said, "I can't go ahead while the car is in reverse" . .

And that is a fact about decision making . . To move forward . . we must have our mind geared to move forward . . You have the opportunity to choose what you want to experience in life . . But it is your responsibility to make the decisions . . You have the wisdom . . the ability and the opportunity to make decisions wisely . . knowing that the immutable Laws of the Universe are in your favor . .

You are intelligent . . You are capable . . You are effective . . You are self-confident . . You are self-reliant . . You are self-assured . . And you have the ability to completely relax . . You have the ability to be comfortable and CONFIDENT in any situation . . And you're going to allow all of this to happen . . Easily happen . . during this moment of silence, which begins . . now . . (Pause one minute)

Regardless of what comes up in your life . . you will be in control of your emotions and feelings . . That is what will cause success to be yours . . more and more . . And soon you will have all that you want in your life . .

Now, I am going to count from 1 to 5 . . and on the count of 5 . . you will open your eyes . . to an alert, waking state . . feeling clear of mind, relaxed and wonderful . . For you are a decisive and confident person . . I will begin my count now . .

One.   You will remember everything you have experienced today with complete understanding . .
Two.   You are now connected with your spiritual, inner supporting strength . .
Three. Everything I have told you is true . . and is already happening . .

Four.   Beginning to be more aware of your body as it fully awakens and wants to stir . .
Five.   Let your hands and feet move now . .   Stir and stretch as you open your eyes, feeling clear, rested and wonderful.

DEEPENING THE HYPNOTIC STATE
(Client is in a difficult light trance)

In just a moment, I will count from ten down to one . . You will feel as though you are in the middle of a dream . . You are in a department store . . riding down an escalator . . As I say each number . . you will keep descending downward . . into a deeper . . more peaceful . . hypnotic state . .

Things in the department store will keep becoming hazier . . and the dream will soon fade away . . as you drift further . . into a deep peaceful . . hypnotic state . .

I will begin counting now . .

TEN. You are getting on the escalator now . . It is slowly moving downward . . You can see everything in the store and all of the people around you . .

NINE. As you drift slowly downward . . you feel yourself becoming drowsier . . sleepier . . But you also feel peaceful and calm . . completely at ease . . and letting go . .

EIGHT. You are experiencing a wonderful feeling all through your body . . as you keep going down . . DOWN . . You are experiencing a more peaceful, more detached feeling . .

SEVEN. You are becoming sleepier . . drowsier . . Drifting into a DEEPER, sleepier state . . Completely effortless . . and natural . .

SIX. You are beginning to feel as though you are floating . . Easily and gently . . Experiencing perfect peace of mind . . Peaceful and calm . . Comfort all through your body . .

FIVE. All other sounds and noises are fading away . . Everything around you is fading away now . . You are continuing to move into a deeper hypnotic state . . Your awareness is narrowing down and you listen only to my voice . . totally at ease . . totally comfortable . .

FOUR. The people are fading away . . becoming less and less noticeable . . as the escalator continues to go DOWN . . You are letting go completely . . Each time you exhale, you go into a DEEPER and DEEPER Hypnotic state . .

THREE. Your conscious mind is relaxing completely . . You are experiencing perfect peace of mind . . Feeling calm . . Feeling relaxed . . drowsy and comfortable . . Completely effortless . . Comfortable . .

TWO. You are very near the basement of relaxation . . You are becoming less and less aware of things around you . . You feel very drowsy . . very relaxed . . You feel like you don't want to move or talk unless I tell you to . . You are really enjoying this wonderful experience of relaxation . . in a DEEP . . DEEP . . hypnotic trance . .

ONE. You are in a DEEP . . very comfortable state now . . Your subconscious mind is very sensitive to the words I am saying to you . . Your mind is absorbing every suggestion and instruction I am giving you . . as every fiber of your body continues to relax more and more . .

Now, you are where you want to be . . Now, we are ready to begin . .

(Proceed with Prescription.)

(Follow Relaxation)

You are rested and relaxed . . Your mind is open to receive what I am about to share with you . .

There is an Oriental fable about some ancient Gods . . who were trying to decide where they should hide . . what they considered to be . . the greatest power in the universe . . So that man would not be able to find it and . . use it destructively . .

One of the Gods said, "Let's hide it on top of the highest mountain." They discussed that idea and decided it would not do . . because man would eventually climb the highest mountain . . and find that great power . .

A second God came up with the idea of . . hiding the greatest power at the bottom of the ocean . .

After another discussion between the Gods . . it was decided that man would . . someday . . find a way to investigate the bottom of the oceans, as well . .

Finally, a third God said, "I know what to do . . Why don't we hide, the greatest power in the universe, within the mind of man . . He will never think to look for it there" . .

And so, according to that old fable . . they hid the greatest power in the universe . . in the mind of man . .

Even though it was just a fable . . scientific research reveals . . that the mind of man is truly . . one of the greatest powers in the universe . .

Another very wise teacher, named Jesus, once said, "The Kingdom of God is within you" . . In making that statement, He was telling us that we have, within each of us, a tremendous source of energy, power and strength . . To accomplish anything we wish to achieve . .

That is made even more clear through other similar words from the Bible . . "As we think with our minds, so we are" . .

Those words are informing us that . . our own power of thought . . can bring us anything we want or need . . as we put our thoughts into actions . .

Most of the situations that come up in our life . . are created as the result of thoughts or ideas from our own mind . .

That means, if your life has been unpleasant . . there is something you can do about it . . You have a wonderful, almost magical, transforming power within you . . which can free you from your inner fears . . and can liberate you completely . . from the limitations of failure, misery and frustration . .

That's one of the meanings of the words in the Bible, that says, "You can be transformed by the renewing of your mind" . .

As your mind is renewed, by having good thoughts . . it brings harmony and peace into your life . . And the creativity of your mind responds accordingly . .

By now, you are realizing that . . feelings of depression . . are caused by thoughts, ideas, beliefs, opinions, theories or . . unpleasant experiences . . that have made an impression in your mind . .

But that can be changed by reprogramming your mind . . in a positive, helpful way . . as we are doing now . .

Think about this . . Your subconscious mind accepts . . whatever your conscious mind focuses on . . An example of that is the way you are directing your attention . . to the words I am saying to you now . . Positive words . . Bringing you positive thoughts . .

Everything I am saying is going directly into the storehouse of your subconscious mind . . And your subconscious mind is responding . . by causing you to put my words into your own actions . .

And you will notice the rapid improvement . . in all areas of your life . . physically, mentally, emotionally and spiritually . .

You are now releasing all tensions and anxieties from your body . . All stresses in your life are gradually slipping away . . as you continue relaxing and feeling more at ease . .

From this moment on . . any time circumstances or conditions in your home . . in your work . . or in any social situation of your life . . becomes unpleasant or too pressing . . you will take the time to go to a quiet place where you can privately relax . .

I am going to give you some instructions now . . Instructions that will enable you to relax yourself easily . . And the more closely you follow my instructions . . the more calm and relaxed you will be, during your daily life activities . .

By following my instructions . . it will be easy for you to completely relax yourself . . All you need to do is to sit down or find a place to lie down . . in a comfortable position . . Close your eyes and breath deeply . . Then, exhale slowly . . five times . . Breathing deeply and exhaling slowly . . will bring more oxygen into your body . . Inhaling oxygen into your body, restores your energy . .

And each time you exhale . . your muscles, nerves, ligaments and tendons will keep relaxing more completely . .

After breathing deeply and exhaling slowly, five times . . begin counting backward in your mind . . starting at one hundred . . Each time you think a number in your mind . . your whole body will continue to feel more calm . . and more relaxed . . You will continue to feel a more peaceful . . soothing calmness . . throughout your entire body . .

During these moments when you are relaxing . . all of the suggestions and instructions I have given you . . will become more deeply reinforced in your mind . . And they will cause you to feel more peaceful . . more calm and more . . at ease . . with yourself and . . with your private world . .

You are continuing to relax even more now . . Feel the peace and love of God, flowing through every part of your being . . You are relaxing and letting go completely now . .

Notice the muscles around your eyes, relaxing even more now . . All of the muscles around your eyes are relaxing completely . . And that relaxation is spreading, over your face . . into your forehead . . your scalp . . and down the back of your head . . and into your neck muscles . .

You are feeling more calm and peaceful . . as the relaxation moves into your shoulders . . Into your arms and down into your hands . . You are feeling a slow, soothing drowsiness . . coming over your whole body now . . Just let the feeling continue . . as you relax . .

That soothing, peaceful relaxation is moving into your spine and back muscles now . . And now, it is coming around into your chest . . You are feeling more peaceful and your thoughts are becoming more harmonious and pleasant . .

Your stomach is relaxing . . And you can feel that easy relaxation moving into your abdomen . . You are experiencing a sense of joy and contentment . . And a feeling of happiness comes over you, as you realize . . how easily you can be relaxed . . and made to feel so completely calm . .

Your hips are relaxing now . . And the calmness is moving gently into your thighs and further down into your legs . . and on . . into your feet and toes . . And now you know that you can completely relax your entire body . . And you can use these same principles of relaxation . . on yourself . . during your daily life . .

Relaxation enables you to think more clearly . . It makes it easier for you to concentrate . . And from now on . . any time it seems that people around you are . . being difficult to get along with. . . you will remain calm and relaxed . . And you will be able to handle the situation in a calm, peaceful and loving way . . If your plans don't go the way you expect them to . . you will remain peaceful and serene . . Even during those times when everything . . seems to be in total confusion . . You remain calm and relaxed . . You will be able to think clearly . . and handle every situation with poise, confidence and dignity . . Regardless of where you are or what you are doing . . you will find that, more and more, day by day . . you will remain calm and relaxed . . And you will be able to cope . . with all of your everyday, changing circumstances . .

You are realizing that it is a waste of time . . to worry about things that happen . . Instead of worrying . . you will use your ability to think . . And you will work out a peaceful solution . . to any problem that comes up in your life . .

You are understanding that you are a spiritual being, created by God . . And, as a spiritual being . . you are blessed with intelligence and wisdom that can release you from anxiety and confusion . .

You will trust the love and goodness of God to help solve every problem in your life . . You feel the love and goodness of God, setting you free, from all mistakes of the past . . The love of God is releasing you from guilt and is cleansing your mind, your body and your soul . . You are blessed . .

What you are feeling now is a pure stream of God's love . . flowing through you . . Cleansing, healing, purifying and restoring your mind and body . . A divine order is being established in all of your activities and concerns . .

You are feeling a good response in your body . . as you are being strengthened and renewed with energy, vitality and enthusiasm . . It is because you are needed . . You are important to many . . And you are fulfilling God's plan and purpose . . in your own . . very special way . .

Every day your self-confidence keeps increasing . . And you continue living your life with a greater feeling of poise, peacefulness and joy . . You are open and receptive to all of the good that flows into your life . . You are becoming more perfectly attuned . . to the beauty . . and to the harmony . . of the universe . . You are filled with a sense of well-being and joy . . And I am so proud to know you as . . my friend . .

EMERGE

You are rested and relaxed . . Your mind is open to receive what I
am about to share with you . . Now, as you continue to relax . . I
want you to be aware of the harmful thing you have been doing to
yourself . . I want you to realize that you have attached an
undesirable label on yourself . . You stuck it on yourself just like
you would stick a label onto a bottle . . And the label you have
placed on yourself is named . . Depressed . . You've been calling
yourself, 'depressed' . . You have been allowing yourself to be
depressed . . And you realize that every time you have repeated the
word, depressed, to yourself . . you increase the belief that you truly
are depressed . . Sometimes we forget that people tend to believe the
things that they say about themselves . . In other words, you are
basically what you believe yourself to be . . And when you tell
yourself that you are a certain thing . . or you act in a certain way . .
that is what you must believe . . It is simply, human nature . .

Now, that's a very simple concept . . I want you to see it . . It's a
real simple concept . . For you understand that an American acts like
an American . . because he believes himself to be an American . .
And if you thought of yourself as belonging to any other nationality,
then you would act like that . . Because we are all what we believe
ourselves to be . . Those of us who are doctors . . will act like
doctors . . Just as lawyers act like lawyers . . And those who believe
themselves to be depressed . . will act as though they are depressed . .

Every once in a while we have people, just like yourself, who place
labels on themselves . .

Somewhere in your past, you have labeled yourself . . depressed . .
for whatever reason . . But now, you are going to tear off that label
of depression . . and you're going to replace it . . That's right . .
Now, you're going to label yourself . . Happy . . And you know
what ? We tend to live up to the labels that we place on ourselves
. . For you realize that all of your actions . . stem from the image
you have of yourself . . in your subconscious mind . . And those
images come from the many labels . . that you have in place right now . .

Now, I want you to begin thinking about . . what you want to
replace those old labels with . . Right now, you are holding a good
image of yourself . . See yourself, standing proud . . See yourself

with a new confidence in yourself . . See yourself, really happy, for a change . . It feels good, doesn't it? . . You want to label yourself, full of happiness . . You want to label yourself, truly joyful . . You're going to experience a new thrill of excitement . . with all of your new labels . . because you know that you will no longer allow depression to overcome you . . You know that you are no longer going to let sadness fill your heart . . These are going to be the times when you do have the joy of good fellowship . . Not only with yourself but with people around you . . whom you love . . and who love you . . You are about to enter the time of your enlightenment . .

But first, I want you to be very aware of the harmful thing . . that you've done to yourself in the past . . For you see, in the past . . you have accepted the label of depression . . In fact, you even said to yourself . . "I just can't overcome my sadness" . . You've said to yourself, "I feel completely inadequate . . in trying to remain happy and joyful . . And I have difficulty in looking on the bright side of anything" . . Now, I am telling you, this is serious . . because it doesn't take very long for you to believe it . . once you start those thoughts in motion . . And, you know . . once you've given yourself the suggestion . . that you can't get out of your depression . . Once you've given yourself the suggestion that you have to feel sad and empty . . Once you start thinking that your confidence is slipping . . Once you begin to think your ability to resist becoming depressed is slipping . . It's just a step away from thinking, "I wonder if I'm really worthy of being successful at anything?" . . Yes, only a step away from thinking, "I'm just not worthy enough to have anything good happen to me" . . Now, do you understand how subtle that is ? How harmful it is to you ? . .

Now, you are going to hold tightly to your new labels . . You're going to hold onto that label called, happiness . . And the label called, joy . . And the label of brightness . . and success . . and reality . . The truth of the matter is . . most people who fail, are failures because they have labeled themselves as failures . . They have convinced themselves that they are failures . . And, you know what else . . They are merely acting out the part of the label that they, themselves, have placed on themselves . . Do you understand this ? . . They are acting out the label of 'failure' . . They are acting out the label called, 'depressed' . . These are not their conditions . .

These are merely the labels they have placed upon themselves . . As though, for all time, this is how they have to be . .

So, right now, you are going to accept the suggestion that you will develop the habit of being happy . . You will let yourself look for the silver lining, so to speak . . You are going to look for the good in everything . . that happens in your life . . from now on . .

You are going to begin by ripping off that label of depression . . that you have placed on yourself . . You are going to rip off that label of sadness . . that you have placed on yourself in the past . . So, in your mind's eye, right now, as you hear the words of my voice . . I want you to let that label be seen, in your mind's eye . . I want you to visualize yourself, with the label, Depression . . I want you to imagine yourself with that label, Depression, on you, right now . . Visualize it ! And now, I want you to reach up, in your mind's eye, and TEAR that label off ! Completely . . Tear it off ! Right now !

You don't need it any more . . In fact, you never did need that label of 'Depression' . . And if you ever thought that you did need that label . . you now realize that the need for that label, Depression, has long outlived its usefulness . . You realize that it hasn't helped you at all, in the past . . In fact, it's only been holding you back . . You're the one being punished! . . by keeping yourself in depression . . You're the one that is being punished by keeping yourself in sadness . . And you realize that your depression is what causes you to perform inadequately . . So, now, you refuse to identify, any longer, in any way, with depression, or with sadness . . And even if you feel completely empty of the ability to be happy . . I want you to label yourself FULL of that ability, right now ! And begin filling yourself with determination to be happy . . Fill yourself with the will and determination to succeed . . And you are going to succeed . . Every day, in every way . .

You'll allow yourself to become more disciplined . . You are what you believe yourself to be . . And whatever you think, in secret, will come to pass . . And since the picture you hold of yourself, dominates your behavior . . you must have confidence in your ability to get along . . without the depression or the sadness . . And you know that you can . .

242

And now, you are going to set a goal for yourself . . The goal you are setting for yourself . . right now . . is to be happy, in every situation, within yourself . . And . . Hear me now . . If you don't pursue that goal . . to be happy . . you realize that you will soon fall prey to negative thoughts . . and negative actions . . The perfect set up for feeling unworthy . . for fear of failure . . And for self-pity . . You see how self destructive this becomes . . But you can be up on top of all this . . By setting that goal . . to be happy . . and never losing sight of that goal . . You can be that happy person . . that you have always wanted yourself to become . .

Now, listen carefully . . Your determination to be happy . . is the promise you have given yourself . . Allow yourself to accept that promise . . as absolute truth, to yourself . . Understand that these are not merely some nice sounding words that I am speaking to you . . This is not just a dream . . or a means of escape, or to merely pass the time . . It is a FACT ! . . Believe it ! Say it over to yourself . . Say it to yourself, right now . . "My determination to be happy within myself, can never be changed" Say it to yourself again . . "My determination to be happy within myself, can never, never be changed" . . I want you to set your goals . . and to Sense your goals . . so you can allow yourself to become . . what you really want yourself to be . .

Now, I am going to give you a moment of silence . . And during this moment of silence . . I want you to contemplate all of the labels . . which you have placed on yourself . . The ones that really should not be there . . You know what they are . . During this moment of silence, you are going to see all of those labels on your body and you are going to rip them right off, without question . . And you are going to replace those old labels with all new labels . . Good, positive labels that you will place on yourself . . Labels of confidence . . Labels of self-assurance . . Labels of self-reliance and labels of love . . Labels of kindness and generosity . . And labels of skillful and artistic ability . .

You're going to let all those harmful labels be gone . . All of the harmful identifications are now gone from your life . . You're going to put good labels all over yourself . . because you are intelligent . . You are capable . . You are effective . . You are self-confident . . You are self-reliant . . You are self-assured . . You have the ability to completely relax . . You have the ability to be comfortable in any

243

situation . . And you're going to allow all of this to happen . . Easily happen, as you tear off those negative labels and replace them all, with positive labels . . during this moment of silence, which begins . . now . .   (Pause one minute)

In a moment, you will awaken feeling good, feeling refreshed and feeling alive . . Now, I am going to count from ONE to FIVE . . and when you hear the number, FIVE . . you will open your eyes and be wide awake . . feeling refreshed and wonderful . . For you are a wonderful person . .

ONE   -   Coming up now . . Feeling rested and refreshed . . You will remember everything with clear understanding . .

TWO - Coming up a little higher now . . You are connected to your inner strength . . Supporting your best interest . .

THREE - Everything I have told you is true . . And is happening now . . You will benefit greatly from this experience . .

FOUR - Becoming more aware of your body . . Move your hands and feet . . Let them stir a little . .

FIVE - You may open your eyes now. Inhale and stretch a bit . .
Tell me, "How do you feel ?"

057 Prescript.   DISC - SPINE PROBLEM
(Follow Relaxation-Deep)
Ref. : Back Ache

You are rested and relaxed . . Your mind is open to receive the suggestions and instructions I am about to give you . .

The doctor has indicated that you have been experiencing Disc Disease of the Cervical Spine . .

This is the doctor's term for the problem you have been experiencing . . with the disc of the cervical spine . . However, your subconscious mind is aware of the fact that your body . . possesses every chemical, every mineral . . and all the healing energies needed . . to rejuvenate and restore those discs perfectly . .

Your subconscious mind controls and directs . . every part of your body . . including your muscles, nerves, ligaments, bones . . and all of the organs and glands . . as well as every atom, every molecule and every cell, of your body . . From the top of your head to the bottom of your feet . .

And your subconscious mind knows . . how to cause the processes of your body . . to function properly . . and repair and rejuvenate discs that have been damaged . . Just as easily as your body processes . . repair your skin, when it has been cut . . or bones that have been broken . . Every part of your body is capable of repairing itself . . including your spinal discs . .

Scientists have discovered that your entire body is in a constant process of . . producing new cells to replace those . . that have been damaged or . . have completed their purpose . . Those new cells are strong and perfect . . They are pure energy . . And the truth is, your spinal discs are made up of cells . . that can be replaced with these new . . and perfect cells . .

Your subconscious mind is understanding everything I am telling you . . and is causing you to continue experiencing changes . . that are restoring those discs . . And getting rid of all pain and discomfort . .

Permitting yourself to be hypnotized . . lets your subconscious mind know . . that you are determined . . to achieve the complete and perfect healing . . of those discs . . That problem has controlled your way of life, long enough . . and you are determined that it will not control your way of life . . any longer . .

The Bible says, "You can be transformed by the renewing of your mind" . . And that is what you are doing now . . You are being released from those improper imprints and impressions that have gone into your mind . . that have been causing the problem . . And those improper imprints and impressions are being replaced . . with the true knowledge . . that those discs are already in the process of healing . . and being restored, perfectly . .

It is normal for every part of your body to be healthy . . It is normal for your discs to be whole . . and provide proper cushioning between the bones . . so you can move your head, your neck . . your arms and shoulders . . and all other parts of your body . . freely and comfortably . .

It is normal for your spine to be in perfect alignment . . And for the muscles in your neck and back to be strong . . And keep your neck and your cervical spine . . in perfect alignment . . And you will be pleased to find that your subconscious mind . . is causing the healing energies of your body . . to function properly . . and heal those discs perfectly . . and rapidly . .

In the past, you may have had some doubts . . But now, those doubts are leaving . . And they are being replaced with a strong sense of confidence . . And a sense of sureness . . That the healing processes of your body . . are functioning properly . .

It may be two weeks . . or even three weeks . . before those discs are healed completely . . But you will be pleased to find that your subconscious mind knows . . what needs to be done . . And is causing the proper adjustments to occur . . as rapidly as your body is ready for it . .

Your subconscious mind knows how fast it can work . . in correcting that improper information . . that has been causing the problem . . And you will begin noticing changes taking place . . in the perfect healing of those discs . .

As you continue moving into a deeper . . DEEPER and more comfortable hypnotic state . . you may notice a pleasant . . healing warmth . . flowing through that area of your spine . . Letting you know that you are already going through a corrective . . healing experience . . Feel the healing warmth . . permeating your spinal column . . Relax . . and just let it continue . . (pause)

246

At this very moment . . your systems are making comfortable adjustments . . Your systems are synthesizing new proteins, nutrients . . and other chemicals and substances needed in your body . . And rejuvenation is taking place . .

You may not consciously understand . . the processes your subconscious mind is using . . to produce the proper healing of those discs . . But that's okay . . You can be pleasantly surprised . . and very happy . . as you become aware of the progress you are making . .

Your expectations are increasing . . and you will be sensing the pleasant changes taking place . . within you . . Relax . . and feel the warmth of healing energies flowing through your spinal column . . From the top of your neck . . right on through to your lower body . .
(pause)

You are pleased and proud of what you are accomplishing . . And the feeling of knowing . . it is being done . . carries with it . . a strong sense of satisfaction and contentment . .

Continue relaxing, just as you are . . for a little longer . . Giving your subconscious mind the time to absorb everything we have talked about today . . Adjustments are being made . . as you relax . .
(pause)

When your subconscious mind knows the changes have started . . and all of the healing processes of your body . . are functioning properly . . and will continue working properly . . you will then, awaken yourself from your hypnotic state . . After you awaken from the hypnotic state . . your subconscious mind will cause your eyes to open . . and you will be back in a wide-awake, fully alert, state . . Feeling good . . feeling confident and feeling happy . . with the beneficial processes that are taking place . .

(Allow client to awaken self.)

(Follow Relaxation)

As you continue to relax . . more deeply and peacefully . . the suggestions and instructions I give you are being completely understood . . by your subconscious mind . . And your mind will cause them to become more and more effective each day . . Your subconscious mind can understand things . . that you do not, consciously, understand . . And your subconscious mind can work out solutions to problems . . that you do not know the answers for . .

I do not know what caused you to start taking drugs in the beginning . . And it's not necessary for me to know . . Nor is it necessary for you to know . . what actually caused you to start . .

Whatever caused you to start taking _____ is past now . . And your subconscious mind is understanding that there is no reason that it needs to continue . . causing you difficulty . . Your subconscious mind can review all of the imprints, impressions, thoughts, ideas and memories in your mind . . that have caused you to continue taking _____, and can assess that information . . And cause you to realize that there is no reason you need to continue . . taking _____ . .

When your subconscious mind understands what caused you to start taking _____, and realizes, there is no reason you need to continue taking _____ . . your subconscious mind will cause one of the fingers on your right hand to lift up towards the ceiling . . And your finger will remain up until I tell it to go back down . .

While I am waiting for your subconscious mind to review . . what has been causing you to take _____ . . and understands the causes and affects . . And causes you to realize that you can now be free from ever again taking _____ . . I want to tell you a story that your subconscious mind will understand . . And it will give you the confidence and courage that you need . . to say no . . to _____ . . to say NO . . to _____, from now on . .

There was a little porcupine who lived out in the woods . . He was a strange looking animal with a small body that was covered, from head to feet, with long, fierce looking quills . . that stuck up all around his tiny little body . .

248

Whenever he was walking around in the forest, he noticed that other animals, much larger than he . . would stop when they saw him . . and give him plenty of room to go by . . No other animal would ever come near him . .

It caused the porcupine to feel very sad and lonely . . because he didn't know any other porcupines . . to associate with . . Yet, any time another animal got near him, he would get scared . . And his fear would cause his quills to stand straight out . . making him appear to be ten times larger . . than he actually was . . And the other animals would usually get out of his way . .

However, once in a while . . some foolish animal would get too close and the porcupine's quills would stick in him . . and he would run off, screaming and crying . . And poor Mr. Porcupine didn't understand any of it . . Because all he had done was stand still and quiver in his fright . .

The other animals accused him of attacking them . . And that puzzled Mister Porcupine . . because he was afraid of almost all of the other animals . . He was quite lonely and confused . . and very bored . . Because he couldn't think of anything to do by himself . . to keep his life interesting . .

One day, as Mr. Porcupine was walking through the forest . . being avoided by all the animals he came close to . . he met a large turtle . . And the turtle stopped . . and looked at him . . and said, "That is amazing! You can make yourself ten times larger than your actual size . . And all I can do is pull in my head and feet to make myself smaller."

Oh, yeah"?, cried Mr. Porcupine. "Let me see you make yourself smaller!" And so the turtle pulled in his head and his feet . . And he really was so much smaller than he first looked . . Much like the rocks and stones around him . . And Mr. Porcupine had to look very closely . . to see which one was the real turtle . .

"Oh, my," said the porcupine, "I wish I could pull in my head and feet and turn myself into a stone". . The turtle peeked out from under his shell and replied, "And I wish I could make myself ten times as big . . And have those fierce looking spears all over me, instead of having to pull myself into this thing . . It's dark and lonely in here . . And it really gets . . boring" . .

"Well, I'm bored too," answered the porcupine . . "Because making myself ten times bigger looking . . and sticking out my fierce looking quills . . causes all the other animals to avoid me" . .

The turtle laughed and said, "I can come near you . . I can even touch you." And he did touch Mr. Porcupine . . And Mr. Porcupine began to shake with fear . . because he was not used to being touched . . And Mr. Porcupine said, "You touched me and my quills didn't stick into you" . .

"That's right," said the turtle, "Because I have my shell to protect me . . You have your quills and I have my shell and they protect us because . . deep down inside, we are both . . really scared" . .

And Mr. Porcupine began to laugh because he had finally found a friend who understood exactly how he felt . . and was not afraid of his quills . . And he was not afraid of the turtle because . . the turtle was not afraid of him . . And so, they became good friends . .

One day, a big, ugly animal came into the forest . . He seemed very mean . . When he laughed, it sounded like a snarl . . And when he snarled, he sounded even worse . . He had ugly fur that was rough and patchy . . He had a long, mean looking nose and long, snagly teeth . . And bad breath . .

Well, now . . That mean, ugly looking creature came walking right up to where Mr. Porcupine was standing . . And Mr. Porcupine said, "Hello," in a quavering voice . . The creature sneered and laughed his ugly laugh . . The one that sounded like a snarl . . And the little porcupine timidly asked, "What's your name" ?

"What's it to ya?" responded the creature . . "Oh," said Mr. Porcupine, "My name is Porky and I just wondered what to call you" . .

"All right, nosy Porky. My name is Laughing . . Hyena, that is. Har Har Wooopp ? . .

"Okay," said Porky. "That's an interesting name" . .

"You're making fun of me, aren't you?" snarled the hyena . . Porky quickly replied, "Oh, no. I'm not making fun of you at all" . .

"Well, you'd better not be," laughed the hyena, "Because I could make mincemeat out of you in one bite. Har Har Wooopp ?" . .

And when he said that, Mr. Porcupine's quills stood straight up . . And the laughing hyena said, "Oh, so you want to fight, do ya? Well, I'll show you a fight" . .

And he jumped at little Porky . . But little Porky was so scared, he just stood there, shaking all over . . like tree leaves in the wind . .

Then, the mean tempered, Laughing Hyena . . got his long, mean snout and his tasseled ears, shot full of quills . . He put his tail between his legs . . and ran into the woods, howling . .

And as Mr. Turtle applauded him . . Mr. Porcupine realized that he had learned the difference between simply, making friends . . and . . protecting himself . .

And now, you are learning the difference between making friends . . and protecting yourself . . You are realizing that . . anyone who offers you _____ is not being a friend . . And you will have the confidence in yourself . . And will say, "NO" . . NO to _____ .
(pause)

One day, while riding as a passenger, in a car . . going through a large city, during the rush hour . . the driver got into a lane that I didn't usually use . . And I asked why she had chosen that lane . .

And she said, "This is the best lane . . I always take this one" . .

I noticed that cars kept passing us on both sides and that our lane was moving more slowly than the other lanes . . So I pointed to a blue truck next to us, one lane over, and said to the driver . . "See that blue truck? Just stay in the lane you're in now and try to beat it across the bridge" . .

The blue truck began to edge out in front of us . . but the driver was still defending the lane she had chosen . . The blue truck kept getting farther and farther ahead of us . . soon disappearing out of sight . . Finally, the driver had to admit she had chosen the wrong lane . .

By permitting yourself to be hypnotized . . to get rid of the habit of taking _____ . . you have shown that you realize that you . . had taken a wrong lane . . And now, you desire to make the adjustments . . and are getting your life straightened out . .

A lot of people, who take drugs, continue insisting that they are right . . even in the face of overwhelming evidence . . But you have now admitted that you were wrong . . And you have taken a big step in overcoming the habit . . that you had acquired . .

Each day, your self-confidence, self-acceptance and self-reliance keep getting stronger . . And you have the confidence and the courage you need . . to refuse . . to have anything more to do with _____, from now on . .

Your subconscious mind understands that you have been absorbing countless impressions . . learning many facts and adding ideas, symbols and all kinds of information . . into the storehouse of your mind . . ever since you first came into existence . . Some good. Some, not so good . . And your mind possesses great amounts and varieties of wisdom . . Far beyond what your conscious mind has been aware of knowing . .

All of that knowledge and wisdom is in the storehouse of your mind . . And is there to be used . . and is a part of your own personal development . . And you are now using that knowledge to enable you to continue advancing and progressing . . in all areas of your life . .

You are setting up goals for yourself, knowing that you have the ability to achieve your goals . .

You are rapidly developing stronger, good qualities and characteristics . . that give you the confidence and courage to remain free from ever taking _____ again . .

NOTE : IF THE CLIENT'S FINGER DOES NOT RAISE BY THE TIME YOU COMPLETE THE SESSION, GO TO "THERAPY BETWEEN SESSIONS" PRESCRIPTION. GIVE THOSE SUGGESTIONS TO CLIENT BEFORE AWAKENING FROM HYPNOTIC STATE. OTHERWISE, EMERG.

EAR NOISE

You will continue relaxing as I am talking with you . . Your subconscious mind is receiving everything I say . . And that will give you a better understanding of what you are achieving . .

We all learn things in different ways . . Sometimes we learn in unusual ways . . Ways that we may not even be aware of . .

I heard about a man who went to work in a steel mill, many years ago . . The first time he went into the mill, the furnaces were going full blast . . The overhead cranes were running . . And all departments were operating . . with hammers, pounding out steel and pounding in rivets . .

The noise was so loud that he couldn't hear anyone talk . . Yet, as he looked around, he could see various employees talking to each other . . and they seemed to understand what was being said . .

He thought they must have learned how to read lips because . . the foreman was standing right next to him . . and he couldn't understand a word the foreman was saying . . The foreman finally took him outside so he could hear the instructions he was being given . .

He told the foreman . . he didn't think he would be able to perform his work because . . on the job he was suppose to do, he would be working together with a partner . . about ten feet away, across the table . . And they would have to talk to each other to do their work properly . .

The foreman said, "Don't worry about that . . It will only take a day or two for your ears to adjust . . You'll soon be hearing clearly . . even when a person speaks in an ordinary tone of voice . .

He said it was difficult for him to believe that could be possible . . But the second day on the job . . he discovered the foreman was right . . And he could hear his partner talking from ten feet away . .

Somehow, his subconscious mind blocked out the noises of the hammers, the cranes, the blast furnaces . . and he could hear ordinary voices . .

All of us are capable of blocking out some sounds and . . attuning our hearing for those sounds we desire to hear . .

Mothers have reported being able to sleep soundly and peacefully near train tracks . . with trains going by . . Or near airports with jet airplanes flying over . . Yet, a child can get sick in another room in the middle of the night . . and they hear their child, easily and instantly . .

The subconscious level of the mind has learned to adjust . . our sensory perceptual functioning's . . in an adaptive manner . . So that we can hear what we want and need to hear . . and shut out sounds we do not want to hear . .

A person working in an onion factory . . where they made onion rings . . had become so sensitized to the smell . . that she hardly noticed it, after working there for only a few days . . Yet, other people going into the factory for the first time . . could hardly stand the odor . .

We get so used to certain sounds and smells that we become unaware of them . . We don't consciously realize the different adjustments . . our sensory organs . . are capable of making . .

NOTE : IF YOU HAVEN'T HAD CLIENT GET NUMBNESS IN HAND, DO SO NOW.

You probably didn't know you were capable of . . getting numbness in your hand . . until you did it . . Now you know that your mind controls your body . . and just as your mind made changes . . so that your hand became numb . . your mind can also cause pleasant changes . . that will get rid of the problem you are having . . with your hearing . .

A lot of people have come to me . . after being told by a doctor . . that nothing can be done to get rid of the Tinnitus . . or ringing . . in their ears . . Yet, after being hypnotized, and having their mind clear up the misconceptions . . many have discovered their doctors had been wrong . . And, you too, can tune out the ringing sounds from your ears . .

Continue relaxing now . . There is nothing you need to do . . You can enjoy the wonderful, comfortable feeling of relaxation . . And you don't need to try to do anything . . Just let it happen . .

As you think back, you realize . . there have been many times during the day . . when you were not hearing the ringing in your ears . . It's not easy to notice things that don't happen . . But there have been times when the ringing sound in your ears did stop . . And because there were no sounds there . . you did not notice it . . So, the important thing for you to do is to forget about the tinnitus . . and remember the times when there is no buzzing sound . . And that is a process you learn . .

It took only two days for the man in the steel mill . . to learn not to hear all of the loud noises . . and to hear ordinary conversations he had been unable to hear only a few days prior to that . . His foreman was right . . His ears adjusted rapidly . . And now, you are learning to rely upon your own body's ability . . to make adjustments . . You can really enjoy good feelings, good sounds and good quiet . . And you will find the quiet moments keep becoming more noticeable each day . .

Your subconscious mind will cause you to ignore the ringing sounds in your ears . . It will gradually keep fading away, more each day . . And will soon be gone completely . .

You realize that you have many abilities that are not known to your conscious mind . . In the storehouse of your mind is information . . about abilities that your have learned . . and suppressed . . over many years . . But any ability you have discarded . . your mind can examine, fully and completely . . And when you desire . . it can be restored . .

Your subconscious mind can restore the ability of your bodily processes . . to function properly . . And can easily restore your hearing loss, your ear problems . . and all tissues and nerves in your ears . . to their normal functioning . . The main part of this whole learning process is . . that you are learning to be happy . . You are learning to adjust to every situation that comes up in your life . . And you are learning to be calm and relaxed at all times, whether you are alone or with others . .

When your subconscious mind knows that changes have begun . . and your hearing loss will continue improving . . one of the fingers on your right hand will raise up . . And it will remain up until I tell it to go back down . . I don't know what is happening, but you can sense something good happening . . So, let it continue . .

It must be pleasing for you to realize . . that your own mind is resolving that problem, in a very pleasant way . . At this very moment, you are experiencing some changes taking place . . As soon as your subconscious mind knows, changes have started . . one of the fingers on your right hand will lift up . . and will remain up until I tell it to go back down . .

NOTE : CONTINUE WITH SUGGESTIONS GIVEN PREVIOUSLY UNTIL FINGER LIFTS. IF THERE ARE NO RESULTS BEFORE TIME TO AWAKEN, GO TO "THERAPY BETWEEN SESSIONS".

You are feeling peaceful and relaxed . . Continue with your relaxation . . while I give you some instructions . . that you will want to follow . .

If a small child becomes excited or hysterical . . we would do our best to calm him down and teach him . . that it is not a proper way to act . . We all need to understand that we should always . . maintain self-control . . But some people have not yet been trained . . and they are overcome by too much excitement . . Or, there may be times when our subconscious mind develops . . a misunderstanding . . So, when something goes wrong . . we lose control . . And sometimes, people even carry this 'lack of control' over . . into their sexual relations . . with their chosen partner . . And perhaps that's what has happened with you . .

We are going to do some experimenting . . I want you to listen to me carefully and follow these instructions . . I want you to hold your left arm straight out in front of you . . Clench your fist tightly and make your left arm rigid and stiff . . Make it as stiff as a board . . Notice how stiff and rigid you have made your left arm . . Okay, make it even stiffer now, Stiffer . . Make it just as stiff and rigid as you possibly can . . And notice, now, how strong and powerful your left arm feels . .

Now, let it relax . . And put it down in a position that feels comfortable to you . . Notice that your left hand and arm feel very comfortable now . .

And now, I want you to lift up your left hand and arm again . . Clench your fist and make your left arm even stiffer than you did before . . Make it so stiff that you feel it aching . . Notice how it keeps aching . . and aching . . more and more . . And as soon as it is aching so much that you dislike the feeling . . Open your fist now . . Now, relax your arm . . and put it down to a position that feels comfortable to you . . Just relax . .

I want to explain something to you . . Now that your subconscious mind is understanding . . You made your left arm rigid and stiff, two times . . The first time, I instructed you to make it just as rigid and stiff as you could possibly make it . . Did you do that ? . . Yes, you did . . And you did not feel any aching in your arm, the first time you made it stiff, did you ? . . (Wait for response)

256

Yet, the second time you made it stiff . . you felt it aching, didn't you ? . . So, why did it ache the second time you made it stiff ? . . (Possible response) It was because I put that suggestion into your subconscious mind . . which caused you to respond to my suggestion . .

Now, I am going to give you another suggestion . . I want you to hold your right arm . . your right arm . . out in front of you . . and make it very rigid and stiff . . Very stiff now . . Notice that it is becoming more NUMB as you keep making it stiffer and stiffer . . More and more numb . . It is becoming so numb . . that all feeling is leaving your right arm . . Tell me when all of the feeling is gone from your right arm . . all the way up through your shoulder . . (Wait for client to say the arm is numb) Good. Now, just hold that position . .

Now, I am going to say something to your subconscious mind . . Something that will make it impossible for you to have an orgasm, prematurely . . You will count these numbers to yourself . .

As you count, slowly, from five down to one . . the normal feeling will come back into your hand, arm and shoulder . . And, with each number you say . . your penis becomes less and less sensitive . . This will make it take much longer . . for you to have an orgasm . . This is something you do not need to remember, consciously . . or even understand, consciously . . Even though your subconscious mind is hearing and understanding it . . and causing it to happen automatically . .

From now on, whenever you make love and want to hold an erection . . count from 5 down to 1 . .

Your subconscious mind is making your penis rigid and stiff . . but less and less sensitive . . so that when you make love with your 'chosen partner' . . it will give your partner the time to have an orgasm . . And then . . you will be able to have an orgasm . .

You will find that you can maintain an erection for a very long time . . as you have intercourse with your chosen partner . . And your partner will have an orgasm . . before you will be able to have your orgasm . . You are remembering clearly, your erection, and how it feels to have an orgasm . . However, your subconscious mind is permitting it to happen . . only after . . your chosen partner . . has had an orgasm . .

Now, your subconscious mind knows what you need to do . . and knows how to cause you to do it right . . So, I want to give you the opportunity . . to carefully review and rehearse, in your mind, every movement . . And experience every sound . . Move with this experience by seeing yourself clearly in your mind . . having intercourse with your chosen partner . . Your subconscious mind is going over it with you now . . You are reviewing it and practicing it . . from the first caress to the orgasm of your chosen partner . . And right up to the final climax of your own orgasm . . All the way through . . So that you know exactly what you will do . . And know that you can do it . . And know that from now on . . you will know how you will do it . . And when the mental intercourse is completed in your mind . . one of the fingers on your right hand will lift up towards the ceiling . . to let me know . .

(Go to one of the prescriptions for building self-confidence)

You are feeling peaceful and relaxed . . Continue with your relaxation . . while I talk about your reason for being here . . You want your eyesight to improve . . That is the reason for permitting yourself to be hypnotized . . And you will find that hypnosis will improve your eyesight . .

The hypnotic state of relaxation is the best condition you can be in . . To enable your subconscious mind to receive suggestions . . and instructions . . that will cause the processes of your body to function properly . . And strengthen the cells and muscles in your eyes . . Causing your vision to become more clear . . Soon, you will be seeing perfectly . .

Continue going into a deeper . . DEEPER, more relaxed state . . Continue to relax . . as you go DEEPER . . Deeper now . . into a restful, pleasant and relaxing state . . You will find this to be the most relaxing, enjoyable and pleasant experience of your life . .

You are aware that the purpose of your eyes is for seeing what is in front of you . . and you want to see those objects, clearly and perfectly . . Your subconscious mind understands that . . and knows exactly what needs to be done to rejuvenate and strengthen your eyes . . But your subconscious mind is not aware of your need to improve your vision . . until it is directed to be made aware of your failing vision . . You see, as you grow older . . the shape of your eyeballs change . . Perhaps, because you look at objects a certain way . . Or because of dryness of you eyes . . Whatever the reason, aging changes the shape of the eyes . . Consequently, light enters at a different angle . . causing you to strain to see things that you used to see easily . .

What we are doing now is making your subconscious mind aware . . that these changes have taken place . . and, we are asking for readjustments to be made . . to reshape your eyes . . Back to the shape they were in when you were younger . . and you could see perfectly . .

The more you use any ability, the more automatic it becomes . . and the more you will continue to improve, in the use of that ability . . That is just as true with using your eyes as it is with any other ability . . But the dis-shaping of your eyeballs may have occurred when you became lazy . . in looking at objects . .

Remember when it was easier looking at things in a 'fuzzy' manner ? . . Perhaps you were tired or overworked . . Eventually, that 'fuzzy' way of looking at things . . became a habit . . And that habit slowly caused your eyeballs to reshape themselves . . Which brings us to where we are today . . restoring the shape of your eyeballs . . to regain the perfect vision you once enjoyed . . And now, your subconscious mind is aware . . of what you want to accomplish . . to regain the youthful shape of your eyes . . and to restore your vision . .

Scientists tell us, the entire body . . is in a constant process of producing new cells . . to replace the ones that have completed their purpose . . Those new cells are strong and perfect . . They are pure energy . . And, of course, your eyes are made up entirely of those new and perfect cells . .

In the past, as your eyes developed those new and perfect cells . . you had already developed the habit of not seeing things clearly . . And when the new cells developed in your eyes . . you held onto the old habit . . of not focusing . . Not seeing as perfectly as you should have . . As a result of holding onto the habit of not seeing clearly . . your eyeballs became misshapen . . Lazy, we call it . . Your vision became blurrier as objects became more and more . . out of focus . . Your subconscious mind has caused your eyes to continue functioning . . the same way they did . . before the new cells were developed . . Your subconscious mind is understanding that now . . and is realizing that there is a reason for your difficulty, in seeing clearly . . And that reason is . . the 'lazy' shape of your eyeballs . .

Like any muscle in your body . . your eyeballs, tendons and ligaments need daily exercise . . Right now, I want you to open your eyes . .Yes, open your eyes, now . . but look at nothing . . Open your eyes but do not look at anything . . Now, roll your eyeballs up . . as high as they will go . . Now, roll them down . . toward the floor . . Now, look toward the left . . high . . and now, low . . Look toward the right . . Both high . . and low . . Very good . . You may close them now and just relax . .

Beginning tomorrow, I want you to do these exercises . . for a few minutes . . faithfully, every day . . I want you to read for a while . . but hold the book a little closer than normal . . and focus . . And then practice looking, in the far distance . . Each time, focusing clearly on some object . . You will improve your eyesight 100 per cent , by practicing this routine for about ten minutes, each and every day . .

By practicing for only ten minutes, every day . . you will free yourself from the old habit of not seeing clearly . . And you will develop a new habit . . That of seeing vividly, clearly and perfectly

. . Your eyes are capable of focusing clearly and distinctly . . So I want you to practice just a short time each day . . After a few weeks . . increase the time to twenty minutes each day . . for a month . .

For the next week . . take your glasses off . . for at least fifteen minutes, each day . . when you are doing something that requires you to use your eyes . . For example . . if you are watching television, take your glasses off for fifteen minutes and watch the program without them . . And do not fixate your stare at the TV for more than an hour at a time . . without doing your eye movement exercises . .

Your eyes will quickly adjust to the new habits you are asking of them . . and the muscles, tendons and ligaments will continue strengthening . . Your vision will become more vivid and more clear . . as the shape of your eyeballs rejuvenate to their old, natural form . .

The second week . . double the time of seeing without your glasses . . And keep doubling the time, each week . . And continue with your eye movement exercises . . for ten to twenty minutes, each day . . In a few weeks . . you will find that your eyesight has improved . . to a point where you will be seeing clearly and distinctly . . without glasses or contact lenses . .

Your eyes are strong and tireless . . And they can be used for long periods of time and still feel relaxed and comfortable . . Your eyes are able to adjust to almost any situation . . And the more you actually use your eyes . . the stronger they become . . But that means, eye movements to each side . . up . . and down . . Not . . continually staring straight ahead for long periods of time . . You may need to divorce your television . .

Each day, your eyesight will continue improving . . And you will be happy with the progress you will make . . as your vision keeps becoming more clear and more perfect each day . .

Continue to relax for a few moments longer . . as your subconscious mind absorbs everything we have talked about today . . (pause)

And now, I am going to count from Five down to One . . And when you hear the count of One . . you will open your eyes, feeling good, feeling wonderful . . For you are a wonderful person . .

FIVE, FOUR, THREE, TWO and ONE . .

You may open your eyes now . .

FAMILY - FUNCTIONAL
Single or Couple - with 'teen Children present
(Follow Relaxation)

Continue to let yourself relax . . Just as you are . . And as you relax . . I am going to give you some suggestions and some insights . . that will help you to function more closely . . as a family . .

Family discipline relies heavily on self-discipline and self-persistence . . In fact, you will find yourself welcoming these suggestions . . and making them a permanent part of your psyche . . Because you realize that they are important to you . . And you realize that they are helpful in maintaining the success that you want to instill . . as a permanent part of your subconscious mind . . You also realize that your immediate success as a family . . is going to be maintained . . through self-discipline and persistence . . (and, the children's future lives will require it, in growing.)

With discipline . . and persistence . . you are going to be able to convert . . your greatest weakness . . whatever that thing is that you believe to be your greatest weakness . . It doesn't make any difference, what it is . . You are going to be able to convert that 'weakness' . . into a strength . . And you are going to convert it to a strength . . through self-discipline and self-persistence . .

These are the necessary traits to create and maintain . . a happy and healthy home environment . .

We have often heard it said, "Oh, if only I had had the patience to wait it out" . . And that's what you have been asking for . . The patience to wait it out . . The persistence to keep plugging away . . The persistence to keep going forward . . and keep striving for the mark, again and again . . and again . . Regardless of failures . . Because we know the system works . . We know that positive suggestions DO have their cumulative effect . . And we know that when we tell ourselves . . we're going to succeed . . then we ARE going to succeed . .

You are much better off by persisting . . than by giving up . . And you are much better off by disciplining yourself . . than by being in a position where others . . must discipline you . . You need self-discipline and self-persistence . . And those are going to be yours today . . Because you realize that, through self-discipline . . and through persistence . . you can transform yourself from, whatever you are, right now . . into a completely and totally successful family member . .

There are many success stories of people . . who have overcome great obstacles . . before finding success . . You will hear about them . . or read about them . . as time goes by . . But yours . . is the success story I am interested in . . Your self-discipline and persistence . . will make it happen . .

So, I would like to ask you . . right now . . What is your main weakness? . . Think about that for a moment . . What is your main weakness ? . . Well, you say . . It might be any number of things . . Fear . . Loss of temper . . Lack of confidence . . Alcohol . . Excessive eating . . Sexual frustrations . . Inhibitions . . Over spending . . Manipulating . . Use of drugs . . Lack of respect . . Giving children money instead of discipline . . Babying the children . . Teaching them to rely only on their parents instead of themselves . . And children, accepting that gift instead of accepting personal responsibility ? . . Only you can recognize your main weakness . . Realize that the weakness . . is only a weakness . . because you focus attention on all the little focal points around it . . But never directly on it . . Even though you are quite aware of it . . You intentionally avoid that one focal point . . or weakness . . And you spend a great deal of effort . . suggesting to yourself that . . because of this weakness . . which you have failed to recognize in the past . . Because of this weakness, you can't succeed . . You can't improve . . You can't get any better . . You've labeled yourself . . inadequate . . Yes, you've exhibited a great deal of effort . . convincing yourself that because of your weakness . . You can't succeed . . You can't do . . any better . .

Now, we need to look for a solution to this dilemma . . for the success and strength of this family . . And that's what we are going to do, right now . . Look for a solution . . But you are not alone . . I am here with you . . to assist and guide you through this . . And together, we will find it . .

You know, when you dwell upon a problem . . the only thing on your mind is, the problem . . But when you concentrate on a solution . . you come up with a solution . . After you get the problem out of the way of your thinking . . So you are going to eliminate concentrating on your problems . . And you're going to start concentrating on solutions . . Right now . . Because the solution for the problem should be resolved . . right now . . And when you resolve it . . that will prove to yourself that you are,

263

indeed, successful . . Right now, you are going to prove to yourself . . literally, beyond belief . . that you can do what others have done . . And you're going to be successful by transforming your greatest weakness . . into your most prized asset . . You choose what your weakness is . . You know it better than anybody else . . And, right now, you're going to transform that weakness into an asset . . by using self-discipline and through your own persistence . .

And when you transform your greatest weakness into a great strength . . what more proof of success can you have, than that ? . . What could be better proof to you, than that ? . . You can do it today . . You can do it, right now . . You can do it, for your family . . You can turn your greatest weakness . . into your greatest strength . . by listening carefully to the following suggestions . .

After you leave here today . . I want you to find a quiet place, where you can be alone . . for some quiet reflection . . I want you to go over your life . . Over your actions . . or lack of actions . . And I want you to consider . . your greatest weakness . . What are you not doing . . that you should be doing . . And what excuses do you give yourself . . for your lack of action . . Realize . . that that excuse is . . your weakness . . I want you to write it down . . Write down . . your greatest weakness. Literally STOP and DO IT . . And I am giving you the suggestion that you will stop . . you will take the time . . you will think about it . . and you will write it down . . And, I suggest you write down any number of other weaknesses you think you have . . And after you write them all down . . study each one of them . . And tell yourself . . as you contemplate that list of weaknesses . . "I am going to transform each one of these weaknesses into strengths . . beginning with my greatest weakness first . . And I am going to begin my transformation, today" . . (Repeat)

Then you can begin . . If you don't like to read . . you'll read three times as much . . If you don't like to cook, you'll take a cooking class . . You'll start making those changes . . And that is what's important to you . . No procrastination here . . DO what you just told yourself you are going to do . .

You have already seen that by saying what you are going to do . . and then doing it . . you'll begin to develop a new habit . . that will counter the old one . . You'll begin to condition yourself to perform . . and successfully . . Now, that's self-discipline . . That's persistence . . And

264

together, they'll put you on the road to success . . Your focus now is to master your weaknesses . . Transform this weakness, that you think you have . . into the strength . . that you will have . .

Because it's true . . that the biggest battle for success . . is to conquer yourself . . The biggest battle . . is conquering one's self . . and you have resolved, right now . . to conquer yourself . . You are resolving, right now, to perform the way you truly want to perform . . for the betterment of the family . . And you'll perform that way, without fail . . Because you're resolved that you're going to perform that way . . This kind of resolution . . once it becomes a habit . . will stick with you forever . . So you're going to resolve to make these changes . . and you'll continue with these changes . . until they become such habits . . that they will stay with you for the rest of your life . .

In the beginning, you'll recall . . you took the easiest way . . And you have been following that way . . out of habit . . Allowing yourself to hold onto the very thing . . that is making you ill, emotionally . . And that is the reason success has evaded you . .

You're going to begin by conquering your greatest weakness, first . . To prove to yourself that everything is possible . . And then, you'll gain the confidence to be successful . . in every other endeavor that you choose . . And you realize, right now . . that the battle against yourself . . begins with the resolution that you're going to change . . And it only ends after self-discipline has become engraved in your mind . . It only ends after self-discipline has become so engraved . . and so conditioned . . into your subconscious mind . . that success is an automatic habit . . that you simply cannot break . .

You're beginning to think 'success' right now, aren't you ? . . So much so . . that you're even willing to allow those thoughts . . of success . . to become habits with you . . Just think . . A habit that you cannot break, no matter how hard you try . . How wonderful it is, to begin to think 'success' . . It's really wonderful, to decide that you really are going to be persistent . . in overcoming your problem . . And you realize that persistence . . is the direct result of habit . . And you are habitually persistent . . when you condition yourself to be . . You understand that . . when you condition yourself to be a failure . . you'll wind up as a failure . . And when you condition yourself to be a coward . . you'll run away . . And you'll end up, running away from life . . Another shortcut to failure . . But realize this . . If you condition yourself to meet life, head on . . If you condition yourself to persist . . over and over, over and over . . and over again . . you will, in fact . . condition yourself to enjoy persisting . . Yes, enjoy it . . even in the face of failure . . Even in the face of depression . . That is when you've conditioned yourself to be persistent . . And that persistence will pay off for you . . You're conditioning yourself to be self-disciplined . . You're conditioning yourself to be alive . . and live abundantly . . And you're conditioning yourself to change those old habits . . into new and positive ones . . The ones that will put you right onto the pathway of success . . (pause)

There are always choices to make . . In this world, we either discipline ourselves . . so that we can handle each situation . . or we discipline ourselves so that we cannot handle them . . You know what your choice is . . And you know you want to be persistent, in setting your goals and then, reaching them . . And you know . . you want and need the discipline in your life . . to cause you to be persistent to be successful, in every way . . The quickest, safest and surest way . . is to turn your greatest weakness into your greatest strength . . And you'll do this through self-discipline and persistence . . including the resolution, that you are going to change . . You are going to make your start, as soon as you can, by writing your list of weaknesses . . Then begin converting them into your greatest strengths . . It feels so good . . to earn the pride and respect . . that you will have in yourself . . And I am already feeling that pride for you . .

Now, I am going to give you a moment of silence . . And during this moment of silence . . I want you to visualize yourself . . in a peaceful and loving . . in-home atmosphere . . resolving to convert those weaknesses . . for the betterment of the family . . During this moment of silence, I want you to reflect on your main, big weakness . . and resolve to change that one first . . Your moment of silence . . begins now . . (pause)

And now, I am going to begin my count, from One up to Five . . And when you hear the count of Five . . you will open your eyes, feeling alert, refreshed and ready to resume your full activities . .

ONE . . Thinking of awakening now . .
TWO . . Your muscles are wanting to stir a little . .
THREE . . Coming up higher now . . feeling good . . Feeling alive . .
FOUR . . Let your arms and legs move a bit now . . and
FIVE . . Open your eyes now and focus on your surroundings . .

FEAR - ELIMINATE
Post Traumatic Stress Disorder

Ref. : Rapid Eye Movement - Induction

The intent of this method is for the immediate alleviation of the client's FEAR. (P T S)

Often times, a client cannot express his or her fear - of having fear. Fear is a constant burden to many people but, generally, it comes in the guise of, "I have a problem"; an abusive spouse, a bully at school, a pervert in the park, an aggressive boss or associate., an automobile accident. There are many reasons for fear, although seldom expressed as actually being a fear of 'something'.

The above mentioned Induction, RAPID EYE MOVEMENT, is the basic process for eliminating fear but with some modifications, as will follow. The client may indicate a high level of stress, hypertension or anxiety due to the fears that they possess. This method should immediately alleviate all fears within the client, followed by a complete relaxation of the nervous system.

The client is awake and alert and is not under hypnosis. Use the following procedure and instructions:

Hold your open hand in an uplifted position, about 18 inches in front of client's face. You will place a bright RED DOT (made with a felt tipped pen) on the center of the end joint of the extended index finger. The other fingers are clenched.

"I want you to concentrate on the person or experience which has caused you to feel this fear that you have. Concentrate your mind on that person. On that situation. Now, DON'T RELAX ! Concentrate your mind on that experience. Watch the red dot. Keep looking at the red dot at all times".

Commence moving the red dot from side to side. Left to right - Left to right - Left to right, gaining speed as you go. Begin slowly but finish, after ten or twelve times, moving very rapidly.

Such eye movement - Left to right - Left to right, very rapidly, has an immediate impact on the frontal lobe of the brain, causing it to 'erase' the vision of fear which has possessed the client.

After 10 or 12 cycles, stop your hand in the upward position. Open your hand, suddenly, and cover the eyes with the palm of your hand, saying, "SLEEP". Lay the center of your palm over the client's chakra (center of forehead just above eyes) about 10 - 15 seconds, applying a firm pressure while placing your opposite hand behind client's head for support.

Now, slowly turn the client's head from side to side in a soft, rolling motion. Do not move the head continuously. With intermittent movement of the head, the client will quickly understand that they must let you move the head. This will allow the client to LET GO.

Next, say, "WHEN I REMOVE MY HANDS, YOU WILL GO TEN TIMES DEEPER".

Now, quickly and decisively, remove your hands and say, "TEN TIMES DEEPER". Or, if a recliner is being used, say, "I AM GOING TO GENTLY TIP THE RECLINER AND YOU WILL GO TEN TIMES DEEPER". You may also tell the client, "WHEN I TURN OFF THE OVERHEAD LIGHT, YOU WILL GO TEN TIMES DEEPER".

Follow this method with a gentle, soothing Relaxation Induction. A leading prescription is not required until further discussion with client, as to their needs, has been completed.

As you are continuing to relax . . you are aware that the subconscious level of your mind . . is going to help you get rid of the problem of having fever blisters . . You are also aware that I don't know . . what has been causing those fever blisters . . and, therefore, I don't know how to cure them . . However . . there is a part of your mind that does know . . what has been causing them . . and it also knows . . exactly what needs to be done to . . eliminate them . .

You will recognize that I am talking to both your conscious mind . . and to the subconscious level of your mind . . And, whether or not I say the right thing . . is not important . . The mere fact that you have permitted yourself to be hypnotized . . and have asked me to help you . . lets the subconscious level of your mind know . . that you are responsive . . And that you want all levels of your mind to cooperate . . and solve the problem . . regardless of what I say or do . .

You want the problem to be corrected, don't you . . But, how ? . . Certainly not by the way you have been attempting to correct it . . consciously . . Nor in any way that I would try to correct it . . If it could be corrected that way, you would not have the problem . . The way you want it corrected . . is by the way your subconscious mind wants to correct it . . And that is in such a way that the healing energies of your body . . are directed towards healing those fever blisters . . Now and forever . . And in a way that is pleasing to you . .

I have been talking to you for some time now . . Specifically, to your subconscious mind . . in order to communicate your need for repair of this condition . . Now that the subconscious level of your mind is aware of your needs . . it can work out the solution to that problem, in its own way . . Because your subconscious mind understands many more things . . than your conscious mind is aware of . . (Pause for a minute or so)

We have the idea that we need to think so many different things . . to resolve this issue . . However, this is not so . . Consider for a moment, the speed of nerve impulses . . traveling at approximately 186,000 miles per second . . Knowing this . . how long would it take to have a whole series of thoughts ? . . Millions of thoughts pass through the subconscious level of your mind . . in only a few seconds

. . Therefore, the subconscious level of your mind . . is resolving that problem . . quite rapidly . .

When the subconscious level of your mind knows . . what has been causing that problem . . And when it knows the problem is resolved and changes have begun . . and . . you are getting rid of the fever blister problem . . for now and forever . . one of the fingers on your (Right / Left) hand will lift up towards the ceiling . . And your finger will remain up . . until I tell it to go back down . .

I want you to keep in mind . . that it isn't necessary for you to consciously listen to me . . The fact that you have allowed yourself to be hypnotized . . lets the subconscious level of your mind know how willing you are . . to absorb the benefits of hypnosis . . By going into a hypnotic state . . you are making use of that part of your mind that knows . . how to work out the solution . . to any problem . . that ever comes up in your life . . And all you need to do is continue relaxing, calmly and quietly . . and rely on the subconscious level of your mind . . to heal you in its own way . . Now, I will remain silent for a time . . as that is being done . . (Pause for a minute or two)

And now, in a few moments . . we will be concluding this session . . and you will be back in a wide awake, fully alert, state . . Feeling confident and happy . . You will feel much better than you did before you were hypnotized . . You will feel better, physically, mentally and spiritually . .

EMERGE

Something most everyone knows . . is that people communicate,
verbally . . We talk to each other by using words . . But we can also
communicate by using sign language . . One very common expression
of sign language . . is when you nod your head, YES . . or shake
your head, NO . . Most everyone does that, from time to time . .
Another kind of sign language is, waving the hand to say good bye or
hello . . Sometimes we lift our hand and motion with our forefinger
. . to signal for someone to come to us . . or we may hold the palm of
our hand, toward a person . . to tell them to stop . . So, we can use our
head . . our hand or our finger . . to communicate with another
person . . And you can communicate with sign language . . even when
you are in a deep, hypnotic state . . There are times when we may be
listening to someone talk . . and we may be nodding our head . . or
shaking our head, in agreement . . or disagreement . . without even
realizing we are doing it . . But it is just as easy to do it with your finger
. . or with your hand . .

I want to ask you some questions . . that can be answered with a
simple YES or a NO . . Questions that your subconscious mind can
answer . . Your subconscious mind can review, examine and explore
. . the information in the storehouse of your mind . . and can give
the correct answer . . to each question I ask . .

Your subconscious mind will answer each question . . by causing one
of your fingers to lift up . . Let's say, your index finger . . The one
next to your thumb . . on your left hand . . It will lift UP for the
answer . .YES . . And the little finger on your right hand will lift up . .
if the answer is NO . .

Your mind has a storehouse . . containing everything you have ever
heard . . everything you have ever seen . . and everything you have
ever experienced . . And will explore, examine and review . . all of
the information in the storehouse of your mind . . and will give the
correct answer to each question I ask you . .

If the correct answer is YES . . your mind will cause your YES
finger to lift up . . If the correct answer is NO . . your mind will
cause your NO finger to lift up . .

Your mind will cause your finger to lift up and give the correct answer . . each time I ask you a Question . . And your finger will remain UP . . until I tell it to go back down . .

(Continue with YES / NO queries and on to required prescription - unless there is no response. To obtain response, please continue.)

TO OBTAIN RESPONSE :

(Note : THESE SUGGESTIONS ARE TO BE USED IF YOU HAVE GIVEN SUGGESTIONS FOR FINGER RESPONSE AND HAVE WAITED FIVE OR MORE MINUTES WITHOUT GAINING ANY RESPONSE.)

I'm going to lift your arm up . . And I'm not going to tell you to put it down . . any faster than you become . . very relaxed . . and learn to allow your other hand and arm . . to float upwards . . towards your face . . automatically . . (Lift hand and arm, of client, up)

Your hand and arm will go down slowly . . while your conscious mind is thinking pleasant thoughts . . and your subconscious mind . . is allowing the other hand and arm to become . . lighter than a feather . . The other hand and arm are becoming so light . . that they feel like floating upward . . toward your face . . One hand and arm goes down . . but only as fast as the other hand and arm continues . . to rise up . . And no faster . .

NOTE : IF THE HAND MOVES DOWN FASTER THAN THE OTHER HAND MOVES UP, SAY, " THAT'S TOO FAST". THAT HAND AND ARM WILL SLOW DOWN AND WILL DROP ONLY AS FAST AS THE OTHER HAND AND ARM CONTINUES TO RISE UP.

Just take your time . . Let your other mind do it . . That's good . . You're learning to do it right now . .

You can enjoy what your subconscious mind can automatically do for you . . You're doing very good now . . Your hand is lifting all the way up to your face . . And when it touches your face . . you will know you are ready . .

You are learning to let your subconscious mind make the movements and the changes . . You are allowing that to happen . . One hand moving one way . . while the other hand moves the other way . . And you can continue . . until your subconscious mind learns to do it perfectly . .

Note: CONTINUE WITH THE SAME OR SIMILAR SUGGESTIONS UNTIL THE HAND HAS TOUCHED THE FACE.   IT'S OKAY TO PAUSE FOR 30 or 40 SECONDS IF THE RESPONSE TIME HAS STARTED AND IS CONTINUING. GIVE WORDS OF ENCOURAGEMENT FROM TIME TO TIME.

It really isn't important right now that your conscious mind knows that this is happening . . It's only important that your subconscious mind, and all other levels of your inner mind, have already started to demonstrate to you, in pleasant ways that you will be noticing . . that wonderful changes have started . . and are continuing . . as you go about your daily activities . .

When you awaken from the hypnotic state . . you will find that your subconscious mind is continuing . . to work out pleasant ways to keep improving you . . physically, mentally, emotionally and spiritually . .

CONTINUE WITH NEXT PRESCRIPTION or EMERGE

HABITS - OVERCOME   I   (smoking)
(USE WHEN MORE THAN ONE SESSION IS NEEDED)
(Follow Relaxation)

Hypnosis works amazingly well . . in helping us to get rid of unwanted habits . . In most cases . . it takes only one session of being hypnotized . . and given helpful suggestions . . to enable us to get rid of the unwanted habit completely . . However . . in some cases, there may be a psychological or emotional reason . . for a person to develop an unwanted habit . .

As you continue to relax . . I want to help you briefly examine . . just what habits are . . and how they work . . This will increase your understanding and will make it easier for you . . to overcome the habit and be rid of it . . completely and permanently . .

To begin with . . all habits are learned . . The first time you (smoke a cigarette / drink an alcoholic beverage / take a drug), it is not a habit . . It becomes a habit only by continuing to do it . . And the more you do it . . the more strongly the habit becomes reinforced in your mind . .

Second . . Habits tend to operate on a subconscious level . . As you begin, you are doing it consciously, at first . . But as you continue . . you are soon doing it without conscious control . .

Third.   It becomes a habit when you are doing it at regular intervals . .

Fourth.   The more you do it, the more it becomes reinforced in your mind . . And soon, you feel compelled . . to continue . .

Fifth.   The habit reaches a point when it begins fulfilling a need . . It becomes a way of coping with other experiences in your life . . Perhaps a way of avoiding those experiences . .

Sixth.   After the habit becomes firmly established . . any attempt to stop it meets with resistance . . And when you do try to stop it . . the need remains unfulfilled . . Harmful habits tend to operate in a circle . . Fueled by the need . . which is not being fulfilled . . The unfulfilled need could be a need for an environmental change . . or a need for companionship . . A need for love or a need for REAL sexual fulfillment . . Or it could be a combination of experiences, which are causing loneliness, anxiety, worry or depression . .

The habit then becomes a substitute . . for attempting to satisfy the emotional need . . But it does not work . . Instead, it fails to accomplish what it was suppose to achieve . . All it does is become a stronger habit . . and causes the body to become less healthy . . And it also contributes to other . . social and family . . problems . .

We know that, consciously, trying to stop the habit . . meets with resistance . . And trying to resist only puts more energy into it . . So, one of the first things you should do . . is to stop trying to fight it . . The change will begin, when you realize . . it is okay to be the way you are . . I'm going to mention something you can do . . Something that will eliminate the need for you to have the habit of (Smoking / Drinking / Doing Drugs).

Continue to relax for a few moments longer . . then I will give you suggestions . . which will help to eliminate this need you have . . to hold onto the habit . . (Pause)

Before you come back for your next session . . I'd like you to do something for yourself . . I want you to take the time to list all of the reasons . . why you want to get rid of that habit . . Make a list of as many reasons as you can . . And then, number the five most important reasons . . for getting rid of that habit . .

After making your list of reasons . . of why you want to get rid of that habit . . make another list of reasons . . that say why you DO NOT want to get rid of that habit . .

And then, make a list of the NEEDS the habit might be fulfilling . . List as many as you can . . and then, narrow it down to one or two of the most important needs . . And then write the different ways that you have available . . that could fulfill those needs . . IF you did not have that habit . .

By doing this . . you will understand the structure of a habit . . and what you get from it . . At the same time . . you will have a better understanding of the problems . . it is causing you . . You will be amazed at how much easier it will be for you . . to get rid of the habit . . And you will have an understanding about the habit . . that will cause your subconscious mind to cooperate . . in getting rid of the habit completely . . and permanently . .

DIRECT CLIENT, HOW TO WRITE OUT LIST WHEN AWAKENED. FROM THIS POINT ON, THE ADDITIONAL SUGGESTIONS ARE FOR SMOKERS ONLY.

You will be aware of how good it feels to walk briskly, up a hill . . and feel clean and strong . . and breathe easily and freely . . You will realize how good it is to feel energetic . . and full of vitality . . Your lungs will feel so much better . . and you will know all of the positive benefits . . once you are free from the habit . . And your mind will make the connections of how you are a much better, all-around person . . Free, at last, from cigarettes . .

There is nothing about smoking that gives you any benefit . . So there is no reason for you to continue smoking . . But, don't try to quit smoking . . If you desire to smoke, it's okay for you to smoke . . because your subconscious mind understands . . that you will soon be a NONSMOKER . . And you will find the craving for a cigarette . . and the desire to smoke . . fading away, automatically . . as the taste of cigarettes turn bitter . . and your need for more oxygen . . increases . . Any time you have a strong urge to smoke . . Go ahead and smoke . . And, enjoy it . .

You are learning to be kind to yourself . . And your subconscious mind is cooperating . . by causing you to desire only what is good . . for your body and for your health . .

You can smoke any time you want to . . And since you are interested in developing a healthier, stronger body . . From now on, you will go through a little ritual . . before each cigarette . . Any time you feel an urge to smoke . . Before you light up a cigarette, step outside and take ten, deep, slow breaths of fresh air . . After doing that, you will be able to choose whether or not you really want to smoke . . And whatever choice you make, is okay . . You will feel good about the choice you make . .

What you are doing is developing . . an interesting, healthy form of substitution . . to replace the habit of smoking . . And you will really be pleased to notice . . the way you keep improving . . in all areas of your life . . physically, mentally, emotionally and spiritually . .

EMERGE

HABITS - OVERCOME II
WHEN MORE THAN ONE SESSION IS NEEDED ,
I.E.. STOP SMOKING, BED-WETTING, NAIL-BITING, THUMB-SUCKING. ETC.
(Follow relaxation)

You are continuing to drift into a more restful . . more peaceful hypnotic state . . Each time you breath . . you are breathing in the energy of life . . And you keep feeling more in tune . . with the harmony and beauty all around you . . And because you recognize that oxygen is the pure energy provider of life . . whether you are working or doing something for fun . . or for relaxation . . or even when you are sleeping . . you will continue to experience a flow of calming sensations . . permeating your entire being . .

These suggestions are going into the storehouse of your subconscious mind . . and they are already working . . to enable you to live your life in a more peaceful, more relaxed way . .

It is highly desirable for everyone to learn to relax . . as you are doing now . . We live in a world that is constantly changing . . And even with all of the turmoil and changes . . going on around you . . you can use these principles of relaxation . . which you are now experiencing . . and they will enable you to cope . . with your everyday changing circumstances . . in a more relaxed way . .

Regardless of where you are . . or what you are doing . . you can be calm and relaxed at all times . . You can continue to experience a happier, more peaceful life . . And you can achieve complete emotional stability . . in all areas of your life . .

The fact that you are here for this appointment . . shows that you have the motivation to overcome the problem we spoke about . . and that, too, will help you to live your life . . in a more relaxed way . . You also have all the desire you need . . to overcome that problem . . Yet, there is still . . one important thing that you need . . and that is . . self-confidence . .

You have probably tried many different things to overcome that problem . . And everything you have tried has been unsuccessful . . And . . you probably expect hypnosis to be unsuccessful, as well . . However, this time, you are going to be pleasantly surprised . . Before this session is over . . you will have all the self-confidence it takes . . to be successful . . All you need to do is to relax . .

Notice how comfortable you are feeling right now . . As you continue to relax . . your body responds by becoming even more comfortable . . Go deeper now . . Relax Deeper . . Deeper . .

Through the many years . . that I have been hypnotizing people . . I've had many clients come to me . . with almost every kind of problem you can think of . . Many have been successful in reducing their bodies . . Most of those who came to stop smoking have stopped . . after only one or two sessions . . Most people who have come with problems of nail biting, thumb sucking or bed wetting . . have also been successful . . Generally, after only one session of hypnosis . .

I remember . . when I was younger . . that I had wanted, so much, to buy a big, beautiful car . . But the price was much more than I could afford . . And so I tried to forget about it . . and yet, I couldn't get it out of my mind . . I imagined myself, driving down the Highway in it . . Or, parking it at the drive-in . . I thought about people seeing it and . . wishing they could have one just like it . . I would be the envy of all the guys in town . . I thought, if I had that big, beautiful car . . I'd have everything I'd ever need to be happy . . But . . I still couldn't afford it . . And, after seeing the same car the next year . . and the next . . it faded in my mind until, finally, I came to realize that . . happiness cannot be found in possessions . . To be really happy, I needed to feel good about myself . . Just as you need to feel good about yourself . . That is where your true happiness lies . .

Now, I understand that no one . . likes to be told what to do . . And so, if I told you . . that you need to stop _____, you would, most likely, resent it . . Especially, since that was the very reason you came here . . And you had already made that decision before coming here . . without me telling you . . I think it's really wonderful that you made your own decision to stop _____ . . So, you don't need to have me telling you what to do . .

And you already know the reasons you want to stop _____ . . So, I don't need to be telling you why it is good . . that you decided to end that _____ problem . . But I do know how proud you are going to be . . now that you have made your own decision . . to be rid of that problem . . And I know how good you are going to feel . . when you leave here today and find . . that you are completely free from that problem . .

Right now, you have NO DESIRE to ever do that again . . You made your own decision to get rid of that habit . . and you decided that you wanted to enjoy the good feeling . . that comes with being free from that problem . . and accepting the responsibility for your own behavior . . You are making a wise decision to just . . let go . . and be rid of that problem, permanently . . Your strong desire, to stop _____ . . is all that is needed . . for your subconscious mind to work out the solution within you . . to make it happen . . And it is happening . . right now . .

Now, I'd prefer that you stop _____ immediately . . but you are the only one who can make that decision . . And you have decided that you are stopping _____ completely (by / at) Insert time client has decided to stop.

Some people wait an hour . . Some wait until after dinner . . And some stop immediately . . And I am proud to know that you have already made the decision to stop _____ . . So, you are feeling good about knowing . . that when you get up from that chair . . you will definitely know the time . . when you will be free from _____ forever . .

GO TO : SELF-CONFIDENCE BUILDING PRESCRIPTION

279

(Follow relaxation)

You are continuing to drift into a more restful . . more peaceful hypnotic state . . Each time you breath . . you are breathing in the energy of life . . And you keep feeling more in tune . . with the harmony and beauty all around you . . And because you recognize that oxygen . . is the pure energy provider of life . . whether you are working or doing something for fun . . or for relaxation . . or even when you are sleeping . . you will continue to experience a flow of calming sensations . . permeating your entire being . .

These suggestions are going into the storehouse of your subconscious mind . . and they are already working . . to enable you to live your life in a more peaceful, more relaxed way . .

It is highly desirable for everyone to learn to relax . . as you are doing now . . We live in a world that is constantly changing . . And even with all of the turmoil and changes . . going on around you . . you can use these principles of relaxation . . which you are now experiencing . . and they will enable you to cope . . with your everyday changing circumstances . . in a more relaxed way . .

Regardless of where you are . . or what you are doing . . you can be calm and relaxed at all times . . You can continue to experience a happier, more peaceful life . . And you can achieve complete emotional stability . . in all areas of your life . .

Today is a very important day for you . . because this is the day you are getting rid of the habit . . of having headaches . . You are going to notice some very pleasant changes in your life . . Beginning today . . you are learning how to live your life . . in a more calm, more relaxed way . .

Hypnosis will help you to be more calm . . more relaxed and feel more peaceful at all times . . during your daily life . .

The fact that you are here for this appointment . . shows that you have the desire and motivation to overcome the problem of headaches . . You will find this to be the most pleasant . . and helpful experience of your life . . and it will also help you to live your life . . in a more relaxed way . .

You have probably tried many different things to overcome this problem . . And everything you have tried has been unsuccessful . . And you probably expect hypnosis to be unsuccessful, as well . . However, this time, you are going to be pleasantly surprised . . Before this session is over . . you will have all the self-confidence it takes . . to be successful . . All you need to do is to relax . . Notice how comfortable you are feeling right now . . As you continue to relax . . your body responds by becoming even more comfortable . . Go deeper now . . Relax Deeper . . Deeper . .

Your mind is accepting all of the concepts I am giving you . . and is using them to help you control . . your emotions and feelings . . They will also help you in developing a greater . . self-confidence . . And enable you to experience improved health . .

You are realizing that this soothing relaxation you are now experiencing . . has been achieved by you . . All I did was give you some suggestions . . And by following my suggestions . . it was YOU who produced the relaxation . . And now you know that you are capable of keeping yourself calm and relaxed . . whenever you wish . . regardless of what is happening around you . .

If you are criticized . . harshly or unjustly . . you will remain calm and completely relaxed . . If you are driving your car . . and another driver does something to slow you down . . or cause you to stop . . you will remain calm and relaxed . . And you will realize that the small delay . . will not change your life . . And the same is true when you are confronted with difficulties . . problems or unpleasant situations . . You will simply remain relaxed, calm and peaceful . .

You can always be in control of your feelings and emotions . . .rather than allow yourself to be controlled . . Regardless of how unpleasant life may seem, at times . . you can always reward yourself by remaining calm and relaxed . . The health of your body and your mind . . will be your real reward . . And your ability to remain in control . . calm and relaxed in every situation . . keeps becoming more automatic each day . .

You will quickly recognize situations which . . in the past . . have caused you to become tense or anxious . . And you will respond to those situations . . by using these principles of relaxation . . which you have learned by permitting yourself to be hypnotized . .

Your nerves will be more relaxed and steady . . Your mind will be calmer and clearer . . You will be more composed . . more tranquil . . and more at peace, within . . Each day, you continue becoming emotionally calmer . . You will be more stable . . more settled . . And you can do every thing in a relaxed manner . .

Your self-confidence, self-reliance, self-acceptance and self-esteem . . will keep increasing . . and you will have a greater sense of personal well-being . .

Each morning, when you awaken . . you will be relaxed and will feel refreshed . . both mentally and physically . . You will relate to your daily circumstances with calmness and confidence . . Knowing that you will remain free . . from any headaches or related problems . .

You are becoming the person you have always wanted to be . . Self-confident, acceptable, capable and strong . .

Your life is becoming more enjoyable . . Your feelings of happiness are increasing . . And your day-to-day living continues to become more pleasurable . .

You have accepted all of the suggestions I have given you . . They are now in the storehouse of your subconscious mind . . And you are adopting them as a normal part of your daily life . . Your subconscious mind will keep your body calm . . and relaxed . . And will enable you to maintain a state of emotional stability . . that is pleasing to you . . (pause)

We determined earlier that oxygen . . is the pure energy provider of life . . I would like you to inhale several times . . deeply, through your nose . . as we shall be ending this session . . in just another moment or two . . (Pause)

And now, I am going to count . . from 5, down to one . . And when you hear me count out the number, one . . you will open your eyes, feeling refreshed and bright . . Aware of your surroundings and ready to take on your next challenge . . I will begin now . .

FIVE . . Becoming aware of your body now . .
FOUR . . Your muscles are wanting to stir a little . . That's okay . .
THREE . . Rising up a little higher now . . Coming up now . .
TWO . . You are becoming more aware of yourself now . . Beginning to waken . . And . .
ONE . . Open your eyes now and tell me, "How do you feel"?

HEADACHE, MIGRAINE

(Follow relaxation)

You have been relaxing for a while now . . and as you continue to relax . . and without even realizing it . . you have gently fallen into a comfortable and restful feeling . . Now, I am wondering if you would like to have . . a really pleasant, surprising experience . . (Pause for response)

In just a moment, I am going to have you awaken from the hypnotic state . . but you will awaken only from the neck up . . Is that all right with you ? . . (Wait for response)

Very good . . In just a moment, when I count to three . . you will awaken from the neck up . . The rest of your body will remain in a deep, peaceful, hypnotic state . . You will awaken for one minute only . . keeping your eyes open, for one minute . . And then, they will become relaxed . . and close again . . And you will go back into an even deeper . . state of hypnosis . .

I am going to count now . . ONE . . You are awakening from the neck up . . TWO . . and THREE . .

You can open your eyes now . . Your mind is alert . . In one minute, your eyes will close again . . and you will be in a much deeper state than you were in before . .

After your eyes close and you are back in a deep, peaceful hypnotic state . . I am going to touch your (L / R) hand . . Each time I touch your hand . . you will notice that it keeps becoming more numb . . Nod your head when you become aware of the numbness that is beginning to develop . . (Keep touching the hand until client nods head)

Now, I'd like you to notice that the skin . . is very numb . . And that numbness is moving into the bones . . Even the tendons and ligaments are becoming numb . . And that numbness is moving into the nerves of your hand . . It is very, very numb now . . Almost as though it is no longer a part of you . . And as you become aware of that . . your head will nod again . . (Pause until head nods)

(Pinch hand on the fatty side and ask client, 'What am I doing?' . . If client says, "Pinching me," say, "By that, do you mean you feel the pressure of your skin between my fingers ?"   (Do not mention the word, 'pain'.)

In just a moment, I'm going to touch your arm . . As soon as I touch your arm . . the numbness in your hand will increase . . And your hand will become ten times more numb than it is now . . as soon as I touch your arm . . (Touch Arm)

Pick up hand by taking skin between thumb and forefinger, with fingernails, and ask, "What does it seem like I am doing now?" (Wait for response.)

Still gripping hand with fingernails, shake hand back and forth and ask again, "Now, what am I doing ?" (Wait for response.) Now, open your eyes and look at what I am doing . .

Have client open eyes and see that you were pinching with your fingernails. Now, pinch arm to show that the arm is not numb. Then pinch the other hand - to show that the other hand is not numb . NOTE : Do not pinch very hard, but as you pinch, tell client, "I'm going to pinch your arm now and you will notice that your arm is not numb . . You'll be able to feel it" . . Then, as you pinch the other hand, say the same thing.

Close your eyes now and continue to relax . . Now, you are realizing that your subconscious mind . . can make changes in your body . . without any conscious effort by you . . You didn't do anything, consciously, to make your hand numb . . I merely put the suggestion in your mind . . and told you I would touch your hand . . Touching your hand was a signal . . and each time I touched your hand . . your subconscious mind caused it to keep becoming more numb . . Your mind responded to that signal . . Then I gave you another signal . . Touching your arm was a signal . . to increase the numbness even more . .

I am going to ask you a question now . . If the answer is YES . . the finger next to your thumb . . will lift up towards the ceiling . . If the answer is NO (spell N - O) . . the little finger on your hand will lift up towards the ceiling . . Which ever finger lifts up, it will stay up until I tell it to go back down . .

As your subconscious mind reviews what has been causing those headaches . . and works out a solution to get rid of them completely . . Is it okay to transfer that numbness to your head ? . . (Response) Lift your hand now and begin touching your head . . with the palm of your hand . . fingers extended . . right where you have noticed the strongest pain . . And now, place your other hand . . on the opposite side of your head . . As you touch your head with your hand . . the numbness is transferred to your head . . And as the numbness goes into your head . . the normal feeling is returning to your hand . . Your head will remain numb as your subconscious mind reviews . . what has been causing that problem . . And works out a solution . . to heal you completely . . and get rid of those headaches . . now and forever . .

Now, you are becoming more and more aware, of the comfort . . That still, quiet, restful and peaceful feeling . . all through your neck and head . . and shoulders . . You are experiencing a feeling of spiritual gratification . . and joy . . That sense of complete comfort and stillness . . All parts of your body are now at rest . . Continue to rest . . Soon, you will be coming back . . to a wide awake . . fully alert state . . Feeling much better than you did . . before you were hypnotized . .

Your subconscious mind has indicated . . that it would be better, right now . . for the numbness NOT to be transferred to your head . . Evidently, your mind needs more time to review . . what has been causing the problem . . So, even after you awaken from the hypnotic state . . your mind will continue exploring . . what has been causing the problem . . and it will work out the solution . . in its own way . . In the meantime . . you will feel much better when you awaken . . from your hypnotic state . . than you have felt in a long, long time . . And your mind will soon understand what has been causing that problem . . and will resolve the problem in a way that is pleasing . .

When you awaken from the hypnotic state . . all the normal feelings will be back in your hand . .

And now, if you are ready . . I am going to count from FIVE . . down to ONE . . And when you hear me count out the number, ONE . . you will open your eyes, feeling refreshed and bright . . aware of your surroundings and ready to take on your next challenge . . I will begin now . .

FIVE . . Becoming aware of your body now . .

FOUR . . Your muscles are wanting to stir a little . . That's okay . .

THREE . .Rising up a little higher now . . Coming up now . .

TWO . . You are becoming more aware of yourself now . . Beginning to awaken . . And . .

ONE . . Open your eyes now and tell me, "How do you feel"?

(Follow DEEP Relaxation)

I am going to give you some suggestions now . . that will enable you to keep improving . . in all areas of your life . . physically . . mentally . . emotionally . . and spiritually . .

I want you to be peaceful and DEEPLY relaxed . . while your subconscious mind is accepting my suggestions . . Each time you inhale . . you move into a deeper . . and DEEPER . . hypnotic state . . And each time you exhale . . you continue relaxing more . . and more . . Relax . . Just relax . . Your conscious awareness is narrowing down . . and that is good . . Your subconscious mind is focusing . . only on the words I am saying to you . .

Each suggestion and instruction I give you. . . will begin working immediately . . and will become more and more effective with each day . .

You can consciously listen to the soothing sounds in the room . . while your subconscious mind listens to the words I speak . . All other sounds and noises keep fading away . . into the distance . . Any other sounds you hear will not distract you . . Hear only the sounds of my voice . .

There may be brief moments . . at first . . when other thoughts come into your conscious mind . . But that will not interfere . . because your subconscious mind is listening only to my voice . . and will absorb the true meaning of each word I say . .

A wonderful drowsiness is coming over your whole body . . And you are experiencing a deep . . and profound relaxation as you become more calm . . and more settled . . Such a peaceful feeling . .

You are drifting into a deep . . dreaming state . . And in a short time . . you will experience something that . . for thousands of years . . has been one of the most important . . and most beneficial . . of all human experiences . . Something that can be experienced . . only . . in a deep hypnotic state of relaxation . . such as you are in now . .

You will experience a kind of healing . . that has been used for centuries . . And it has been proven to heal every kind of illness . . disease . . and physical handicap, known to mankind . .

In fact, it does much more than improve your health . . It also increases your self-confidence . . It multiplies your self-acceptance . .

And it provides your mind with an understanding . . that leads to expanded spiritual growth and advancement . .

For thousands of years, people went into a temple . . whenever they were ill . . And history reveals how the temple priests would help them . . to go into a hypnotic state . . similar to the one you are in now . . They would be left in that state throughout the night . . And they would be aware . . of some entity . . coming to them, sometime during the night . . They believed that the entity who came to them . . while they were in that deep state . . was a God, who possessed great wisdom and powers . . far beyond normal human powers . . And the person in that deep state . . for the purpose of being healed . . would experience many different sensations during those nights . . They believed those Gods were examining them . . but were also causing healing forces in their body to be activated . . to heal the body . . so it would function properly from that time on . . When the person awakened the next morning . . they would be transformed . . The mind and body would function properly to complete the healing . . and restore the body to perfect health . .

That was a common practice for thousands of years . . And the amazing thing about it was . . that it worked . . There were always beneficial results . . for anyone who went into the temple . . to undergo a deep state of meditation and relaxation . .

We understand even more about it today . . Today, we realize, that it was not some kind of a God, who produced the healing . . Instead, we have found that the human body . . was created with its own healing power . . And being in a state of relaxation . . as you are in now . . activates those natural healing energies and enables them to work properly . .

Science has found that the cells of your body . . can receive directions from your mind . . to produce the healing vibrations your body needs . . to heal itself perfectly . . So, it is not other Gods who produce the healing . . It is done, as the Bible says . . "Through the renewing of your mind" . .

Continue inhaling DEEPLY . . and exhaling, slowly now . . I want you to drift into an even DEEPER . . DEEPER . . state of relaxation . . By permitting your mind and body to relax . . through your own ability to concentrate . . you will notice . . after the session is over . . that you will feel much better . . mentally, physically and spiritually . . Right now, you can feel the power of your own mind working . . And you can feel that energy, surging up within you . . (pause)

You are realizing that your body was created . . with an innate ability to heal itself . . If your skin gets cut . . the cells of your body know exactly what to do . . to cause the skin to grow back together again . . and heal perfectly . . If you get a bruise . . the cells of your body will function properly . . and heal the area that was bruised . . If you break a bone . . the cells of your body do what needs to be done . . to cause the bone to mend itself and heal completely . .

Every cell, atom and molecule of your body . . contains life and energy . . Every cell of your body has a specific purpose . . And each cell has the wisdom to know how to function in a perfect way . .

All of the energies that produce healing in your body . . are already in place . . You have tremendous healing powers in your body . . And you are allowing yourself to exercise that healing power, right now . . as you continue to relax . . Perfect order . . Perfect harmony . . And perfect health . . are being established throughout your entire bodily system . .

Focus your mind, now, on where you want the healing energies to flow . . Your mind is concentric on peaceful, health restoring thoughts and ideas . . that are causing all of your body processes . . to function properly now . . And will continue the same . . after you are out of your hypnotic state . .

Each day, you will become more aware of love . . all around you . . Ready for you to share . . And you will find that, as you express yourself to others . . in a loving way . . you will experience more love and harmony, flowing into your life . . And you will be filled with a wonderful, harmonious feeling of love and peace . . and perfect health . .

You are placing yourself, and all that concerns you, in the love and care of God . . And you are realizing that, what you cannot do, God can do . . You are being strengthened and rejuvenated . . by the divine healing power . . of love . .

You are getting ready to awaken from the hypnotic state now . . And you will continue experiencing a surge of energy and enthusiasm . . And know that life on Earth is a wonderful experience . . to be enjoyed . . Your health and happiness will continue improving more each day . .

EMERGE

Now, I would like you to close your eyes and . . begin breathing deeply . . slowly . . and deeply . . So that you will become very calm and relaxed . . Before you let go completely . . and slip into a deep hypnotic state . . just let yourself listen to everything I say to you . .

Right now, there is nothing you need to be concerned about . . Whatever is going to happen, will happen, automatically . . So you don't need to think about that now . . And you have no conscious control over what has already happened . . I understand, you have recently suffered a great loss in your life . . I am deeply sorry . . There are many affects from such a loss . . as you have had . . And you will not find them to be troublesome . . Indeed, they will serve as reminders . . of the love and the joy you shared . . while you were together . .

You are doing very well . . Breathe deeply . . Slowly and deeply . . You will notice the muscles . . in and around your eyes, relaxing all by themselves . . as you continue breathing deeply . . Easily and freely . . Breathe deeply now . . through your nose . . and slowly exhale . . Do that three or four more times . . Notice the cosmic energy coming into your mind and your body . . Relaxing energy filling your lungs with life . .

Without thinking about it . . you will soon enter a deep, peaceful, hypnotic trance . . without any effort . . There is nothing important for your conscious mind to do . . There is nothing really important except the activities of your subconscious mind . . And that is where all events will take place . . But you will notice many events taking place . . on a higher plane . . after this event has passed . .

You are responding very well, without even noticing it . . You have already altered your rate of breathing . . You are breathing much more easily and freely now . . And you are revealing signs that indicate you are beginning to drift . . into a very restful state of being . .

You can enjoy relaxing more and more now . . And your subconscious mind will listen to each word I say . . And will guide you through the steps of your journey . . So it becomes less important for you to consciously listen to my voice . . Simply relax . . Relax . .

I want to take you . . to a restful . . quiet place, deep in the forest . . where you will find peace and comfort . . in a totally relaxing world of your own . . We will only stay for a little while . . You're going to take a short journey . . up a mountain trail . . where tall trees nestle high up . . in the rain clouds . . The clouds bump and mesh together . . swirling . . in shades of pink and soft azure blue . . Occasional drops of rain settle softly . . on your face . . And you smile because . . the rain drops make you feel excited and . . happy inside . .

It is time now to let go . . Let yourself go . . To be free to slowly drift up . . up . . to the tops of the trees . . High above the trees . . Where you are free to sail on the wind . . Look away and you will see the far mountain ranges . . covered in white snow caps . . many miles away . . You can see them clearly in the distance . . Beautiful patches of white snow . . against the blue and green background . . of the Earth . . But you are not going there now . . Perhaps, another time . .

Let yourself slowly drift through the branches of the elm trees . . and the oak trees . . Tall and majestic . . You are settling down into the top of . . a great elm tree, with its mighty . . spreading branches . . Where birds flutter past in darting flashes . . Chipmunks and squirrels . . find food to store for the winter . . And there . . far below . . you can hear and see where a gurgling brook trickles . . with singing waters . . Winding through the forest grasses . . far, far below . .

You are drifting freely now . . Slowly rocking on the winds . . like the leaves . . Drifting slowly, to the left . . then to the right . . Back and forth, as you slowly, gently, sail down . . down Deep . . deeper . . Look down, to the green grasses of the forest . . far below . . Slowly you are turning . . Circling . . through the huge branches of the trees . . Drifting in high circles . . Swaying to the right . . Sailing upward, with the leaves in the wind, around you . . Then to the left . . Circling . . circling . . among the drifting leaves . . The winds carry you gently in a downward motion . . Drifting and circling . . Down . . down . . Deep . . Very Deep . . Until at last . . your feet touch the soft, green grasses . . covering the earth . . Here, you will find peace and tranquility . . Complete relaxation . . Here, you are as one, with all that God has created . . for your absolute enjoyment . .

There are no sounds . . besides my voice . . and the noise of rushing waters in the distant brook . . flowing through the forest . . Any other sounds will only support you . . in your relaxed state . . Your mind and body are open to complete trust . . Trust in the power of God . . Your mind is very relaxed now . . and open to receive the beneficial suggestions I will soon give you . . We will stay . . in this beautiful place, for a while . . For here, there is much to experience . . and later, to recall . .

Enjoy this time . . here in this beautiful garden . . where birds chatter happily in the trees . . The animals roam freely . . without fear . . with nothing to disturb their natural way of life . . The swaying grasses in the meadow are filled with colorful flowers . . blown by the soft winds of springtime . . The high alpine peaks glisten on the distant horizon . . A peaceful love is in your heart . . and in your memories . . You are not alone . . You are sharing this moment . . with that one special person . . whom you have recently lost . . Love is here . . with you now . . I want you to take this time . . to share . . together . . Just the two of you . . before we continue . . (take 3 minutes)

Continue inhaling DEEPLY . . and exhaling, slowly now . . I want you to drift into an even DEEPER . . DEEPER . . state of relaxation . . By permitting your mind and body to relax . . through your own ability to concentrate . . you will notice . . after the session is over . . that you feel much better . . mentally, physically and spiritually . . Right now, you can feel the power of your own mind working . . And you can feel that energy, surging up within you . . (pause)

You know that you are a spiritual being, created by God . . And, as such . . you are blessed with intelligence and wisdom that can release you from anxiety and confusion . . You will trust the love and goodness of God to help solve every problem in your life . . You feel the love and goodness of God, setting you free, from all mistakes of the past . . The love of God is releasing you from guilt and is cleansing your mind, your body and your soul . . You are blessed . . What you are feeling now is a pure stream of God's love . . flowing through you . . Cleansing, healing, purifying and restoring your mind and body . . A divine order is being established in all of your concerns . . Concentrate on that pleasant feeling of relaxation . . Your mind and body are relaxing more and more . . You are learning to be relaxed and calm . . and will continue using these principles of relaxation . . during your daily life . . By learning to relax . . as you are doing now . . you will experience a happier, healthier, more enjoyable life . . than ever before . . You are noticing a feeling of energy and vitality . . flowing through your entire body . . Cleansing . . healing . . purifying and rejuvenating your body . . gradually and perfectly . . You are

291

feeling a good response in your body . . as you are being strengthened and renewed with energy, vitality and enthusiasm . . It is because you are needed . . You are important to many . . You are loved . . And you are fulfilling God's plan and purpose . . in your own . . very special way . . Every day your self-confidence keeps increasing . . And you continue living your life with a greater feeling of poise, peacefulness and joy . . You are open and receptive to all of the good that flows into your life . . You are becoming more perfectly attuned . . to the beauty . . and to the harmony . . of the universe . . You are filled with a sense of well-being and joy . . And I am so proud to know you as . . my friend . .

EMERGE

HEALING WITH MIND POWER

You will continue drifting into a deeper, DEEPER . . more peaceful, hypnotic state . . of relaxation . . as I give you suggestions and instructions . . that will cause you to experience a continuous improvement . . physically . . mentally . . and spiritually . .

As you submerge yourself, going deeper . . and DEEPER . . You can notice how you are becoming . . even more relaxed and settled now . . Concentrate on that pleasant feeling of relaxation . . Your mind and body are relaxing more and more . .

All tension is leaving your body . . And all stress and strain are moving out of your system . . as though they are being drawn out of your body . . with a powerful magnetic energy . .

You are learning to be relaxed and calm . . and will continue using these principles of relaxation . . during your daily life . . By learning to relax . . as you are doing now . . you will experience a happier, healthier, more enjoyable life . . and a more productive life . . than ever before . .

You will soon notice a feeling of energy and vitality . . flowing through your entire body . . Cleansing . . healing . . purifying and rejuvenating your body . . gradually and perfectly . .

We keep hearing on radio and television . . about 'Faith Healers' . . as though they are the chosen few . . who have been granted special powers from God . . to heal the sick and the handicapped . . But in reality . . we all have that 'special' power and energy within each of us . . to be healed completely . . from any illness, disease and physical handicap . . from within ourselves . .

There are some words that are credited to Jesus, in which he said . . "The Kingdom of God . . is within you" . .

Perhaps that gives us an explanation . . for the fact that we all have a power within us . . that is capable of cleansing, healing, purifying and restoring our body . . in a perfect way . .

The more research we do . . the more we find that it is our own mind . . that directs the healing energies of our body . . So, the important thing for you to realize is . . that you have a tremendous power within you . . that can renew, restore and heal your body . . completely and perfectly . . And all those healing energies are all directed . . by your mind . .

293

Your subconscious mind has capabilities . . far beyond what you have been consciously aware of . . And your mind is remembering everything it needs to remember . . to cause the healing energies of your body to function properly . . to heal your body completely . .

All limitations are being lifted . . And you are being revitalized with increased energy and inner strength . . Your body, mind and soul are continuing to function . . in a more harmonious way . .

Self-realization and understanding are opening up within you . . A feeling of peace is moving through every part of your being . . instilling greater awareness of the power of God within you . .

You are letting go completely now . . And you are more aware of the feeling of peacefulness . . blanketing your whole body . . A feeling of complete calm . . like a blessing from God . . That calmness and peacefulness will continue . . to enshroud you . . during your daily life . .

When you were young, you played a game with other children . . drawing squares on the sidewalk with chalk . . Pretending the chalk marks were big walls . . and no one could touch you because you were 'safe' . . once you were inside your boxed-in area . .

Many people do similar things . . which cause them to develop illness' and physical problems . . They allow negative ideas into their conscious mind . . Those negative thoughts and ideas cause them to become ill . . or physically handicapped . . And they believe they cannot be healed . .

During the time Jesus was on Earth . . He met many people who had become imprisoned . . in their own minds . . by physical problems . . until He helped them to understand . . that they didn't need to remain imprisoned by their physical defects . . He met blind people, deaf people, cripples and sufferers . . from all types of diseases and illnesses . . And he taught them to understand the healing powers . . of their own minds . . And taught them to replace their negative, unloving thoughts and ideas . . with thoughts and ideas of love . . and joy . . and peace . .

As they developed love and understanding . . and a good, positive way of thinking . . the healing powers of their bodies were able to function properly . . and they were healed completely . . They discovered there was nothing keeping them from being healed . . They had merely been imprisoned by the negative thoughts and ideas . . that had entered their minds . . And it were those thoughts, ideas and beliefs . . which had caused them to become sick . . paralyzed or blind . . or to experience other types of diseases and physical handicaps . .

Jesus understood the powers of the mind . . and He realized that their illness' and handicaps . . were caused by their own beliefs . . He taught them how they could be released . . from their self-made prisons . . As they began to believe that healing was possible . . with positive thoughts of love . . the natural healing powers of their own bodies were released . . and they were cured . .

Many people today yet suffer from various types of diseases and physical problems . . because they do not understand the operations of the mind . . The flow of the mind can cause illness . . just as it can cause them to be healed . . Without sufficient teaching . . it is hard to understand that improper information entering the mind . . causes disharmony in the body . . And that renewing their mind with good, uplifting thoughts . . instills harmony in the body . . and enables the body to heal itself . .

Healing your body is simple . . once you understand these true facts . . So, I am going to give you some suggestions now . . that will change the improper information in your mind . . and renew your mind with thoughts of health, joy, happiness and love . .

Your subconscious mind understands that your body . . was intended to be healthy . . And that it only becomes unhealthy . . because of misunderstandings in your mind . . Your mind is reviewing that misunderstood information . . Assessing it . . And is realizing there is no need for you to continue experiencing that problem . . Because there is no need for you . . to retain that negative information . . which you have absorbed . . into your conscious mind . . in your past . .

As soon as your mind has resolved that problem . . and knows the changes have started . . that will cause you to be healed completely . . one of the fingers on your right hand will lift up towards the ceiling . . and will remain up until I tell it to go back down . . (Wait for response)

You are feeling the healing processes of your body at work . . And you are realizing that you . . are in control . . of those healing energies . . The power which is flowing . . within your own body . . You have seen healing powers at work . . The mysterious curing power . . that heals cuts and broken bones . . So, you know that your body has the power to heal . . But more than just the obvious . . it can heal any damage, disease or sickness you ever experience . . And you are letting that healing energy flow freely now . . Let it continue . . (Pause)

295

As you continue drifting . . into a DEEPER and DEEPER hypnotic state . . I want you to visualize yourself with a healthy, strong and beautiful body . . Exactly the way you want your body to be . . See yourself clearly . . Project that image of yourself . . with a perfect body . . Exactly the way you want your body to be . . in every way . . As you continue to think of yourself . . the way you want your body to be . . your subconscious mind is accepting that image . . and is causing all of your body processes to function perfectly . . And is healing your body completely . .

Each night, just before you go to sleep . . Close your eyes and think of yourself . . just the way you want yourself to be . . with a healthy, strong and perfect body . . As you continue to do that . . each night . . you keep reinforcing that image in your mind . . And your own mind causes you . . to develop . . a perfectly healthy body . . You will also find your self-confidence and self-acceptance . . growing stronger . . And you will continue improving in all areas of your life . . physically, mentally, emotionally and spiritually . .

You will have the knowledge to solve every problem that comes up in your life . . You will look forward to each day of your life with anticipation . . And you will find that each day will bring you greater happiness and joy . . You will arise each morning, feeling rested and refreshed . . And you'll continue having more energy, more strength . . and more vitality . .

All of the suggestions and instructions I have given you . . are now in the storehouse of your mind . . And they are already working to keep improving your health . . and your way of life . . They are intended to influence your thoughts, your feelings and your actions . . in a positive, helpful way . . You will notice some very positive improvements . . And you will be very pleased . . with your continuing progress . . (pause)

In a moment, you will be, once again, in a normal state of mind . . Now, I am going to count from ONE to FIVE . . and when you hear the number, FIVE . . you will open your eyes and be wide awake . . feeling refreshed and wonderful . . For you are a very wonderful person . .

EMERG

You are deeply relaxed now and I want to talk with you . . about your health . . Both physical and mental . . There has been a tremendous amount of research in recent years . . with regard to the affects the mind has on the physical body . . The results of that research has caused . . the opening of many holistic health centers . . and hypnotherapy clinics . . all over the country . .

Research in medical schools and universities has shown . . there are better ways of overcoming illness and physical problems . . than has ever been achieved with medicine or surgery . . The researchers have found . . that there are approximately ten natural methods . . that can help to cure . . all types of disease and illness . . which can realign and rejuvenate every part of the body . . And it has been found that . . hypnotherapy . . is one of the best techniques . . for getting those various natural methods to function, automatically . .

I am going to mention those ten natural methods . . for achieving and maintaining perfect health . . And then I will give you suggestions . . that will get your subconscious mind to cooperate . . and cause you to use them to heal your body completely . . Thus, keeping you healthy and strong . .

The first method for attaining natural health is, simply, to eat properly . . The second is taking the right vitamins for your body . . And third is getting the minerals your body needs . . Fourth is getting the proper proteins . . And fifth is the importance of getting sufficient potassium . . Sixth is getting the right kind of exercise . . Seventh is achieving adequate sexual fulfillment . . Eighth is getting enough laughter, yes . . Ninth is having plenty of time for relaxation . . And the Tenth method for attaining natural health is . . getting the proper amount of sleep . . that your body requires . . All ten of these items are important . . not only for healing the body . . but for keeping it healthy . .

Eating properly, of course, helps provide the nourishment your body needs . . to strengthen muscles, ligaments and bones . . And since it is important for your health . . to eat properly . . your subconscious mind is causing you . . to desire, select and eat foods . . that are beneficial to you . .

You will eat lean meats, eggs . . and other foods each day . . that provide your body with the correct amount of proteins that it needs . . You will also want to eat fresh vegetables, fruits . . and other foods that supply the vitamins and minerals needed . . to keep your body healthy . . And you will take the time to learn more about . . vitamins and minerals . . so you will know and understand about the proper supplements you need to take each day . . And to get the proper amounts your body needs . . to keep it healthy . . You will also enjoy eating bran and other dietary fibers . . which will cause your elimination system to always function properly . . And will keep waste materials cleansed out of your body . . through the natural processes of your elimination system . . Along with eating properly . . and getting the vitamins, minerals, proteins and potassium . . your body needs each day . . you will want to be sure to drink plenty of water . . to maintain a good fluid content in your body . . Water aids your digestive and elimination systems . . It helps regulate your body temperature . . It keeps your kidneys healthy . . Keeps your urinary tract clean . . and washes bacteria and other impurities out of your body . . through the normal processes of your elimination system . . So, you will enjoy drinking lots of water each day . .

Many medical researchers have come to the conclusion that . . exercise is absolutely necessary . . to maintain a healthy body . . That's one of the reasons so many people are out jogging . . Of course, it isn't necessary to go out jogging . . to get the exercise your body needs . . Walking also produces good results . . Square dancing, regularly . . Bowling, regularly . . Playing golf, playing tennis, swimming . . and many of the other comparable activities . . are all very beneficial for your overall health improvement and maintenance . . Good things happen in your body during exercise . . It causes your metabolism to function better . . The movements of your muscles help pump the blood through your circulatory system . . It strengthens your heart . . It enables your muscles to absorb more oxygen by increasing your lung capacity . . And, exercise helps your entire physical structure to function better . . So, you want to take part in a good exercise program that is enjoyable to you . . And you will find that it will rejuvenate your body . . to continue becoming healthier, firmer and more youthful . .

You are born with sexual needs . . and those needs continue throughout your life . . Most people have no idea of the importance . . of achieving sexual fulfillment . . in order to maintain a healthy body and mind . . Your sexual urges are normal and natural . . And, for your well being, they should not be suppressed . . God created your body so that it can function, sexually . . And God doesn't create something . . and then forbid it from being used . . So, you will be pleased, as your natural sexual urges and desires come into your conscious awareness . . And you

298

will enjoy the pleasures of fulfilling those desires . . in a normal, natural way . . with your chosen partner . . Expressing sexual urges and desires . . releases tension in your body . . And it causes your body activities to keep becoming healthier . . Functioning more perfectly . . Your subconscious mind is causing you to come up with creative ways . . of achieving sexual satisfaction and enjoyment . . with your chosen partner . . Another reason that sexual satisfaction improves your health . . is that it provides a way of expressing love and affection that is very special . . Especially when there is a strong emotional attachment . . or a bonding, of emotional love . . It is one of the means that God has made available . . to experience a union of oneness . . with your chosen partner . . So, you will continue enjoying sexual relations . . more and more . . And you'll be pleasantly surprised . . at the way it will cause your health to continue improving . .

Medical researchers have also found that laughter . . is very important for the health of your body . . And it is interesting to note . . that even the bible says . . "Laughter is a good medicine" . . Scientifically conducted experiments have revealed that . . laughter causes the brain to produce hormones called, catecholamines . . And that causes a release of endorphins into the system . . which is a natural healing agent . . Laughter also exercises the chest and improves the heartbeat . . so the heart can more easily pump blood . . and oxygen . . into the circulatory system . . Some have gone so far as to claim . . that laughter increases the life span . . I believe that is true . .

And next we come to relaxation and sleep . . It is a fact that relaxation . . and sleep . . helps the body to rejuvenate itself . . You will be wise to set aside some time each day to relax . . Meditating is a good way to relax . . And vacationing away from your normal work routine . . is a way of relaxing . . And you will want to get a proper amount of sleep . . Breathing deeply and exhaling slowly a few times after lying down . . will help your body to relax . . Making it easier for you to drift into a comfortable state of sleep . . You should also keep regular bed time hours . . And even though it is good to take time each day to relax . . it has been found that you will have more energy and vitality . . and will sleep better at night . . if you avoid taking a nap during the day . .

All of these methods will cause your health to keep improving . . You will be pleasantly surprised at the way they will all work together . . Doing one makes the others easier . . Doing one causes you to automatically do the others . . following a program to a healthier, happier life . . EMERGE

DEMONSTRATE 'HEALING HANDS' PROCESS PRIOR TO HYPNOSIS.
REF. 096 Prescript.

You will continue drifting into a deeper, DEEPER . . more peaceful, relaxing hypnotic state . . As you continue relaxing now . . your conscious awareness will keep narrowing down . . and your subconscious mind will be hearing . . only to the words I am saying to you . .

You can hear the soothing sounds in the room . . but they will not distract you . . and it becomes less and less important . . to consciously try to listen to the words I am saying to you . . Your subconscious mind is receiving my suggestions and instructions . . as other sounds and noises gradually fade away . . into the distance . . And it is easy for your mind to listen to what I say . .

The suggestions and instructions I am giving you . . will cause your subconscious mind to work out a solution . . to that problem . . But for now you are waiting . . and continuing to relax even more . . And you are continuing to experience a more pleasant and calm feeling of relaxation . . moving slowly through your body . .

As you go deeper now . . deeper and DEEPER . . you are approaching a perfect level of relaxation . . that is enabling your subconscious mind to review . . examine and explore . . the information in the storehouse of your mind . . that has been causing you to have that problem . . And then, your subconscious mind can assess and understand that information . . from a different point of view . . than what you had . . when the information first went into your mind . . And your mind can resolve that problem completely . . and cause the changes to be made . . that are needed . . to heal your body perfectly . .

You are realizing that being hypnotized . . can be one of the most pleasant and most helpful . . experiences of your life . . And it can automatically help you in many different ways . .

Being in a state of relaxation . . automatically causes your body processes to function at a higher level . . And that enables the healing energies of your body . . to function perfectly . . And it magnifies the power to remedy many ailments . . that you may not even be aware of . . So, you will find that your health keeps improving . . more and more each day . .

Being hypnotized will also improve your character . . by removing any features of your character that you wish to have removed . . And by strengthening those features of your character . . which you feel are more desirable . . This will enable you to direct all of your future efforts more effectively . . And will enable you to be more successful . . and more prosperous . . in all other areas of your life . . And it will enable you to live a happier, healthier, more full and more productive life . . than ever before . . So you are really happy that you decided to have these hypnotic sessions . .

Each time I hypnotize you . . you will go into a deeper . . DEEPER . . more peaceful and more detached state . . The suggestions I give you . . will go into the storehouse of your subconscious mind . . and your mind will cause them to begin to work automatically . . And you will continue improving more and more each day . .

Now, it is time for you to think about the problem we are concerned with today . . Concentrate on the area of your body . . that you want to be healed . . (Pause and observe)

I want you to use your imagination now . . I want you to visualize that area of your body . . the way you want it to be . . after it is healed perfectly . . (Pause) Now, if you can reach that part of your body with your hands . .
I want you to open your eyes long enough to energize your hands . . the way I instructed you to . . (PAUSE) . . Now, place the palms (finger tips) of your hands . . on that part of your body . . which is to be healed . . You can feel the energy flow . . from the palms of your hands . . into your body . . You will gradually feel a healing warmth . . flowing through your skin . . The healing processes of your body are working . . right now . . And will continue functioning properly . . to heal your body completely . . You may also do this at home . . Close your eyes now . .

Your muscles, tendons, ligaments and nerves . . are relaxing more and more . . as the healing energies permeate your body . . where it is needed the most . . You are continuing to feel more comfortable and more at ease . . Your body is responding to the normal, natural healing energies . . that are working . . to restore and rejuvenate . . and strengthen your body . . in a perfect way . .

The cells of your body are alive . . and know how to perform their tasks . . of sending nourishment to every part of your body, where it is needed . . They cause your fingernails and toenails to continue growing . . They cause your hair to continue growing . . And they keep all other parts of your body functioning properly . . The cells of your body know how to cooperate with each other . . and conduct their activities properly . . to restore your body to its normal, healthy condition . . Your subconscious mind is directing the mind of each cell . . to cooperate in full harmony and unison . . with all other cells . . to heal your body completely and perfectly . .

Your mind is being renewed with positive thoughts and ideas . . that are causing you to become stronger and healthier each day . . Each day, your nerves will be more relaxed and steady . . You will continue developing more strength . . more energy . . and more vitality . . And your thinking will be more stable, more settled . . And you will find that your conditions are greatly improved . . in all areas of your life . .

Continue to relax a few minutes longer . . Relax . . while your subconscious mind absorbs . . everything we have discussed here today . .
(Pause)

I am going to begin my count now . . And when you hear the count of FIVE . . you will open your eyes and be wide awake . . feeling refreshed and rejuvenated . . And ready for your next challenge . . In a moment, you will be . . once again . . in a normal state of mind . .

Now, I am going to count from ONE to FIVE . .

ONE - Coming up now . . Feeling rested and refreshed . . You will remember everything with a clear understanding . .
TWO - Coming up a little higher now . . You are connected to your inner strength . . Supporting only your best interest . .
THREE - Everything I have told you is true . . And is happening now . . You will benefit greatly from this experience . .
FOUR - Becoming more aware of your body . . Let your hands and feet move a little now . . And . .
FIVE - You may open your eyes now . . Inhale and stretch . . You are doing very well . .

075 Prescript.   HEALTH - RESTORE
(Follow DEEP Relaxation)

NOTE : IN WORKING WITH A CLIENT TO HELP HIM OR HER TO OVERCOME ANY KIND OF ILLNESS, DISEASE OR HANDICAP, YOU WANT TO USE ONE OF THE TECHNIQUES FOR UNCOVERING THE UNCONSCIOUS CAUSE (S) OF THE PROBLEM. ONCE THE CAUSE HAS BEEN IDENTIFIED, YOU THEN ASK THE SUBCONSCIOUS MIND IF THERE IS ANY REASON THE PROBLEM NEEDS TO CONTINUE. ONCE YOU GET A "NO" ANSWER, THEN ASK FOR A FINGER TO LIFT UP, WHEN THE SUBCONSCIOUS MIND KNOWS CHANGES HAVE STARTED AND THE CLIENT IS GOING TO BE HEALED COMPLETELY. THE PRESCRIPTIONS THAT FOLLOW WILL WORK BEST AFTER THE CLIENT HAS BEEN RELEASED FROM THE UNDERLYING CAUSE OF THE PROBLEM. BUT THEY ALSO CAN BE USED DURING THE SESSIONS IN WHICH THE CAUSE IS BEING UNCOVERED.

The suggestions and instructions that I am giving you now . . are going into the storehouse of your mind . . And your own subconscious mind will cause them . . to begin working immediately . . wherever they are needed in your body . .

Even though you are not consciously aware of it . . the healing processes of your body continue functioning at all times . . They are continuously; nourishing tissues, strengthening muscles, repairing and replacing cells . . keeping your body temperatures stabilized . . keeping your heart pumping and causing your blood to continue circulating . . cleansing waste materials and impurities out from your body . . through the natural processes of your elimination system . . And conducting many other activities . . that we normally take for granted . .

Those processes are continuously working . . to keep your body healthy and strong . . They are normal and natural . . They keep functioning, twenty four hours a day . . causing all organs, glands, cells, atoms and molecules within your body . . to continue working in perfect harmony with each other . .

Scientists have found that each cell of your body . . performs functions that the world's most outstanding chemists, scientists and physicians . . have not been able to duplicate . . And all of those activities in your body . . are being guided and directed . . by your own subconscious mind . .

Imprints, impressions, thoughts and ideas . . have been entering your mind . . since your soul first came into existence . . And your mind

303

operates from the accumulation of . . all the information . . that is stored there . . Whether the information is correct . . or is . . incorrect . . If the information is incorrect . . your mind can review it . . and understand it better now . . from a more knowledgeable, more mature point of view . . And with such information corrected . . it can restore your body to perfect health . . This means that your own mind . . can cause your body processes to function properly . . And produce healing energies that heal your body perfectly . . And you will help your mind to produce these healing energies . . by thinking positive, pleasant, uplifting thoughts about yourself . . And by imagining yourself as being vital, healthy and strong . . That causes your mind to activate the processes of your body . . And to renew and rejuvenate every cell, every atom and every molecule . . so they all function perfectly . .

The fact that your mind controls your body is not a new concept . . Thomas Edison did research on the subject, many years ago . . And he concluded that, "Every cell of the body, thinks" . . He realized that every cell of the body is in possession of its own mind . . And receives directions from . . the subconscious mind . .

And the bible says the same thing . . It says, "As we think in our mind, so we are." In other words . . thoughts and ideas, impressions and imprints, made in our mind, cause our body to respond . . And they can cause us to be sickly . . or healthy . . depending on the way our mind has received the information . .

And that is the reason why . . your own mind . . can generate every medicine needed by your body . . And can restore, rebuild, strengthen and heal . . every part of your body in a perfect way . .

If your body was solid flesh and bone . . it might be difficult to understand that the mind has control over it . . and can heal it completely and perfectly . . But your body is not solid . . Scientists tell us that it is more than eighty per cent liquid . . Even your bones are soft . . and pliable and porous . . And are penetrated by capillaries of blood . . And scientists tell us that . . if the body was condensed into actual, solid mass . . it would be no larger than the head of a pin . .

Since your body is more than 80 percent liquid . . your subconscious mind has the power to direct the flow of healing energies . . wherever they are needed . . to restore your body to perfect health . .

The strongest force of energy your body possesses . . is your own mind . . And when you have been experiencing illness or disease . . or any kind of physical handicap . . it can be changed . .

And your body can be transformed into a healthy body . . by renewing your mind . . with thoughts and feelings of confidence, good health, happiness and spiritual love . . That is one of the meanings of the words . . in the bible . . that say, "You can be transformed . . by the renewing of your mind" . . And that is what you are doing now . . The sessions that we are having . . are permitting your mind to be renewed . . with healthy thoughts and positive impressions . . that restore your body to perfect health . .

Sometimes, people get the idea that God . . made them sick . . It's his way of punishing them . . Or He has some other reason for wanting them to be sick . . They don't realize that . . having thoughts like that in their mind . . may be one of the causes for their illness . . God is not a neurotic being . . with a split personality . . wanting some people to be healthy and others, to be sick . . If God wanted people to be sick . . it would be useless to take an aspirin, to get rid of a headache . . If God wanted us to have a headache, and we got rid of it by taking the aspirin . . it would mean, we must have outsmarted God . . There would be nothing we could do . . And nothing any physician could do . . to make us well or keep us from getting sick . . if God wanted us to be sick . .

So, sickness, disease, cancer, polio, aids and other physical handicaps . . are not caused by God . . They are caused by imprints, impressions and beliefs . . that go into our mind . . And you can be well by changing those thoughts and beliefs . . to thoughts of good health, happiness and love . .

And that is one of the meanings of the words in the bible that say . . "Do not be conformed to this world . . but be transformed . . by the renewal of your mind . . that you may prove what is the will of God . . What is good and acceptable and perfect" . . Romans 12 : 2.

So, your mind is being renewed by good thoughts and ideas . . that are causing the processes of your body to function properly . .

Every cell of your body is learning to do its work . . in a more perfect way . . And will continue rejuvenating . . and strengthening . . every part of your body . .

You feel yourself growing stronger and healthier . . The improvements are progressive . . Each day, your health keeps improving . . Your self-confidence, self-acceptance and self-esteem continue increasing . . Your energy is increasing . . Your nerves are becoming more relaxed and steady . . You will be more stable, more settled . . and will be doing everything in a relaxed way . . This is already working in your body because . . you want it to work . . And your subconscious mind is cooperating with your conscious desire to be healthy and strong . .

Your entire organism is responding well . . And you will be happy as you notice how your life changes for the better . . And how your health . . is continuing to show improvement . .

Take some time each day to sit down or . . lie down in a comfortable position . . And then concentrate your mind on good, uplifting thoughts . . of health, happiness, success and prosperity . . Imagine your body as being perfectly healthy and strong . . And your mind will cause your health to continue improving, more and more . . every day . . Each day, your nerves will be more relaxed and steady . . You will continue developing more strength . . more energy . . and more vitality . . And your thinking will be more stable, more settled . . more calm . . And you will find that you are greatly improved . . in all areas of your life . .

Continue to relax a few minutes longer . . while your subconscious mind absorbs everything we have discussed here today . . (Pause)

I am going to begin my count now . . And when you hear the count of FIVE . . you will open your eyes and be wide awake . . feeling refreshed and rejuvenated . . and ready for your next challenge . . In a moment, you will be, once again, in a normal state of mind . .

Now, I am going to count from ONE to FIVE . . When you hear the count of five, you may open your eyes . .

ONE - TWO - THREE - FOUR - FIVE -

You are feeling very relaxed now . . and you are doing very well . . I want you to go a little deeper . . With each breath you breath in, you will go deeper . . DEEPER . . and DEEPER . . As you exhale . . you will relax more . . Every breath you exhale . . you will relax more . . as you go deeper . . and DEEPER . . Just relax . . RELAX . .

It is your God-given, rightful ability to hear perfectly . . The Bible tells us that your body is a temple of God . . And God did not create anything . . with the intention of . . not having it work perfectly . . Your ears were created for the purpose of hearing . . Therefore, you have a God-given right to be able to hear clearly and distinctly . .

Every part of your body has a specific purpose . . Your heart pumps blood through your circulatory system . . Your circulatory system carries oxygen and nourishment . . into every part of your body, where it is needed . . and keeps impurities cleansed out of your system . . Your digestive system processes the food you eat . . separating the nourishment from the waste materials . . Your elimination system cleanses the waste materials out of your body . . in an easy, natural way . . And all of your glands, organs, muscles, nerves, ligaments, tendons, bones and other parts of your body . . have their own specific purposes . . And they all function properly . .

Just as other parts of your body have their own specific purposes . . your ears are made for hearing . . And just as you want all of your other body processes to function properly . . you want your ears to function properly . .

Your subconscious mind has the important job of . . directing the various activities of your body . . Any time some part of your body is not functioning the way it should . . your subconscious mind can review the information in your mind . . and understand it from a different perspective . . than what it had when the information first went into your mind . . And your subconscious mind can work out the proper solution . . and cause you to experience very pleasant changes . . And restore the various parts of your ears . . that may be damaged . . so that you hear perfectly . .

Your subconscious mind is accepting the suggestions and instructions I am giving you . . and is causing them to begin working immediately . . And is directing the living cells in your ears to function properly . . Restoring and rejuvenating the condition of your ears . . beginning at the level of cells . .

and molecules . . So that all parts of your ears are restored to perfection . . And you will notice your hearing continuing to improve . .

Medical scientists have found that . . ideas implanted in the mind . . can cause various types of physical problems . . to develop in the body . . They call that 'psychosomatic' illness . . It has also been found, through extensive research . . that hypnosis is a method which can be used . . to help correct those misunderstandings in the mind . . And with those corrections . . the mind then causes the processes of the body . . to function properly . . And heal and restore that part of the body perfectly . .

You understand that your body was created to keep itself healthy . . If you get a bruise on your body or cut your skin . . or break a bone . . the normal processes of your body function properly to heal the skin or bone . .

Your ears are made up of some very intricate parts . . And your mind knows how to cause the parts of your ears to function properly . . Your mind directs the functioning processes to heal your body . . and will cause your hearing to continue improving . . until it is perfect, as it should be . .

Every time you look at water . . you will become relaxed and calm . . When you are calm . . and peaceful inside . . that will enable your body processes to continue functioning more perfectly . . and will restore your ability to hear more perfectly . .

Even the nerves and tiny bone tissues that may have been damaged . . are being repaired and restored . . Just as easily as your skin is restored . . when it becomes damaged . .

Your subconscious mind is accepting these suggestions and instructions . . to heal your ears . . You are experiencing the processes of your body changing . . in a pleasant way . . And your hearing is improving rapidly . . You will experience a continuous improvement in your hearing . . The progress in your ability to hear clearly . . will become more noticeable each day . . You will be aware of the improvements . . no matter how slight they may seem, at first . . And your confidence will continue growing stronger . . as you become more aware of your ability to hear, clearly and distinctly . .

Each day, you will keep hearing more and more clearly . . It will give you a feeling of personal satisfaction . . You will be very pleased and happy as you become more aware . . of what you are accomplishing . .

The Bible says . . "You can be transformed by the renewing of your mind" . . That is what you are doing . . by permitting yourself to be hypnotized . . Your thoughts and ideas about hearing . . are becoming more positive . . And your subconscious mind is causing the processes of your body . . to function properly . . and will restore your hearing perfectly . . And so . . your hearing will continue improving . . until it is clear and perfect . .

When you awaken from the hypnotic state . . you will feel relaxed and well . . You will have confidence that your hearing is already improving . . You will know that your subconscious mind is cooperating . . By causing these suggestions and instructions to work . . And your ears are already in the process . . of being completely . . and perfectly healed . .

It is a cycle of progress that keeps increasing . . Each day your hearing will improve noticeably . . and you will soon be hearing clearly and perfectly . .

I want you to continue to relax a little longer . . as your subconscious mind absorbs all that we have talked about . . Just relax . . and in a moment we will end this session . . And soon, you will be wide awake, feeling refreshed and ready for a new challenge . . Just relax now . . (Pause)

I am going to begin my count now, from ONE to FIVE . . And when you hear the count of FIVE . . you will open your eyes, feeling aware of everything . . You will be fully awake and alert . . Rested and relaxed . . And you will become more fully awake with each number that I say . .

ONE . . TWO . . THREE . .FOUR . . and FIVE . . Open your eyes now and . . take a deep breath . .

The fact that you are permitting yourself to be hypnotized . . indicates that you believe hypnosis can help you . . And that's one of the keys to improving your heart condition . . Permitting yourself to be hypnotized . . enables your subconscious mind to review . . examine and explore . . the information in your mind . . that has been causing the problem . . And then, your subconscious mind can work out the solution . . and resolve the problem . . and heal your heart perfectly . .

For many years . . specialists have studied, what affects . . the mind has on the body . . and they have found that the subconscious level of the mind . . controls every activity of the body . . They have found that negative thoughts or ideas . . or misunderstood information . . can go into the mind . . and cause various types of physical problems to develop in the body . . They call that, Psychosomatic illness . . And they have also found that what the mind can cause . . the mind can also cure . . by replacing the negative thoughts with positive suggestions . .

Hypnosis provides a means of renewing your mind . . with good suggestions . . that cause the processes of the body to function harmoniously . . And that causes your heart to keep functioning more perfectly each day . . Your subconscious mind is a storehouse of information . . that has gone into your mind since your soul came into existence . . And it can use that information to work out a solution to your problem . . and heal your heart completely . .

You have within you . . all the information needed . . to resolve that problem with your heart . . and to heal your heart completely . . So, I want your subconscious mind to begin reviewing . . examining and recalling . . from the storehouse of your mind . . all information that is related to the problem with your heart . . Specifically, that which may be the cause . . for the problem . .

Your mind has accumulated much more information since that first dose of misinformation occurred . . and can understand it better now . . from a different point of view . . And your mind can realize . . that there is no reason for you to need . . to continue experiencing that problem . .

Your mind can work out a solution . . that is pleasing to you . . and can cause the processes of your body to . . once again, function properly . . and heal your heart completely . .

As your mind is reviewing that information . . you are continuing to drift deeper . . and DEEPER . . into a hypnotic state . . And as you go even deeper, and become even more relaxed . . you are feeling powerful energies flowing throughout your body . . as the healing processes of your body begin working . . Let those feelings of energy continue . . Let them permeate your entire being . .

Your subconscious mind knows exactly what is needed . . to heal your heart . . and is causing those changes that are needed . . to take place . . You will notice the improvements . . and you will be pleased . . as your heart continues to function more perfectly . . each day . . And you will look forward to each new day . . with great anticipation . . For each day will be filled with radiance . . with joy . . with love and . . with happiness . .

Relax a few more minutes as your subconscious mind absorbs . . all that we have talked about . . (Pause)

(CONTINUE WITH ANOTHER 'HEALING' PRESCRIPTION.)

You are responding very well to everything I am saying . . And now you are ready for your inner mind . . to begin making proper adjustments in your body . . which will give you far greater pleasure and enjoyment . . than you have ever experienced before . .

Permitting yourself to be hypnotized lets your subconscious mind know . . that you sincerely want every part of your body to function properly . . so you will be healthy, virile and strong . . And will be able to experience true sexual satisfaction . . with your chosen partner . . You have made a wise decision . . And you will be pleased and happy . . that you have asked me to help you . . to overcome this sexual problem . .

You realize that the subconscious level of your mind controls all of the functions and activities of your body . . So the conscious level of your mind can continue relaxing . . as your subconscious mind responds . . to everything I say . .

Just relax . . and continue to listen to the soothing sounds . . from the tape recorder (Air Conditioner) . . You don't need to make any effort to listen to my voice . . because your subconscious mind will hear everything I say . . And will cause you to automatically respond . .

You know what it's like to daydream about something . . and not really be looking at anything . . And not really listening to anything . . And as you are daydreaming . . someone in the room may be talking . . but you don't notice what is being said . . Just as easily . . you can enjoy the comfort of being . . in a deep hypnotic state . . And later on, when you awaken . . you don't need to remember anything that happened . . while you were hypnotized . . And so, you will not . . remember anything that happened . . while you were hypnotized . .

Relax deeper now . . DEEPER . . Relax . . DEEPER and DEEPER . . Listen, easily, to the soothing sounds . . coming from the tape player . . And you can experience the feeling of drifting away . . Much like when you drift into a natural state of sleep . . Your subconscious mind will be hearing each word I say . . as your conscious mind relaxes . . enjoying the restful . . peaceful feeling . . of drifting . . floating your body . . just above your chair . . Just relax . . RELAX . .

There may be some sounds that you are not familiar with . . but you will find yourself enjoying it . . It feels good . . to let yourself go completely

312

. . Gently and easily . . you continue drifting into a deeper . . and DEEPER . . more comfortable state . . The music continues to play in the far background . . and an enchanting aroma . . comes to your senses . . Breath in that pleasant aroma . . It is sensual . . and pleasing . . As you hear one part of the music . . another piece may come to mind . . A piece . . that you can enjoy, over and over again . .

You don't need to pay attention to me . . Just give your attention to the enchanting aroma . . and the beautiful music . . in the background . . And you will begin to notice the wonderful sensations, pulsing . . all through your body . . It will seem like they are caressing . . every part of your body . . And it keeps becoming more enjoyable, more pleasurable . .

Just relax . . because your subconscious mind understands everything I say . . Even things that you don't understand . . Just relax and flow with it . . Your subconscious mind is going to give you some really wonderful . . sensual vibrations . . and sensations . . all over your body . . (pause)

Your entire body and organism is cooperating . . with everything I tell you . . Your subconscious mind understands . . that your sexual urges and desires . . are normal and natural . . It is one of the ways God has provided for you . . to experience a union of oneness . . and express yourself . . through love and affection . . You will be pleased . . as the natural urges of your body keep increasing . . and you will continue to enjoy these sensations . . and a greater love-sex relationship . . with your chosen partner . .

We are going to help you, once again, be in total control . . of your sex life . . providing you with the support you need . . to get . . and to keep . . an erection of your penis . . Allowing you and your partner to enjoy long lasting . . sexual relations . . The problems you have experienced may have been physical . . or psychological . . Where even attempting to have sexual relations . . may have caused stress and anxiety . . But now, your past problems will be eliminated . .

Your conscious mind is very busy now . . listening to the sounds of the music . . While your subconscious mind is listening . . to everything . . that I say to it . .

And everything I say is very meaningful to your subconscious mind . . (pause) Your conscious mind is hearing only the music . . and your subconscious mind is free . . to limit itself . . to everything that I say . .

Whether you only experience erectile problems from time to time . . or you have chronic erectile failure . . all of the time . . If you cannot control . . when you ejaculate . . it will diminish your sexual drive . . And your libido will be depressed . . Causing you to feel more stressed . .

Your subconscious mind already has a complete understanding . . of how it fully supports your normal erectile function . . But it is not aware that you are having this problem . . Which is the reason we are here now . . To discuss the problem so that your subconscious mind . . can absorb your cause for concern . . and make the adjustments needed . . So that your body will function normally, once again . .

All erections begin in the brain . . in response to sexual stimulation . . Triggering the release of 'Dopamine' in the brain . . And sending neurotransmitters . . or signals . . to the penile nerves . . A chemical, Nitric Oxide . . is then released . . hydrolyzing the activation of chemical intermediaries . . This causes the smooth muscles inside the penis to relax . . The arteries widen . . and the penis fills with blood . . and becomes fully erect, firm and rigid . . for sexual intercourse . . And it remains that way until ejaculation takes place . . or until relations are completed . . Allowing you and your partner, opportunity to enjoy . . satisfying sexual relations, whenever you want . .

Your subconscious mind is now aware . . of your needs and desires . . and is making the adjustments needed . . to bring about the changes you desire . . Not only will you have the confidence to maintain strong and hard erections . . but your sexual drive and desire . . your libido . . will dramatically increase . . As will your ability to control the timing of your orgasm . . Your improved performance and staying power . . will surely amaze both you and your chosen sexual partner . .

From now on . . you will be in complete control of your sexual activities . . in a natural and satisfying way . . Weak, flimsy erections . . even full erection failure . . will be a thing of the past . .

Now you will benefit . . from the pleasures of extra-strong and long lasting erections . . Such as you are experiencing now . .

Your subconscious mind is really taking over control now . . And it will be very pleasing for you to experience . . And now, you are beginning to feel a sense of confidence . . and a sense of competence . . and sureness . . as sensations pulsate and flow . . all through your body . . that you haven't experienced for a long time . . You are feeling strong and . .

excited . . about it . . And you will be pleased that it will continue . . even after you awaken from the hypnotic state . .

I want you to do something for me now . . I want you to hold your (L/R) arm, straight out in front of you . . and make it rigid and stiff . . Make it just as stiff as you can make it . . Now, notice the feeling of energy and strength in that arm . . Okay, now, let the arm relax and feel very comfortable . . Put your hand on your lap again . .

Now, just by deciding . . to make your arm, rigid and stiff . . you were able to do that . . You controlled it easily . . just by listening to what I suggested, and responding . . Because you were willing to respond . . And just as easily . . you can control any other part of your body . . including your penis . . Okay, now I want you to hold your penis, straight out in front of you . . and make it rigid and stiff . . Just like you made your arm rigid and stiff . . Make it just as stiff as you possibly can . .

You understand that your sexual urges are normal . . Having sexual relations with your chosen partner . . is a body-soul expression . . of love and affection . . It is one of the ways God has granted us . . for the uniting of your body and soul . . with the body and soul of your chosen partner . .

Even after you awaken from the hypnotic state . . you will continue experiencing these wonderful feelings and sensations . . that accompany the powerful penile erections you will enjoy . . as your body is responding, normally and naturally . .

The cells of your body are alive . . and they know how to function properly . . The cells of your body know how . . to conduct their activities, normally . . and restore every part of your body . . to normal functioning . . The cells of your body are continuing . . to work in perfect harmony . . causing your metabolism . . your hormones . . and all of your glands and organs . . to function perfectly . .

You will continue experiencing . . pleasant physical sensations . . and very masculine erections . . of your penis . . resulting in a plentiful supply of semen . . to flow . . upon ejaculation . . Restoring, rejuvenating and revitalizing . . every part of your body . .

You want your body to function properly . . You want to enjoy, normal and natural, sexual sensations and stimulations . . You want to enjoy . . sexual satisfaction and fulfillment . . And your subconscious mind . . is cooperating . . with your wants and desires . . And is causing you to

315

experience . . arousing changes . . that are increasing your pleasure and enjoyment . . of sexual relations . . with the partner of your choice . .

Every time you are with the partner of your choice . . those wonderful feelings and sensations . . will keep growing stronger . . And you will realize that they are normal and natural . .

As the sexual parts of your body become more responsive and stronger . . this will cause all other parts of your body . . to keep becoming healthier . . and continue functioning, more perfectly . .

You will always enjoy having me hypnotize you . . Every time I hypnotize you . . you will enjoy it even more . . You will enjoy the wonderful, sensuous feelings of comfort, peacefulness . . tenderness . . and love . .

ERECT

As I am talking with you now . . you continue moving into a deeper
. . more peaceful . . more comfortable . . state of relaxation . . Deeper
. . Go DEEPER now . . and just relax . . RELAX . .

You subconscious mind is sensitive to everything I am saying to you . .
and is causing each suggestion to begin working immediately . . And
continue working automatically . . as you go about your daily affairs . .

Your eating habits . . and patterns of eating . . are improving more
each day . . You have an appetite that enables you . . to enjoy the
foods you eat . . So much that you are completely satisfied . . with
just a small amount of food . . And you eat only what your body
needs . . to keep you healthy and slender . . You eat just the right
amount needed by your body . . at that time . . then you stop . .
You know, intuitively . . when you've eaten the right amount . . to keep
your body slim and trim and healthy . .

You always chew your food thoroughly . . and then swallow it . . Your
food will always digest properly . . and your assimilation system
functions properly . . causing your body to make the best use of the
foods you eat . . to create blood, muscles, strength, energy and vitality . .

Digesting your food properly . . also causes your elimination system
to function normally . . so you have a normal, natural cleansing process
. . of the waste materials from your body . .

Every night, when you want to sleep . . you can easily drift into a deep,
peaceful state of sleep . . And sleep comfortably, until the time for you to
awaken . . You will always feel calm, peaceful and relaxed when you are
sleeping . . And you will awaken each morning, rested and refreshed . .

When you dream . . your dreams will always be pleasant . . And
when you awaken . . your mind will be alert . . You will feel healthy
and strong . . and look forward to the activities of the day . .

You will continue experiencing many other benefits . . Your will
power and self control keep increasing . . You will be happy and
cheerful . . You will be calm and relaxed in every situation or
circumstance . . that comes into your life . .

All of your body organs do their work correctly . . Your heart keeps
pumping properly . . And your circulatory system keeps functioning
perfectly . . Your lungs continue becoming cleaner and healthier . . and

doing their work better . . enabling you to always breath easily and freely . . Your stomach, intestines, liver, kidneys, your bladder and all of your glands . . perform their activities correctly . . Your digestive system, your metabolism and all other processes of your body . . are continuing to function as they should . .

Your self-esteem, self-reliance, self-acceptance and self-confidence . . keep growing stronger each day . . You'll have the needed confidence in yourself . . at work or in other activities . . And you're becoming more aware of the tremendous power, which is within you . . You realize that you are capable of accomplishing anything you decide to do . . You can set goals for yourself, and you have the ability to achieve those goals . . Whenever you have a task to perform . . you will think of it as being easy . . And you will work out the wisest way to accomplish it . . easily . .

(Follow this with another prescription with specific suggestions on what client wants to accomplish)

Now that you are calm and relaxed . . I want you to take three deep breaths . . and drift into a level of hypnosis that is similar to sleep . . Go ahead . . take your first deep breath . . You can reach that level by listening to the soothing sounds . . coming from the air conditioner (or tape player) . .

The subconscious level of your mind will listen only to my voice . . until we have completed this therapy session . . At that time, you will drift into a peaceful, natural state of sleep . . for five minutes . . Breathe deeply now . .

Because you want to sleep peacefully and calmly . . you will follow this routine, each night, when you are ready to go to sleep . . and you will awaken each morning, feeling rested and refreshed . .

You will begin by closing your eyes . . Then let the muscles in your upper eyelids relax . . to the best of your ability . . Let them keep relaxing . . until your eyelids feel like they want to remain shut . . When you have them completely relaxed . . test them to be sure they remain shut . . Then let them relax even more . . Let every muscle and every nerve in your eyelids . . become even more relaxed . . And then, allow that feeling of complete relaxation . . move through your entire body . . From your eyelids . . all the way down to the tips of your toes . .

As your eyelids . . and the muscles, tendons and ligaments in your body . . continue becoming more relaxed . . without even noticing it . . you will drift into a deep and peaceful . . restful . . very comfortable . . state of sleep . . While you are sleeping . . you will be relaxed and calm . . You will sleep, naturally . . until your set time to awaken . .

It is easy for you to relax and go to sleep . . by using this technique . . of closing your eyelids . . and allowing them to become so relaxed . . that they feel like they want to remain shut . . and then, by letting that relaxation move through your entire body . . from your eyelids, down to the tips of your toes . . Whenever you use this technique . . you will continue drifting into a natural, peaceful state of sleep . . More smoothly . . more easily and more quickly . .

You will sleep more calmly and peacefully . . until it is time for you to awaken . . Unless some emergency arises, and you need to awaken . . If an emergency arises, during the night . . you will awaken easily

. . You will take care of the situation . . Then, when you are ready to return to sleep . . you'll use the same technique . . to reach that level of restful sleep you had before . . Emergencies are rare, so you will, normally, sleep calmly and peacefully . . throughout the night . .

When you awaken, each morning . . you will feel refreshed and eager to begin another day . . During the day, you will be energetic and strong . . You will enjoy the activities of the day . . You will be enthusiastic about all of the activities . . you participate in each day . . And you'll look forward to a pleasant evening . . Your routine will be normal . . just as it has been in the past . .

Each night, when you are ready for sleep . . the moment you close your eyes . . you will think only about the peacefulness . . of letting the muscles and tendons . . in and around your eyelids relax . . You will experience the calming flow of God's peace . . moving throughout your entire being . . And you will feel the easy, smooth flow of spiritual currents . . soothing you into a peaceful state of sleep . . Without even noticing it . . you will quickly drift into a normal, natural state of sleep . . throughout the night . . You will remain completely at ease . . knowing that you are always in the protective care of God's loving presence . .

If you have any thoughts going through your mind . . after you close your eyes . . I want you to, first, concentrate on relaxing the muscles around your eyelids . . And your thoughts, to be of love and calmness . . and the beauty of Gods creation . . You will realize that you are an important part of that creation . . and that you are not alone in the universe . . Your mind will be set at ease . . And you will sleep peacefully and calmly . . under the grace of God . . throughout the night . .

You are responding well to the suggestions I have given you . . And now you will sleep . . (Allow six to eight minutes of silence or soothing music)

In just a moment, I will begin my count, from ONE to FIVE . . When you hear the count of FIVE . . you will open your eyes and be wide awake . . feeling refreshed and invigorated . . Ready ? . . ONE . . TWO . . THREE . . FOUR . . FIVE . . Open your eyes now . .

081 Prescript.   INSOMNIA OVERCOME

(Follow Relaxation)   *** Numb Hand

I understand that you are having a problem . . getting enough rest and sleep at night . . . We are going to talk about that problem now . . And your subconscious mind is receptive to the suggestions and instructions I am about to give you . . Just continue to relax . . Deeply . . Relax . .

You were born with the ability to sleep . . whenever you needed sleep . . When you were a baby . . you didn't think about sleeping or staying awake . . Whenever you needed sleep . . you would automatically go to sleep . . That was an ability you were born with . . and you still have that ability . . You have the natural ability to go to sleep . . easily and quickly . . You can sleep comfortably, in any environment . . You can sleep . . even when it is noisy . . or if there is a light in the room . . And you can sleep comfortably . . regardless of your emotional state . . at the time you go to bed . .

There are millions of grown people who go to sleep, almost instantly . . as soon as they close their eyes . . And you are just as capable of going to sleep . . easily and quickly . . But perhaps, you have temporarily forgotten how to . . And so, I will give you some simple reminders . .

From this session, you can see that it keeps becoming easier . . for you to relax . . And that is the key for you to go into a deep, relaxing sleep . . any time you go to bed . . for the purpose of sleeping . . You can fall asleep just as easily . . as you did when you were a baby . .

You can go to sleep, easily, in any position . . and in any surroundings . . You can go to sleep, even when it is noisy . . And you can sleep comfortably . . even if there is a light shining in your face . . or even if it is totally dark . .

(***) Your subconscious mind has an amazing capacity for learning . . You proved that when you got the numbness in your hand, even though you had never done that before . . And just as your mind already knew what to do to cause the changes and make your hand numb . . Your mind already knows what to do . . to enable you to go to sleep, quickly and easily . . and can enable you to sleep comfortably and soundly . .

You will be so calm and peaceful, when you are sleeping . . that nothing but an emergency will waken you . . until it is time for you to awaken . .

If something happens during the night, while you are sleeping . . that makes it necessary for you to awaken . . you will awaken immediately . . And when you are ready to go back to sleep . . you will be able to do so . . rapidly and gently . . You can sleep for as long as you wish to . . And you will awaken at the time you wish to awaken . .

Right now, you are relaxing in a gentle hypnotic state . . And you are learning that it is easy for you . . to go to sleep . . and that you can sleep peacefully and calmly . . You have rapidly learned to go into a deep hypnotic state of relaxation . . And you are realizing that it is just as easy for you . . to go into a deep state of natural sleep . . any time you go to bed . . for the purpose of sleeping . .

Whenever you want to go to sleep . . you will simply close your eyes . . Breath deeply, through your nose . . and exhale slowly . . Four or five times . . Each time you inhale, you will feel yourself becoming drowsier . . And each time you exhale . . you will continue to become more relaxed . . Clear your mind of your daily affairs . . and concentrate on relaxing the muscles around your eyes . . Let them relax . . and let that relaxation flow . . all through your entire body . . After breathing deeply . . and exhaling slowly . . four or five times . . begin counting backward . . in your mind, slowly . . starting from one hundred . . Each time you think of the next number . . your mind will become drowsier . . and the numbers will keep fading away . . until they disappear . . And you will drift into a deep, sound, restful sleep . .

That's how easy it will be . . To go into a deep, sound, peaceful sleep . . You will breath deeply and exhale slowly, five times . . and then begin counting slowly . . back from one hundred . . in your mind . .

As you continue doing that each night . . you will automatically keep going to sleep . . more quickly and easily . . The numbers will keep fading away more rapidly . . each time you use this method . . to go to sleep . . And you will always go into a peaceful, calm, restful sleep state . . as the numbers fade away . .

While you are sleeping . . your body will be relaxed and comfortable . . You will sleep comfortably, until it is time for you to awaken . .

Emergencies are rare . . But if something makes it necessary for you to awaken . . you will awaken easily and you will be fully alert . . You will do what is necessary and then . . when you are ready to go back to sleep . . you will do so even more easily than you did before you were awakened . .

Each time you are ready to go to sleep . . it keeps becoming easier . . night after night . . And it will always be easy for you to awaken . . when it is time for you to awaken . .

During the day . . you will feel more energetic . . more cheerful . . And you will experience increased vitality . . Your energy level will increase . . and your health will continue to improve . . more and more every day . .

In just a moment, I will begin my count, from ONE to FIVE . . When you hear the count of FIVE . . you will open your eyes and be wide awake . . feeling refreshed and invigorated . .

ONE . .

TWO . .

THREE . .

FOUR . .

FIVE . . You may open your eyes now . .

And now, as you continue to relax . . I want you to go even deeper . . and DEEPER . . DEEPER and DEEPER . . into relaxation . . with every breath you take . . All of the sounds have faded away into the far distance . . and you pay attention only . . to the sounds of my voice . . You are sinking . . deeper and DEEPER . . into complete relaxation . . And you are letting go . . completely . . Relaxing your entire body and mind . . in every way . . Your arms and legs grow heavy . . like lumps of lead . . Your body grows heavy . . like a huge lump of lead . . You sink DEEPER and DEEPER . . DEEPER and DEEPER . . Completely relaxed, so that your arms become so heavy that you cannot move . . And your legs become so heavy . . that you cannot move a muscle . . And they grow heavier and . . HEAVIER . . with every breath you take . . You are going DEEPER now . . Much DEEPER . . Very deep now . .

I want you to use your imagination now . . I want you to imagine . . that we are covering your entire body . . with a layer of ICE . . Very cold material . . Very cold, freezing material . . And we are spraying this freezing material over your entire body . . When we spray this material on . . you are wearing no clothing . . And this material freezes instantly . . We are just spraying it on . . Right now, we are spraying it on your arms . . On your legs . . We are spraying it all over your body . . Your back . . Your chest . . We are spraying it all over your head . . Your eyes, your nose and your mouth . . Your ears and your neck . . All of your skin is receiving this very . . ICE COLD spray . . It feels very cooling and comforting . . and we are spraying it all over your bare body . .

Your entire body is being completely covered with misty spray . . And it is just freezing . . FREEZING . . all over your body . . Small pieces of ice are forming . . Clinging to your skin . . The freezing cold spray is making your skin feel cool and numb . . COOL . . and . . NUMB . .

All discomforts and all feelings of itching goes away . . Dissolving . . because your skin feels so calm and cool . . and numb . . And you are relaxed completely . . And the frozen feeling penetrates . . as though there is caked-on ice . . all over your body . . Very cold and very numbing . . You can feel that cake of ice forming . . Just layer upon layer of cold, freezing ice . . as this material is sprayed all over you

. . You feel these layers of ice that cool your skin and numb it completely . . Cooling and numbing . . all across your back . . Up and down your arms and legs . . All over your abdomen . . All over your chest . . And over every bit of bare skin on your entire body . . Everywhere is made to feel cold and numb . . COLD and NUMB . . Completely in every way . . And you can see the layers of ice forming . . One layer upon the next . . Forming the freezing layers, right over your bare skin . . Relaxing and cooling the skin . . Cooling the skin . . Cooling the skin completely . . And you feel relaxed completely . . You feel very comfortable . . and very, very calm . . and very, very cool and relaxed . .

And as you relax . . you let go more . . And as you let go more and more . . all of these feelings of smoothness and calmness . . and coolness . . permeates every cell of your body . . And you relax . . as you go DEEPER . . and DEEPER . . Go DEEPER and DEEPER . . You are getting HEAVIER and HEAVIER . . And you sink farther and farther into a very deep . . DEEPENING hypnosis . .

And you feel . . above all . . a TREMENDOUS letting go . . And a tremendous feeling of relief . . A TREMENDOUS RELIEF . . as all of the symptoms vanish from your body . . And all of the symptoms disappear . . They vanish . . as you sink DEEPER and DEEPER . . And you go farther and farther into a DEEPENING hypnosis . . Sinking DEEPER and DEEPER now . . Letting go and relaxing DEEPER and DEEPER . . with every breath you take . . (pause for a moment)

Your body is warming a little now . . causing that cold, smooth ice to melt from your skin . . So, we are spraying on new layers of freezing ice . . over the old layers now . . And as a layer of ice melts and cools and calms you . . and smoothes out your skin . . we are replacing it with a new layer over the old one . . We are spraying on new layers all the time . . to maintain your skin . . so it is cool and comfortable for you . . Your skin is feeling so cool and relaxed . . and comfortable in every way . . Feeling wonderful . . You feel so wonderful . . You feel more and more calm . . and more and more relaxed . . and you are pleased to go deeper and DEEPER . . And most of all, you simply feel . . RELIEF . . Relief, that the itching is gone . . Relief that the symptoms have dissolved . . Relief that you can really relax . . and enjoy . . relaxing . .

And you are relaxing . . because you are relieved . . And you are relieved because you are relaxing . . And you say this to yourself . . over and over again . . It goes round and round . . Round and round . . Just like a circle . . "I am relieved because I am relaxing . . And I am relaxing because I am relieved" . . "I am relieved because I am relaxing . . And I am relaxing because I am relieved" . . "I am relieved because I am relaxing" . . "And I am relaxing because I am relieved" . .

As you repeat this to yourself . . you can feel the effect of the cool ice upon your skin . . Relaxing your skin and relieving it of the symptoms . . Relieving it of the symptoms and relaxing it in every way . . As you go deeper and . . DEEPER . . you become cooler and cooler . . And feeling wonderful all over . . And this feeling of coolness, or numbness and relaxation and relief . . is going to last . . And last a long, long time . . After you have awakened, it will last a long, long time . . because you will feel so calm and so smooth and so relaxed in every way . . Even after all the ice melts . . Even after all the spraying is done . . That feeling of coolness and calmness and relaxation and relief . . will just last on and on and on and on and on . . And nothing disturbs you in any way . . Now as you sink deeper . . Much deeper . . DEEPER and DEEPER and DEEPER and DEEPER and DEEPER . . RELAX . . Relaxed and relieved and you go DEEPER and DEEPER . . Feeling this relief and this tremendous relaxation . . as you become more and more comfortable . . in every way . . Realizing that this state of wonderful comfort is going to last and last and last . .

I am going to give you a period of silence now . . as all of these suggestions seal themselves . . into the deepest part of your subconscious mind . . And they will reinforce themselves, over and over again in your mind . .

Your subconscious mind is absorbing everything I am saying . . Continue to relax now . . as this period of silence begins . .
(2 to 3 minutes of silence)

(Client is now prepped for psychosis or for Regression - Continue with . . or EMERGE)

I am going to begin my count, from TEN down to ONE . . etc.

The fact that you are having this session indicates . . that you realize . . jealousy or, envy, of other people . . or objects . . is an undesirable characteristic to possess . . And you sincerely want to overcome that characteristic . . Most everyone has some characteristics, which are undesirable . . Even harmful . . And it is good that you recognize that your jealousy . . is a harmful quality . . And that you have the determination to eliminate it from your life . .

One of the things I have learned . . as the result of hypnotizing many, many people . . is that your subconscious mind knows how to examine, review and further explore . . the impressions, imprints, thoughts and concepts . . that have gone into the storehouse of your mind . . And it knows how to assess them and understand them . . And to work out a solution to the problems they have been causing you . .

Another thing I have learned is how easily your subconscious mind can hear . . and understand everything that I say . . And remember what I say . . And you don't even need to pay attention to me, consciously . . We know very little about what the subconscious mind can comprehend . . But we do know . . beginning right now . . your subconscious mind can review, examine and explore all of the imprints, impressions, thoughts and ideas . . as well as the experiences you have had . . which may have caused you to develop the characteristic that we know as, jealousy . . And your mind can then work out the proper solution to rid you of . . that unwanted quality . .

Continue relaxing now, with your eyes closed, hearing nothing but the sound of my voice . . as you experience a wonderful feeling of drifting . . Drifting away . . to a peaceful place . . Drifting into a state that is similar to . . deeply dreaming . . deep . . deeply dreaming . .

You are ready to make some very important changes in your life . . that will bring you greater happiness . . And you will be pleased that your subconscious mind is receiving . . everything that I say . . And you'll be surprised at your ability to make true . . everything I am saying . . I am telling you only those things I know you can do . . You'll be able to do everything that I present to you . . I want you to take your time now . . as you are relaxing . . Mentally and silently and to yourself . .

I want you to begin counting down from the number, Ten . . back down to the number One . . And as you count each number to yourself . . you will continue moving into a deeper, more relaxed hypnotic state . . Begin counting to yourself now . . as I continue talking to you . . I want you to really enjoy this experience . .

For your subconscious mind to review the memories that caused you to become jealous in the first place . . may take some time . . And to be completely free of being jealous . . is not likely to occur all at once . . What is likely to happen is, that you will be rid of some of it today . . And part of it tomorrow . . And the following day, a little more of it will be gone . . And soon, all feelings of jealousy and envy will be gone completely . . It keeps fading away, a little more each day . .

And the great thing about it is . . that you will notice your own self-confidence and self-acceptance increasing more, each day . . This is comparable to any other learning process . . That's how the mind works . . It learns a little bit at a time . .

You know, that's the same way babies learn certain words first . . And each day they keep learning more and more words . . until the day comes when they put together, their first sentence . . And then longer sentences . . And then paragraphs . .

In your own experience of learning, that's the way it is, isn't it . . Day by day, you continue progressing . . It is hard to know, at this point . . how long it will take for you to be completely free of your jealousy . . or envy . . It may be a week . . It may take two weeks or even a month . . before those feelings are completely gone . . All you really know, right now, is that you will keep progressing more and more, each and every day . . until it is gone from your life . .

You can continue relaxing even more now . . And you don't need to talk . . And you don't need to move . . unless you are uncomfortable . . You don't even need to pay any attention to what I am saying to you . . Your subconscious mind is aware . . and is absorbing everything I say . . And that's the only important thing right now . .

I heard a story one time about . . a ragpicker's son . . He lived just down the road from a huge castle, high on a hill, overlooking the town . . Inside the castle lived a king and his son, the duke . .

The duke was quite young and so, had a nurse, who took care of him . . He was quite well off and, of course, had far more than the ragpicker's son . .

The duke had everything that the poor ragpicker's son didn't have . . Fine clothing to wear, good food to eat . . and a pedigreed dog, named . . Hubert . .

Ironically, except for the differences in wealth and material things . . the two boys looked like identical twins . . And when the nurse took the duke out walking by the river one day . . they happened to meet the ragpicker's son . . And you couldn't tell which was the duke and which was the ragpicker's son . . except that the duke wore fine satin and the other boy . . was dressed in rags . .

The little duke used to look longingly . . Wishing he could go swimming in the river . . like the poor boy did . . for it was the most beautiful river in all of France . . But it was against the nurse's rules to let the little duke play in the water . . And she had to keep her rules, even though she felt sorry for the little duke . . He was, simply, not allowed to play in the river . .

One day, as she and the duke were out walking . . the duke's pedigreed dog, Hubert, ran up to the ragpicker's son's mutt, Barffer . . They touched noses and quickly became friends . . The duke and the poor boy smiled at each other and said, "Hello" . . After that, whenever they met, the boys always greeted each other with some sign of friendship . .

And one day, the ragpicker's son pointed at the river and offered, "Let's go in and play" . . The little duke looked at his nurse and she shook her head, "No" . . And he was angry with her for the rest of the day . .

The next morning, the little duke had disappeared . . And everybody around the castle was all stirred up . . His nurse, his guardian and all of his attendants, went into the town to find him . .

Asking everyone they met if they had seen him . . Finally, they went to the old ragpicker . . Yes, he said . . He had seen him, an hour or so earlier, going to the river with his son . . Hurriedly, they all headed down to the river . . including the old ragpicker . .

After walking about a mile along the banks, they spied the two boys . . playing in the river . . As naked as the day they were born . . And on the shore lay a heap of clothing . . Rags and fine linens were piled in a heap . . All tousled together . .

The nurse and the duke's attendants were all very angry . . and shouted for them to come out of the water . . But they were laughing and having so much fun . . All of the shouting was ignored . .

Finally, the old ragpicker waded into the water and brought them back to shore . . And they stood before all of the people . . naked . . and grinning . .

The duke's guardian was going to scold the duke . . And the old ragpicker was going to scold his son . . But they couldn't tell which boy was which . . Without their clothes on, standing naked in the sunlight . . they were identical . . And as the boys realized that no one could tell them apart . . they grinned more than ever . .

Someone got the idea of having the boys put on their clothes . . thinking that would settle the matter . . But the two boys picked up pieces of clothing as they came to them . . One of them put on the ragged shirt and the velvet coat . . And the other put on the fine linen shirt with the ragged coat . . And the people still couldn't tell them apart . .

"This is dreadful", cried the duke's guardian . . "For all we know, we may take the ragpicker's son back to the castle . . And the duke may grow up to be . . a ragpicker's son" . .

And now you know . . why . . you are getting rid of jealousy and envy . . And you know why your self-confidence and self-realization keeps increasing . . more and more . . You are realizing that you were created by the same creator . . who created everyone else on this earth . . And therefore, you are just as good as everyone else . . And you have no reason to be jealous . .

You do not yet fully understand . . what caused you to become jealous . . But you are realizing that it has been caused by . . misunderstandings . . that formed in your subconscious mind . . Things long since forgotten . . And you know now that they are things of the past . . And you are enjoying the pleasure of understanding . . that they do not need to cause you any more difficulty . . And doing it this way . . will give you a great feeling of accomplishment . . as you keep becoming more . . and more aware . . of your own self-confidence and self-acceptance . .

Your subconscious mind knows how fast it can work . . in clearing up those improper understandings in your mind . . And your mind knows how to use those past experiences . . to increase your own self-acceptance . . your own self-reliance . . your own self-confidence and self-esteem . .

And there is a great sense of accomplishment . .   and happiness . .
awaiting you . .

I want you to continue to relax for a few more minutes . . And then
I'm going to have you awaken, in a short time . .   So just enjoy what
your subconscious mind is doing for you . .   (pause)

I want you to have a very profound feeling of comfort . . and
accomplishment . .   when you awaken . . A feeling of knowing that
something good is happening . . I want you to enjoy that . . (pause)

And now you can begin thinking about awakening . . I will count up
to FIVE . . And you will progressively awaken, a little more . . with
each number that you hear . .   When I reach the number, FIVE . .
you will open your eyes and awaken . .   feeling calm, peaceful,
confident, well rested and . . very happy . .

ONE

TWO

THREE

FOUR . . and . .

FIVE

I want you to continue to relax now . . just as you are doing . . Relax . . and I will present to you . . information that will be of great benefit to you . . The suggestions that I am giving you . . and the guidance and instructions I am providing . . are going directly into the storehouse of your mind . .

And your subconscious mind . . will cause you to put them into your own actions . . To continue improving your ability . . to remember and recall everything you read, hear, see and learn . .

As you listen to the sound of my voice . . you will continue drifting into . . a deeper . . and DEEPER . . more peaceful state of relaxation . .

Very often, when people are watching television . . or are daydreaming . . they don't notice other things going on around them . . Have you ever done that ? (Wait for answer) Good . . Then you know you have the ability to concentrate, so profoundly . . that you become unaware of other events going on around you . . In fact, in the process of going into this hypnotic state . . you have demonstrated an excellent ability to concentrate . .

Right now, you are concentrating on what I am saying . . And to achieve the hypnotic state of relaxation . . as you have . . you have used your own ability to concentrate . . So, you know that you have excellent concentration powers . .

You are continuing to have more confidence in your ability to concentrate . . The fact that you have been able to concentrate . . well enough to achieve a hypnotic state of relaxation . . indicates that you also have the ability to concentrate . . whenever you are reading, listening and studying . . And without being hypnotized . .

I am going to give you some suggestions and instructions now . . that will improve your ability to concentrate . . and improve your learning skills . . So much that your memory will also keep improving more . . each day . .

From now on . . when you want to read or study . . or listen to a lecture or a speech . . you will get your materials ready . . such as, books or writing materials . . Then when you are ready to begin concentrating . . you will breath deeply and exhale slowly, three times . . And then, think of the numbers 3, 2 and 1 . . As soon as you breath deeply and exhale slowly, three times . . And think, the numbers . . 3 , 2 and 1 . . you will become calm and relaxed . . the way you are now . .

Breathing deeply and exhaling slowly, three times and thinking the numbers 3, 2 and 1 . . will be a signal . . Your subconscious mind will respond to that signal . . and will cause you to become calm and relaxed . . just as you are now . . And your awareness will narrow down . . to absorb the reading . . studying or listening you want to do . . You will be less sensitive to surrounding noises or distractions . . while you are studying . . Your total involvement will be devoted . . to what you are concentrating on . . As you read, study or listen . . in that state of calmness and relaxation . . your close attention will increase to perfection . . and will remain that way for at least One Hour . .

Your concentration will be perfect for at least One Hour . . Unless there is some emergency or other important reason that requires you to stop . . and give your attention to something else . .

Your concentration will be perfect for at least One Hour . . each time you use the signal . . of breathing deeply and exhaling slowly, three times . . while thinking of the numbers 3 , 2 and 1 . .

After One Hour . . if you still have more reading or studying you need to do . . you will take a break for a few minutes . . and then, use the signal again . . And if you are listening to a lecture . . you will continue listening . . while you breath deeply and exhale slowly, three times . . and count in your mind . . from 3 . . down to 1 . .

The more you use this procedure to relax . . and focus your attention on your reading and studying . . the more rapidly your learning skills will improve . . And the knowledge you absorb, by . . reading, studying, observing or listening . . in this way . . will remain in your conscious mind much longer . . You will be able to remember facts, principles, detailed lists, theories, mathematical formulas, equations, general trends . . or any other information . . more perfectly . . Your memory and your recall . . will keep improving more each day . . You are realizing that you have the ability . . to remember and to recall . . everything you learn . .

Your mind is comparable to a computer . . It records everything you see, hear and experience . . And you are capable of recalling everything you learn . . Some of the material you learn is not important enough . . to remain in the conscious level of your mind . . So it goes into the storehouse of your mind . . But the information is always there . . And it is available whenever you need to recall it . . All you need to do is to let the subconscious level of your mind know . . you need to recall something . . And it will permit the information to come into the conscious level of your mind . . whenever you need it . .

Have you ever tried to think of the name of someone you know . . but find yourself unable to recall it ? . . If you have . . nod your head . . When you fail to recall the name right away . . you begin trying harder . . And that sets up a mental block . . which keeps the name from coming into the conscious level of your mind . . So, you finally give up trying . . and you may say . . "Oh, well, I'll think of it later" . . And then you start doing something else . . And in a short time, you suddenly recall the name . . It was there, in the storehouse of your mind, the entire time . . But was blocked, until you relaxed your efforts to recall it . . When you informed your subconscious mind of your need to recall . . and relaxed your thinking by doing something else . . you released the tension . . of trying to force yourself to recall the name . . And when you released the tension . . it enabled the name to come into the conscious level of your mind . .

So, any time you need to recall material that is in your mind . . or to answer questions on a test or exam . . and you do not recall the answers immediately . . Just think to yourself . . "I know the answer to that question . . And I will recall it, in a minute or two" . . Then move on to the next question . . And as you are studying the next question or two . . all of a sudden, you will recall the answer . . And then you can go back and write it down . .

Now you understand what real concentration is . . and that will cause your attentiveness to continue improving . . Your ability to recall . . will improve more each day . . Memories will stay in your conscious mind much longer . . And your ability to bring information out . . from the storehouse of your mind, more quickly . . will also improve greatly . . You will become a memory giant . . and your future career . . will depend on it . .

I am going to give you a period of silence now . . as all of these suggestions seal themselves . . into the deepest part of your subconscious mind . . And they will reinforce themselves, over and over again in your mind . . Your subconscious mind is absorbing everything I am saying . . Continue to relax now . . as this period of silence begins . . (2 to 3 minutes of silence)

I am going to begin my count from FIVE down to ONE . . And when you hear the number ONE . . You will open your eyes and be wide awake, feeling alert and ready to face your next challenge . .

FIVE, FOUR, THREE, TWO, ONE . . You may open your eyes now .

334

LETTING GO Of LOVE - PAIN

As you are relaxing comfortably . . I want to talk with you about . . what you have been going through recently . . in your personal life . . But first, I want to tell you about . . a friend of mine . .

When Jason, one of my associates, heard the cries of two robins in the yard . . outside of his office . . he had no idea that it would lead to . . one of the most difficult decisions of his life . .

When he first saw the two birds in the yard . . he thought they were fighting . . They were flapping their wings and tumbling over each other . . He continued watching for a few minutes and finally realized . . that somehow . . they were tangled together with some kind of string . . And, that was how I became involved . . He came into my office and asked if he could borrow a towel from my laundry room . . Then he went back out in the yard, threw the towel over the birds and, gingerly, picked them up . . He noticed that their legs were all tangled together with a thin, fishing line . . He borrowed the smallest scissors he could find . . and began snipping the fishing line off their legs . .

After getting the line off the bird's legs . . he noticed that one of the bird's legs was injured quite severely . . He wrapped it in the towel and . . took the other bird out to the edge of the porch and . . released it . . He began talking to the bird saying, everything was going to be okay . . and that, he was going to take good care of him . . He asked me if he could keep the towel . . to keep the bird wrapped in . . so he could take it home with him . .

At home, he cared for the bird . . feeding it several times daily and, generally, nursing it back to health . . He wasn't really sure if it was a male . . or a female . . But it didn't matter to him . . He called his newfound friend, Charley . .

Day after day, he fed the bird . . talked to it, sang to it and continued nursing it . . And the leg kept healing more and more . . He was thinking about buying a cage . . fearing that it may fly away after its recovery . . And then, he began thinking how, it would not be fair to the bird . . to keep it caged . . After all, it was born free . . And he asked himself, What right did he have to cage it ? . .

He began to realize that . . everyone has their own path they must follow . . And of how he would feel if someone were to put him in a cage . . He appreciated being free . . and making his own decisions . . Having the freedom to go about his business, with no one to answer to . . Doing what he wanted to do, saying what he wanted to say . . Eating what he wanted and when . . Making all of his own choices . .

He decided that the bird needed his help . . and protection . . for a while . . Just like we all need love and protection from certain things . . that are beyond our ability to handle . .

Then, he remembered that he was coming to my office when he found the bird . . He wanted my advise about a problem he was having . . And although he knew I would gladly help him . . he certainly didn't want to be held captive . . just because he needed some temporary assistance . . So, the day arrived when Jason knew . . the bird was well enough . . And needed to be set free . .

He had really become attached to the bird . . And when you have to make this kind of decision . . it stirs up all kinds of feelings . . And you remember a line from a song . . "Fish got to swim . . Birds got to fly" . . Again, you think to yourself . . It would not be right to keep the bird . . after it's ready to leave . . So, you take the bird and you move towards the door . . A few tears dampen your cheeks . . You feel the lump in your throat . . and the ache in your chest . . Yet, through the tears, you experience a warm, glowing feeling, coming over you . . Because you know in your heart . . that you took good care of Charley when he needed you . . And you recall that someone once said . . "Absence makes the heart grow fonder" . . So, you open the door . . and walk over to the edge of the porch . . You hold Charley up to the sky and . . open your hands . .

Charley flew out, for a moment . . then turned and came back toward you . . As though he wanted to say, Thanks . . He swooped by, then went on his way . . Jason stood there a few moments . . wondering if he would ever see Charley again . .

Several months went by . . Occasionally, Jason would find himself thinking about Charley . . Wondering how he was getting along . . Time went on and he had nearly forgotten about Charley . . when one morning, he awakened . . and saw Charley . . sitting on his window ledge . . He jumped up quickly and opened the window . . He stuck his hand out and Charley hopped onto his hand . . and he drew Charley in with a smile . . And he realized that . . someone you love never leaves forever . . Jason felt a great sense of relief . . Almost a sense of closure . . Then he put his hand back out the window . . and Charley flew into the distance . . And Jason thought to himself . . There is a bonding unity . . and a oneness, to all of life . . And in reality, there is no separation . .

I want you to continue relaxing now . . And allow your subconscious mind to absorb . . what you have heard here today . . I believe your problem will resolve itself . . very soon . . as you come to realize that love . . is never gone from your heart . . It is always there . . for as long as you wish to hold it . . (pause)

I am going to count now, from ONE up to FIVE . . And when you hear me say the number FIVE . . you will awaken, feeling refreshed, and relieved . . that you have reached a resolution . .

ONE . . You are coming up now . . Soon you will awaken . .

TWO . . Your fingers and toes want to wiggle now . . Let them move . .

THREE . . Feeling refreshed and wonderful . . for you are, truly, a wonderful person . .

FOUR . . You're almost there . . Take a deep breath now . . and . .

FIVE . . You can open your eyes now . .

HYPNOSIS CAN HELP EASE A PERSON'S ANXIETY ABOUT LOST OR
MISPLACED ITEMS. IT CAN ALSO HELP TO SPEED UP THE PROCESS OF
LOCATING THE MISSING OBJECTS, IF THE INFORMATION OF WHERE THE
OBJECTS ARE LOCATED IS IN THE PERSON'S MIND.

Continue relaxing easily and gently now . . You are listening only to
my words . . All other sounds and noises are faded into the
background . . You are not trying to think of anything in particular . .

You may experience brief intrusions of fleeting thoughts . . entering
your mind . . from time to time . . but they will soon fade away
completely . . And you will be concentrating only . . on my Words . .
and on what I want you to think about . .

Just relax, as you are doing . . and I will take you to the place . .
where you want to be . . Take a deep breath now and . . let it out slowly . .
Relax . .

Imagine yourself in a cool, quiet place now . . resting gently in a
DEEP recliner . . Settle into that DEEP recliner . . all the way down
into it . . In just a moment, you will experience a feeling of floating
away . . as though a fluffy, white cloud is moving under your body .
. and lifting you up . . easily and gently . . You can experience the
feeling of floating away . . Moving out, beyond space and time . . Your
mind and body are relaxing peacefully . . and comfortably . .

You are rising up now . . Gently drifting . . And you are moving
slowly, to that familiar place where you last had _____ . .
I am going to count from FIVE down to ONE . . When I reach the
count of ONE . . you will be at the place where you last had the
_____ . . You will see yourself as having already found it . .
You will find it right where you last had it . . Or where someone else
moved it . .

All that is important in your mind now . . . is that you reunite yourself with
the missing _____ . .

See it right where it was left . . Feel it back in your possession . .
Sense that you already have it . . Take your time now . . And when
I reach the count of ONE . . you'll be at the place where you last
had _____ . .

FIVE . . You are moving toward it now . . FOUR . . You're feeling very happy about locating it . . THREE . . You're moving closer and closer to the place where it is located . . TWO . . When I say the next numbers, you will be there . . You will see it and sense it, clearly and vividly . . ONE . . As soon as you see _____, tell me where you found it . .

IF CLIENT DOESN'T LOCATE IT, CONTINUE AS FOLLOWS :
It's all right . . We will locate _____ from a different angle . . I want you to move aside now . . And you will be responding . . as though you are merely observing what is happening . .

You are going back in time . . to a period before _____ was misplaced . . It is easy and very enjoyable for you to do this . . Reliving an experience is always interesting . . and enjoyable . . You are slowly moving back in time . . to a period just before _____ was misplaced . . You are retracing your actions . . exactly as they happened . . You are in a deep level of relaxation . . And you are moving into a higher level of self-awareness . . It is very easy for you to relive this experience . . And to recall the exact whereabouts of _____ . .

Take your time now . . You have plenty of time . . You have all the time you need . . You are reliving the events that led up to the misplacement of _____ . .

You are understanding that . . some people see a memory while others . . hear a memory . . Some people sense a memory and still, others, relive it as a new experience . . It doesn't matter how it comes to you . . The thing that is important now . . is for you to enjoy recalling . . or reliving . . exactly what happened . . when you last saw _____ . .

Your mind is focusing in on the exact scene and activity . . It keeps becoming more vivid and clear . . And more real . . (Ad Lib as needed)

You are understanding now . . what happened to _____ . . How you did what you did . . and why . .

After you awaken from the hypnotic state . . the exact location of _____ will remain clear in your mind . . And, perhaps, you will be able to go directly to its location . .

You may be amazed to find that _____ will not be in the first place you look for it . . But at the second place . . you will find it . .

And you will be very happy and pleased with your success . . You will be grateful to have found the _____ . .

In a moment, I will count to FIVE . . and you will awaken feeling refreshed and wonderful . . You will awaken a little more with each count you hear . . You will remember everything you have experienced and . . everything you have learned is true . . I will begin my count now . .

ONE . .   You are coming up now . . Soon you will awaken . .

TWO . .   Your fingers and toes want to wiggle now . . Let them move a little . .

THREE . . Feeling refreshed and wonderful . . for you are, truly, a wonderful person . .

FOUR . . You're almost there . . Take a deep breath now . . and . .

FIVE . .   Open your eyes . . and let me see a big smile . .

Love . . Love . . More and more . . and more love . . Everywhere, in everything . . For everyone . . That is the one great need that we all have . . Who can supply that love to a person . . when love is so lacking ? . . Or, there never seems to be enough . . when it is given . . No life is complete without love . . Needing love is the great driving force within us . . It is one of our greatest needs . .

I am going to help you to overcome this problem you are having . . with your marriage . . But I would like to tell you . . first . . about another client I once had, who I will call, Joan . . Her situation was similar to yours so . . you can relate to it very well . .

When Joan came to my office complaining about . . ten years of being in . . an abusive marriage . . and having been beaten more times than she could count . . I asked her why she put up with it . . Why doesn't she get a divorce . .

She explained her fears . . If she divorced, she said . . she wouldn't be able to support her children . . In addition to that . . her husband threatened to kill her . . and her children . . if she ever left him . . He ascribed his great love for her, saying that he couldn't live without her . . And if he couldn't have her . . no one else would . . Yet, with all of the love he professed to have for her . . he continued to beat her, with no mercy . .

Further discussion with Joan revealed . . that she had been sexually and physically abused . . as a child . . She recognized that her father was unstable . . and that her mother would not defend her . .

She recalled, one day when she was about five years old . . that she had been beaten by her father . . And then, he sexually molested her . . to show her his love . . And that was the first time she decided to leave home . . She felt sure that neither her father . . nor her mother . . loved her . . so, she was going to leave and try to find someone who would love her . . She got her doll buggy . . and her doll . . and all the clothes she could put into the buggy . . and started walking down the street . . Determined to leave her father and her mother behind her . . She was going to find the love she deserved . . She knew she deserved to be treated better than that . . even as a child . .

Words don't really express true love . . Joan's husband told her many times . . that he loved her and couldn't live without her . . Yet, he continued to beat her . . His words were not backed up by his actions . . As I know you understand, real love brings joy . . and happiness . . and harmony into the home . . And to the individual lives of those living in the home . . There is no greater joy than to give happiness . . to give true love, serenity and security . . to one who needs it so desperately . . This was what Joan was needing . . This was what she had been looking for, all of her life . . I wondered . . What could I do? How could I help her? . . She had never told her story before, to anyone . . And now, she had come to me . . seeking help with this . .

I decided to go ahead and hypnotize her . . Inducing the hypnotic state, I thought . . would give me time to figure a way . . of helping her . .

After getting her into an hypnotic state . . I suggested that she use her imagination . . And to see herself standing . . completely nude . . in front of a full length mirror . . And to notice that she is a very beautiful woman, with a very good figure . . And she really was a very attractive woman . .

So, all she had to was to see herself . . as she really was . . And then I told her to tell me what she was seeing . . as she looked in the mirror . .

The first thing she noticed was the reflection of her own face . . Then I asked her if she would really look closely at the face . . To notice everything about the face . . very clearly . . And I suggested that . . when she became aware of the fact that she had . . a very attractive face . . one of the fingers on her right hand would lift up . . and then I told her to look closely at her breasts . . And to notice that her breasts were very nicely developed . . And to notice . . all the rest of her torso . . closely . . And when she recognized the fact that she had . . a very pleasant, attractive body . . A finger on her right hand would lift up . . I continued on . . Having her see that she was a loving, caring person . . That she deserved to be loved and treated respectfully . . It took a little time but her finger lifted after each thing that I mentioned . . until I said, "Now, I want you to see . . that you are a forgiving person" . .

I knew Joan had a lot of anger within her . . And I knew that the anger would do her more harm . . than those who had caused the anger . . So, I wanted her to release all of that built-up anger . .

Joan had been mistreated for many years . . and had suffered all those years in silence . . with no one to turn to for help . . And everyone needs to express whatever feelings they have . . She had never been given opportunity to express her feelings and emotions . . I explained to her that she had a right to be angry . . and to go ahead and express her anger . . And so, she did . . and during that episode, she also experienced a lot of pain . . And by experiencing all of the pain . . she came to realize that . . she is a human being . . And she is alive . . And she has a good, healthy nervous system . . And, more than anything . . she wanted to be loved . .

I reminded her that it would have been a shame . . if she hardened up . . so that she no longer had any feelings . . Her feelings were letting her know that she had still retained the ability . . to be sensitive and caring about others . . And by being an understanding, caring and loving person . . she would know a much happier, more enjoyable life . . than she had ever experienced before . .

As she continued looking into the mirror . . tears began streaming down her face . . Tears that she had held in for a long, long time . . She was finally letting go . . Letting it all out . . And through those tears, I could see the kindness . . the compassion . . the signs of loving and caring . . And all of the other good qualities . . that she had stored up within herself . .

I asked her to walk away from the mirror . . and to remember all of the good she had seen in herself . . And then I asked her to move over to the video player . . and put in a video tape that was showing her life . . I asked her to move it a little forward in time . . And it would show, how she was going to make the necessary changes in her life . . that would release her . . from her unhappy plight . . And replace that anguish with love . . joy, happiness, kindness and . . more love . . And then I mentioned to her that . . her finger would lift up . . to let me know when the solution to the problem had been worked out . .

It is really amazing . . how your subconscious mind can review . . what has been causing a problem . . and work out a solution . . And help to resolve the problem . . in a very pleasant way . .

And just as easily as Joan's mind worked out her solution . . your own mind is now reviewing, examining and exploring . . what has caused your problem . . that you are now experiencing . . and it is working out the solution . . Enabling you to have the confidence to make the changes . . that are needed to get your problem resolved . .

Even after you awaken from the hypnotic state . . your inner mind will continue reviewing everything . . that had to do with causing that problem . . The reviewing can continue in your dreams . . And when your subconscious mind understands . . there is no reason the problem needs to continue . . and it finds a way . . your inner mind will help you work out the best solution . . And you will soon be completely free . . from that problem . . May God be with you . . (pause)

EMERGE

MEDITATION

(Follow Relaxation)

One of the most inspiring statements . . attributed to Jesus . . in the entire New Testament, are the words . . "The Kingdom of God . . is within you" . . Just think of the tremendous meaning . . contained in those seven words . . The Kingdom of God . . is within you . . (Pause for one minute)

Those words mean that there is a power within you . . that can keep you strong at all times . . They mean that there is a source of wisdom within you . . that can provide you with guidance . . in every situation of your life . . Those words by Jesus also mean . . you have within you . . a source of knowledge . . which can free you from all confusion . . and from all conflicts . . and can give you complete peace of mind and happiness . .

They also mean that you have within you . . the transforming power of love . . And that your life can be enhanced . . by letting that love come through . . The more you let that love come through . . in your daily activities . . the greater inflow of love you will experience . . coming into your own life . . You can give that touch of love to every challenge . . and the challenge will be easier to overcome . .

Those words by Jesus also mean . . that there is a good reason for meditating . . Because meditation is the best way of getting your mind attuned . . with the Kingdom of God, within you . .

Your inner mind may be compared to a radio . . A radio cannot produce voices . . or music . . or any other sounds . . unless it is turned on . . and properly tuned in . . to a broadcasting station . . The vibrations of energy . . that bring voices and music to your ears . . through the radio . . are flowing around you all the time . . But you never hear those sounds . . until you turn on your radio . . and permit those vibrations to come through . .

Think about this for a moment . . Those vibrations are in the room with you right now . . whether you turn on a radio or not . . In the same way . . vibrations of love, wisdom, healing energy . . and the power from God, are within you all the time . . Waiting for you to turn them on . .

As Jesus said . . The Kingdom of God is within you . . It is there, right now . . And meditation is an excellent way . . of getting your inner mind tuned in . . to that tremendous source of wisdom and power . .

Let yourself continue to relax now . . as I give you some suggestions . . that will enable you to move into a level of awareness . . that is most conducive . . to meditation . .

The more you listen to my voice . . the deeper your hypnotic state becomes . . You will go deeper and DEEPER and DEEPER . . and find that you are relaxing more and more . . As I talk to you . . it will become less and less important . . for you to consciously listen to my voice . . As you go DEEPER and DEEPER . . you will begin to feel yourself drifting away . . And that is good . . And you will find that, drifting, may occur quite rapidly . . Relax . . and flow with it . . (Pause)

You may drift into a state that is quite similar to a dreaming state . . Much like the way you feel just before sleep . . Relax . . as you drift into a drowsier, more peaceful state of complete relaxation . . Flow with it . . Gently . . RELAX . . relax . . (Pause one minute)

As I talk to you now . . it is not important that you pay any attention to the words I am saying . . I will describe a scene . . which you will gradually come to accept . . And soon, you will feel yourself in the situation . . that I am describing to you . .

You are continuing to drift into a deeper, dreaming state . . And you may begin having a feeling of floating . . as though you are safely floating on a soft . . billowy, white cloud . . Without noticing it . . you are continuing to become more calm and relaxed . . Experiencing a feeling of peace . . and serenity . . Letting yourself go . . to experience and enjoy . . a perfect, peace of mind . . This is such a wonderful, pleasant, soothing experience . . that you are becoming more relaxed . . more calm and more peaceful . . As you float gently and safely . . on your soft, fluffy, white cloud . .

During the night, when you are sleeping . . you can dream . . And in your dreams, you can hear, see, move and experience . . a variety of activities . . In the same way . . you can, now, experience, more and more . . a variety of sensations . . that can be of great value to you . .

As you continue drifting, on your soft, gentle white cloud . . you may begin to notice a beautiful, tall building . . off in the distance . . The cloud is gradually carrying you towards that beautiful building . . (Pause) You are gradually approaching the most beautiful building you have ever seen . .

Your expectations are growing as you move closer to the building . . (Pause) You begin to notice a sign . . in front of the building . . It says, INSTITUTE OF UNIVERSAL KNOWLEDGE . .

When you enter the building . . you will find that conditions are perfect . . for enabling your mind . . to be tuned in to your God Consciousness . . And you will be in direct contact . . not only with universal knowledge . . but also with truth, wisdom and understanding . .

You are gradually approaching the building now . . at your own pace . . There is no need to hurry . . You have plenty of time . . to enjoy this pleasant experience . .

When you are inside the building . . you may notice a variety of wonderful sensations . . You may notice a wonderful aroma . . A feeling of complete peace and contentment . . A pleasant warmth . . A feeling of unconditional love . . And a strong feeling of oneness with God . .

Inside the building . . you will find many wonders . . First of all, you may notice the three large windows . . The first one, that you can look through . . will show experiences from your past . . and enable you to understand them clearly . . A second window exposes future events . . that can be of great value to you . . And a third window . . reveals solutions to your problems . . and answers to your questions . . The windows are there . . inside the building . . And they are available to you . . when you enter the building . . There is also a special room . . It's a healing room . . A room you can enter to improve your health . . You may notice that the door . . to the Institute of Universal Knowledge . . is opening now . . You may select a window to your past, your future, solution to a problem or developing better health . . It is your choice . . And you may enter the building . . as soon as you are ready . . Starting now . . (Pause for 3 to 5 minutes)

Now . . you are beginning to gently float out of the building . . You are leaving the building for now . . But with the knowledge that you can return . . in the future . . any time you desire to do so . .
Before coming back to a wide-awake, fully alert state . . be aware of the experience you have just had . . And feel yourself in perfect harmony . . physically, mentally, emotionally and spiritually . .

In this world, where all is one . . And you are one . . with all that is . .

EMERGE . .

MEMORY IMPROVEMENT

You are relaxing very well . . Now . . you are going into a deeper . . DEEPER state of relaxation . . I want you to continue to relax . . but as you hear my words . . you will go DEEPER and DEEPER . . DEEPER . . into relaxation . . Breath deeper now . . And with each breath you take . . you will sink a little DEEPER each time . . Just flow with it . . and relax . . RELAX . . RELAX DEEPER . .

Now, I am going to give you a few suggestions . . about memory recall . . Memory Recall . .

In the first place . . the art of memory is attention . . You must pay attention to something . . in order to remember it . . People with excellent memories . . that don't pay attention, don't remember . . People with most excellent memories . . heads of state, politicians . . doctors or lawyers . . who are at a party and are introduced to people, may say . . "How do you do, Mr. Jones" . . And one minute later, can't recall what the man's name is . . They don't know . . Why ? Because they paid no attention at the time they were introduced . . To remember something, you must pay attention . . You hear the name and you look at the person . . You associate . . Later, you may see the face . . And you think of the name . . Because you associate one with the other . . Unless you weren't paying attention . .

Some people carry this inattention trait, with them, for the rest of their lives . . Simply, paying no attention . . They don't really care about remembering . . until the time comes . . when they need the information . . Then they want to remember . . That's not good . .

The very first lesson in being able to recall something . . is to remember it in the first place . . You have to put the facts into your memory bank . . before you can recall it . . When you feel excessively fatigued . . When you're tired and really worn out . . Or when you don't feel good . . The tendency is to say . . "Ah, heck with it . . I don't need to pay attention to that" . . And, how quickly your memory fades . . It's not because you don't have a good memory . . You have an excellent memory . . But you're not using it because you are not paying attention . . You must literally Pay Attention . . Then you store the facts, properly, in the memory bank so that it's all ready for you when you need it . . So, the most

348

important point is . . no matter how fatigued you are . . or what difficulties you are stressing under . . or what you may have on your mind . . From this moment on . . you're going to utilize the good memory you have . . by paying attention . . Paying attention to whatever is going on around you . . to what is being said and what you are hearing . . and to what you see . . So that when you need to go into your memory bank . . to make a withdrawal . . you won't need to hold up the bank . .

When you go to the bank . . you fill out a withdrawal slip or write a check . . and have it cashed . . You do the same thing with your memory bank . . You don't force them to give you money . . And you don't force your memory bank . . to give you information . . As soon as you try to force it . . you won't be able to think of it . . You say . . "I've got to know that . . I've got to know the name of that song . . or that name . . or phone number . . What was it ? What was it ? . .

Immediately, your subconscious mind rebels against you . . And the harder you try, the harder it is to remember . . This is true of every living human being . . It doesn't mean you have a bad memory . . It simply means that you are using the good memory that you have . . improperly . .

Just like, if you went to the bank . . with a gun . . you'd be using the bank . . improperly . . You know you'll get more from the bank with a check . . than with a gun . .

That only leads to frustration . . And that same thing is true with your memory bank . . If you try to force it . . It will only lead to . . frustration . .

In order to recall something . . you let the subconscious do the recalling for you . . And it will come to your mind, naturally . . And, if it doesn't come, immediately . . forget it . . It will wash up on the sands of consciousness in a few moments . . when you least expect it . .

One method of recall, known to everyone . . is by simply going through the alphabet . . What was the name of that hotel ? Was it B or C or D ? Oh, D, that's it ! . . It's the Dubuque Hotel . . That is to say . . You had a hook . . A hook which you stretched down into the bank . . and withdrew your memory . . Just like writing a check . . By going through the alphabet . . you gave the letter to the teller of your memory bank . . and out came the right answer . . Now, the same thing can be done in many ways . . besides with the alphabet . .

If you want to remember where you left something . . you simply go through the motions of what you were doing . . the last time you had it . . You retrace your steps, mentally . . Since the memory is 'hooked in' with the action . . Many items that you want to recall . . may be remembered in this way . . By associating an action . . hooked to the memory of what you want to know . . That action . . is the check you write . . to get the withdrawal from your memory bank . .

Your memory has always been good . . So, it isn't a question of needing to improve your memory . . It's a question of properly utilizing the memory bank . . within your subconscious mind . . in order to obtain the maximum recall . . The key word to remember is . . Association . . Associate the word or the name you want . . with something else . . Maybe the man's name is Jones and he has a big nose . . Think of nose and Jones comes with it . . You write that mental check to your memory bank . . by doing something or associating something similar . . to the word or name . . that you want to recall . .

All these suggestions are very important . . for they represent the proper way to begin utilizing . . the good memory that you have . . First, you make the proper deposit in the memory bank by . . paying attention . . Second, when you want to make a withdrawal from the memory bank . . your memory recall is successful . . because you withdraw in the proper manner . . Using association as your check . . You don't force it . . You utilize some association . . that you're familiar with . . to bring it out . . These suggestions alone will improve your memory recall . . by over 200 % . .

Reliability on your memory, from today on . . is improving in every aspect . . You shall always recall what you need to remember . . The impressions received . . in your memory bank . . will be clearer and more definite . . Whatever you wish to recall . . will immediately present itself, in the correct form, in your mind . . You are improving rapidly . . And very soon . . your memory will be better than it has ever been before . . Whatever you need to remember, will be easily and readily recalled . .

Whenever you need something from your memory . . Formulate the question in your mind . . stay relaxed and wait for the answer . . Whatever you need to remember . . will be easily and readily recalled . . Whenever you need some bit of information . . it springs, naturally, into your mind . .

And the very need for that information . . makes you feel calm, easy and self-possessed . . Because you know . . you can trust . . that you have a better recall . . You now, have a greatly improved memory . . for several reasons . . You are more interested in retaining everything . . You want to retain as much as possible . . because it makes a much more interesting life and career . .

All obstacles, which may have diminished your memory recall . . are fading away . . And every day, in every way . . your memory is becoming better and better . . Whatever you have learned and need to recall . . is always there for you . . And you are always at ease, calm and composed . .

The 4 parts of a good memory are : One . . Impression . . Concentrate on what you need to remember. Two . . Association . . Associate something familiar with the memory. Three . . Retention . . Your retention span is steadily increasing. Four . . Recall . . Your memories flow freely and easily thru your mind . .

EMERGE

MENOPAUSE - EASY NATURAL

You are relaxing very well . . Now, you are going into a deeper . . DEEPER state of relaxation . . I want you to continue to relax . . As you hear my words . . you will go DEEPER and DEEPER . . DEEPER . . into relaxation . . Breath deeper now . . And with each breath you take . . you will sink a little DEEPER each time . . Just flow with it . . and relax . . RELAX . . RELAX DEEPER . .

The word, Menopause, literally means, 'Cessation of Menses' . . and refers to that time in a woman's life . . when the reproduction function has ceased . . or has come to an end . . There is a decline in hormonal secretion by the ovary . . and it all occurs in an easy, natural way . . A more common name for the menopause is, "Change of Life" . . This is a wonderful experience . . because it indicates an important progression in a woman's life . . It brings to a woman the freedom from ever getting pregnant again . . It enables her to realize . . that after her children are grown . . she will have much more freedom for doing the things she has looked forward to doing . .

Experiencing that change of life . . also enables the woman to enjoy sexual relations . . with her chosen partner . . without the use of contraceptives or birth control pills . . Knowing that she will never again become pregnant . .

When we were children . . most of us played the game of 'wishing on a star' . . The first star we saw in the evening . . we would make a wish . . Then there was also the wish we made . . when we blew out the birthday candles . . There were other occasions, weren't there . . when we made special wishes . . And many of us have continued making wishes . . right up to the present time . .

You have probably made many wishes through the years . . Actually, we are realizing, more each day . . that what we think in our mind . . can actually happen . . If we want to achieve a goal . . one of the most important key elements for achieving it . . is to close our eyes and visualize it being accomplished . . in our mind . . If we do this enough . . to get it firmly embedded in our mind . . our mind will cause us to perform the proper actions to accomplish our goal . . It changes from merely wishing it would happen to . . actually making it happen . .

When it comes to getting things . . that we seriously want in life . . getting a million dollars is pushed far into the background . . Most of us would

352

much prefer to have good health . . joy in our work . . loving . . and being loved in return . . Having the freedom to be and to do things . . that bring us happiness . . And, advancing the spiritual progress of our soul . .

Many times, when walking down the street . . we greet people by saying . . "It sure is a beautiful day" . . One day, I met a friend and greeted her with these words . . She responded by saying . . "Yes it is, but the flu season is here . . They were warning everyone about it on TV last night" . . True to her words, two days later . . she had the flu . . And had to miss work for a week . .

It is a fact that our health is the result of the thoughts . . we accept in our mind . . If we believe in flu and believe the flu bug is out there . . just waiting for us . . we can easily develop it in our bodies . . Instead of thinking about ill-health . . we need to be aware that our bodies were created to be healthy . . Our bodies are created with the capability of eliminating any kind of bacteria or disease from our system . . and remain healthy at all times . . By holding onto positive thoughts . .

The same is true with women going through the change of life . . By thinking of it as a wonderful experience . . A time of life that God has granted only to a woman . . to experience . . It is an enjoyable time . . and a wonderful experience . .

Think of every month of the year as a healthy season . . April . . February . . September . . Every month is a . . healthy season . . This mental attitude works just as powerfully . . for health . . as thinking about illness does, for producing sickness . . The energies in the body are made to keep the body healthy and strong . . If you have been experiencing any kind of difficulty . . you are reversing that situation now . . By getting your body attuned . . to its natural healing energies . .

Your natural body processes are functioning perfectly . . And the thoughts in your mind are on positive . . good health, issues . . And your good health continues improving . . more and more each day . .

In just a moment now, I will count to FIVE . . and you will awaken . . feeling refreshed . . and wonderful . . You will awaken a little more with each count you hear . . You will remember everything you have experienced and . . everything you have learned at this time . . is true . .

I will begin my count now . .

ONE . .   You are coming up now . . A little at a time . . Soon you will awaken . .

TWO . .   Your fingers and toes want to wiggle now . . Let them move a little . .

THREE . . Feeling more awake, refreshed and wonderful . . for you are, truly, a wonderful person . .

FOUR . . You're almost up now . . Take a deep breath . . and . .

FIVE . .   Open your eyes . . and let me see a big smile . .

091 Prescript.   MORNING SICKNESS - OVERCOME
(Follow Relaxation)

You are very calm and relaxed now . . And you are aware . . that it was really you . . who produced the relaxation, wasn't it . . All I did was give you suggestions . . and you relaxed yourself . . So you know now that you are capable . . of being relaxed and calm at all times . . during your daily life . .

I want you to concentrate on your abdomen now . . And notice that it feels gently warm and relaxed . . And you are now noticing . . that your abdomen is becoming even more relaxed now . . (Pause) Your stomach and abdomen feel so relaxed and comfortable . . that you feel like you can easily . . eat the foods and drink the liquids that your body needs . . to continue improving your strength and good health . .

Each day, as the baby continues to grow . . you will desire to eat foods and drink liquids . . that are perfectly suited for you . . and for the baby . . And you will notice that your stomach and abdomen will adjust perfectly . . so you will always feel comfortable and at ease . .

You are anticipating the birth of your baby . . and your happiness keeps increasing more each day . . You are experiencing such joy and happiness that your entire body is responding . . by continuing to become healthier and stronger . . Each day, you will continue to experience . . a more wonderful feeling of well being . . throughout your entire body . .

Now, visualize a clear pool of water . . Every time you look at water . . that will be a signal to your subconscious mind . . Your subconscious mind will respond . . by causing you to feel relaxed and calm . . and peaceful . . The way you are now . . And you will remain calm . . and relaxed and peaceful . . for at least six hours . . Every time you look at water . . you will be more calm and relaxed . . from now on . . Whether you are awake or sleeping . .

Your breathing will be smooth and easy . . All of your glands, organs, muscles, nerves, ligaments and tendons . . will keep functioning more perfectly . . Your digestive and elimination systems . . are continuing to function more perfectly each day . .

Regardless of what is going on around you . . you will always remain calm and relaxed . . Your nerves will be more relaxed and steady . . and you will be emotionally calmer . . This will enable you to do everything in a very relaxed manner . .

Having a baby is a perfectly normal experience . . And your body knows how to adjust to these conditions perfectly . . And you will always remain calm, healthy, relaxed and peaceful . . You will have all the strength you need . . to continue on with your daily activities . .

At night, when you are ready to go to sleep . . you will close your eyes . . breathe deeply and exhale slowly, five times . . And that will relax the body completely . . so you will go to sleep easily . . You will remember that all you need to do . . to go to sleep easily . . is to get into bed . . close your eyes, breathe deeply . . and exhale slowly, five times . . And when you do that, you will relax and drift into a comforting state of sleep . . calmly and easily . .

While you are sleeping, you will be relaxed, calm and comfortable . . Each morning, when you awaken . . you will feel rested and refreshed . . Your mind will be alert and clear . . And you will feel healthy, strong and energetic . .

All of these suggestions and instructions . . are now embedded in the storehouse of your mind . . They are now a part of you . . And will be used automatically by you . . to enable you to continue living . . a happier, healthier and more enjoyable life . .

You are in a cycle of progress . . that keeps growing stronger each day . . And you will so happy and proud . . to have this opportunity . . to bring your child into a peaceful, loving home . .

You are now able to maintain poise and calmness . . in the midst of changing circumstances . . And you will maintain a state of emotional stability . . that is pleasing to you . .

Each day, you will become more aware of love . . all around you . . Ready for you to share . . And you will find that, as you express yourself to others . . in a loving way . . you will experience more love and harmony, flowing into your life . . And you will be filled with a wonderful, harmonious feeling . . of love and peace . .

You are placing yourself, and all that concerns you, in the love and care of God . . And you are realizing that, what you cannot do, God can do . .

You are being strengthened and rejuvenated . . by a divine healing power . . of love . .

You are getting ready to awaken from the hypnotic state now . . And will continue experiencing a surge of energy and enthusiasm . . And know that life on Earth . . is a wonderful experience . . to be enjoyed . . Your health and happiness will continue improving more each day . .

In a moment, you will be . . once again, in a normal state of mind . . Now, I am going to count from ONE to FIVE . . and when you hear the number, FIVE . . you will open your eyes and be wide awake . . feeling refreshed and wonderful . . for you are . . a wonderful person . .

ONE - Coming up now . . Feeling rested and refreshed . . You will remember everything with a clear understanding . .
TWO - Coming up a little higher now . . You are connected to your inner strength . . Supporting only your best interest . .
THREE - Everything I have told you is true . . And is happening now . . You will benefit greatly from this experience . .
FOUR - Becoming more aware of your body . . Move your hands and feet . . Let them stir a little . .
FIVE - You may open your eyes now . . Inhale and stretch a bit . .
Tell me, "How do you feel ?"

As you go deeper and deeper in your relaxation . . you are aware that you are completely safe and secure . . You are resting . . in a comfortable position and there is no motion . . Nothing to arouse you . . or upset you in any way . . And I want you to know that you are completely safe and secure . . in any situation you encounter . . involving motion . .

The first principle about motion sickness . . whether it is car sickness, air sickness or sea sickness . . Whatever it is caused from . . the feeling you get from it . . creates a fear in you . . And that fear causes an increased amount of neurons to react on the vagus nerve . . thereby causing excessive acid to be released in the stomach . . This, in turn, causes the individual to become sick . .

In addition to that, fear also causes excessive adrenaline . . to flow into the bloodstream . . And the adrenaline causes the stomach muscles to churn around even more . . And so, even those people who remain afraid . . can stop the sickness to some extent . . by keeping a full stomach . .

That is something sailors have known for a long time . . When they suspect the sea is going to be choppy . . they eat a hearty breakfast, before putting out to sea . . This is especially true of fishermen . . who put out to sea for a day . . and return to shore on the same day . . Because, before they ever begin to feel the motion . . they already have a full stomach for the acid . . and the muscles . . to work on . .

Since it is normal to excrete acid . . it is also normal for the stomach muscles to contract . . when there is food in the stomach . . And since we know the contracting will occur . . it is much better if you have your stomach full of food . . before you set sail . . or fly . . or ride in a vehicle . . So, that is the first rule to remember . . Make sure you eat a full meal before the motion ever begins . . The second thing you can do is to . . medicate yourself . . the most common medication is Dramamine . . but there are many others . .

Some people are afraid of any motion at all . . The slow movement of a car or an airplane, taxiing on a runway . . Even a ship on a calm sea can cause it . . With other people, it may take a great deal of commotion . . Like a small plane or small boat . . One that gets tossed around easily . .

And so, the first two rules we have are . . to eat a big meal and fill the stomach . . before setting out . . so that the acid has something to work on . . And the next was to cut down on the muscle stimulation by taking a medication . . such as Dramamine, or some other such medicine . . And the third thing is the removal of the fear, completely . . And that comes through the use of medical hypnosis . . Which is what we are doing now . .

But in any case . . the basic thing is, survival . . There is an urgency to survive . . because of those burning questions that gnaw into the conscious mind . . "What would happen if the boat sank? What would happen if it were a little more rough . . and the airplane went down ? Of course, what would happen . . is that the individual would not survive . . So, basically, it a fear for survival . .

Now, there is another way we can look at this . . If you are on a bucking horse . . and you don't even know how to ride a horse . . you can be pretty sure of . . getting thrown off . . On the other hand . . if you concentrate your entire mind on riding the horse . . there is no mind power left to think about getting thrown off . . even if you knew it was going to happen . . In fact, the cowboys who ride bucking horses . . never worry about being thrown off at all . . They fully expect to be . . and . . so what? . . They have a term that they yell at each other . . that urges them on . . You've heard it before, I'm sure . . It is simply . . "Ride 'em, cowboy!" . .

Now, "Ride 'em, cowboy!" is a very good term . . because it insists that the individual . . do something . . If a student is flying a small plane . . and the instructor realizes that he is frozen at the controls . . frozen with fear . . he may yell at the student, "Ride 'em, cowboy!" "Ride 'em, cowboy!" Meaning, take over the controls . . Don't let the plane fly you . . How wonderful it is . . when you have something to do . . instead of just sitting there . . thinking about your stomach . .

That is also important in a small boat . . Take over the controls and . . do something . . Set the boat into the waves to cut down on the turbulence . . Ride the waves . . just like you ride it in the air . . Ride it out and enjoy it . . Get a big kick out of it! "Whoopee"! . . And the more you concentrate your mind on the, "Whoopee", the better you will feel . . What fun it is that you have some motion . . And that you're not just sitting there with a . . flat tire . . Enjoy the very thing that causes you to have fear in the first place . . And from this moment on . . that is the approach you are going to take . . You are going to really enjoy . . the very thing that turns your stomach into a knot . . You are going to have fun with motion . . like riding a roller coaster . . After all, it IS fun! . . People pay for that

359

privilege . . What a really dead feeling it is . . if the air or the water is so calm . . that you do not even know you are moving . . If that is the case then, why travel ? . . The kick you get from traveling is that you know you are traveling . . What fun is it to travel in a great big bus . . if you can go in a sports car ? . . It is much more fun to fly a fighter plane than a big 747 . .

Motion is fun . . Especially if you really allow yourself to enjoy it . . And, if you get a big splash of water in your face . . Wonderful! . . All the more fun . . It's exhilarating . . and you are really going to enjoy it . .

The more the motion, the more the fun . . And let those thoughts just sink into the deepest part of your subconscious mind . . and register fully, in every way . . "Ride 'em, cowboy!" . . Now, you can show what's really in you . . You can really show how good you are . . Fly that plane . . Steer that boat . . Have the fun you want to have . . Do what you want to do . . and be . . what you really want to be . . Show what a good pilot or sailor you really are . .

Let these phrases burn into your mind . . so you never forget them . . And say them to yourself, every single time you are faced with a situation . . The more the motion . . the more the fun . . "Ride 'em, cowboy!". .

I am going to give you a period of silence now . . as all of these suggestions seal themselves . . into the deepest part of your subconscious mind . . And they will reinforce themselves, over and over again, in your mind . . Your subconscious mind is absorbing everything I am saying . . Continue to relax now . . as this period of silence begins . .

(2 minutes of silence)

In a moment, you will be, once again, in a normal state of mind . . Now, I am going to count from ONE to FIVE . . and when you hear the number, FIVE . . you will open your eyes and be wide awake . . feeling refreshed and wonderful . . for you are . . a wonderful person . .

EMERG

MOTIVATION

You are relaxing very well now . . And so I want to bring to mind . . the purpose of this session . . which is to help you realize that you are very important . . and to increase your motivation . . so your full potential will emerge . .

You are probably not aware of this but . . the truth is . . you are the most important person in the world . . And you already have the capabilities to achieve outstanding accomplishments . .

Some people develop the mistaken idea that it is wrong . . to think of themselves as being . . so important . . And, of course, you wouldn't want to go around telling everyone . . that you're the most important person in the world . . because, like most people . . you have grown up being taught that we should always think of others . . and should always put others first . . But realizing your own importance doesn't mean you are downgrading others . . In fact, you must care for yourself before you can care for others . . Consider what your own needs are and use the information as a barometer . . when considering other people's needs . . We are also taught that people are conceited if they appear to be gloating over their own self-importance . . We certainly don't want to be conceited . . And so, I'm not suggesting that you become that type of person . . But I am interested in helping you to adopt a viewpoint of yourself . . that will increase your self-confidence, your self-respect and your self-acceptance . . You ARE important . . and there is nothing wrong in living your life realizing your own importance . .

You deserve the recognition and status the creator intended for you to have . . You deserve to have a good life . . You deserve a happy life . . And you deserve to attain the success you would like to have for yourself . .

Most everyone is similar in that we all have fundamental urges . . We have desire for friendship . . We have desire for love . . We have desire for self-expression and desire for recognition . . And as those desires and urges are achieved, we recognize our own self-worth . . Our own importance . .

Consider the meaning of the word, IMPORTANCE . . Importance. In this sense, translates into only one factor . . value to others . . You are important . . to yourself and to others . . so your subconscious mind is accepting these suggestions and instructions I am giving you to increase your motivation for success, happiness and . . a lifetime of fulfillment . .

Let me ask you . . Do you know what is really controlling your life ? . . Your first thought may be that you . . control your own life . . But you, In fact, are being controlled . . You have a God-force within you that controls every move you make . .

Think about that for a moment . . When you breath, do you control every breath you take ? . . No. You continue breathing even when you are asleep . . And your subconscious mind keeps your heart pumping blood through your circulatory system whether you are awake or sleeping . . And when you put food in your mouth and chew it, do you consciously control the muscles in your jaws . . or do they function from some unconscious force ? . . What causes those automatic responses ? What causes the automatic movement of your muscles, ligaments and tendons when you brush your teeth, walk down the street or scratch an itch ? . . Why, in fact, did you itch at all ? . . What causes your food to digest ? What causes you to see, when you open your eyes ? What causes you to hear or feel or to even think ? . .

The answer is that there is a God-force within you that controls everything you do and every response you make . . There has never been nor ever will be . . a moment when you are not affected by that unconscious power within you . . It affects you when you are awake and continues to affect you . . when you are sleeping . .

The power that controls you is in your own mind . . You are constantly doing what your subconscious mind influences you to do . . And in reality, many people become slaves of their subconscious mind . . because they don't realize that they can do something about it . . if they are being controlled in an undesirable way . . The good news is . . you don't have to be a slave to your subconscious mind . . You have a conscious mind that enables you to think . . And you have the ability to use your conscious mind to program your subconscious mind . . so that it will operate the way you want it to . . By redirecting your subconscious mind in a good, positive way . . you can live your life the way that you want to live it . . And that is what you are doing by having this session . .

Permitting yourself to be hypnotized reveals that you are open-minded . . And it also reveals how you realize that you are capable of motivating yourself for improvement . . And you are making that effort to improve . . Therefore, you will be successful . . You will be happy that you are taking the time to experience hypnotic relaxation . . Because at the same time, you are learning techniques that will increase your motivation for success . . The ability to motivate yourself is . . one of the most important skills you will ever acquire . . Study various people who have impressed you as being successful . . and you will discover that they are people who have learned to motivate themselves . . Notice people who have self-confidence . . People who are calm and relaxed, who are in control of situations at all times . . People who make decisions with confidence . . and you will find they are all people who have learned self-motivation . . Self-motivated people are successful people . . They have learned to put the power of their mind to work for them . . They determine what they want to achieve . . and then they take action to make things happen . . And to continue advancing towards the goal that drives them on . .

Someone made this statement, on motivation : "Within each of us is a spark of genius . . All that is needed to fan the tiny flame into an inferno of action is strong, affirmative desire" . .

As you continue going into a deeper hypnotic state of relaxation . . I am going to give you suggestions that can increase your motivation for success . . I want you to go deeper now . . Deeper and Deeper . . Continue to relax but continue going deeper . . I want you to go deeper . . so you may fully absorb everything we are discussing here today . . Relax . . (pause)

The first point is to understand the importance of taking . . one step at a time . . Don't be too proud to begin at the bottom of the ladder to achieve success . . Take it one step at a time . .

The second point is to decide on the goal you want to achieve . . So much that you will not be satisfied until you have achieved it . . The next point is to perform some action, each day . . to keep you advancing toward your goal . . Take action today . . The step you take toward your goal today will prepare you to advance even more tomorrow . .

You are developing the attitude of expectancy . . Each day you will decide what you will do to keep moving closer to your goal . .

And you proceed with confidence, knowing that every move forward . . brings you closer to completion of your goal . .

What you are doing right now is really quite valuable in your pursuit towards your goal . . in assisting your progress towards greater success and fulfillment . . You have taken the most important step by permitting yourself . . to learn these principles of hypnotic relaxation . .

Never be content with what you have already accomplished . . Keep telling yourself that you have only started . . and that you want to continue advancing towards even greater accomplishments . . Every step you make towards your goal is an accomplishment . . regardless of how small the step may be . . For example : If your goal is to have a thousand dollars in the bank . . you would be advancing towards that goal even if there were days when . . you added only a penny to your savings . . Keep moving forward at all times . . Never let a day go by that you haven't done something to move towards your goal . . One new fact learned . . or one new contact made . . is making progress . . instilling pride in your accomplishments . . Keep the goal in sight on a daily basis . .

Direct your attention closely now . . and I will describe a number of energy forces that will strengthen your motivation and determination . .

The first force of energy . . that increases your motivation and determination . . is by studying in the area or field . . in which you want to achieve your goal . .

The second is a force of energy called, expansion . . You may already be quite competent in your work . . but there are always ways to improve . . Make a special effort to expand your abilities . . that will speed up your progress . . Always be alert for new ideas that can increase your competence . .

The next force of energy is to make a list of all possible opportunities for advancement . . Take advantage of even the smallest idea or opportunity to advance . .

Another is to find out what other people are doing . . who have the same goal or a similar goal as your own . . Ask advise from the person who has already achieved success . . Most successful people are happy to give advise . .

A fifth force of energy comes from being open to what may seem to be strange ideas, thoughts or discoveries . . Remember that many of the most successful people in history came up with ideas that were considered strange . . when they were first presented . . For example : Many men of science thought the electric light bulb was a very strange idea, indeed . . And they were sure it would never be used . . But today, there are very few homes in our world that are not making use of . . what was once considered strange . . and useless . .

Read challenging books that are related to the field you are striving for . . Learn a new language . . and learn to express yourself fluently and clearly . . There are so many things you can do to improve yourself . . But keep in mind . . Your own motivation is the key to your own success . .

And finally, always be reaching a little beyond your present capabilities . . Never feel that you have reached the limit of your potential . . You can always accomplish . . a little bit more . .

I want you to rest now and absorb all that we have discussed . .
(pause 2 to 3 minutes)

In just a moment I will begin my count from Five . . down to One . . And when you hear me say the number One . . you will open your eyes, feeling refreshed, renewed and ready to take on your next challenge . . You will recall everything, clearly . . that you have learned here today and you will enjoy putting your new knowledge to good use . .

I will begin my count now . .

Five . . Four . . Three . . Two . . and One . . Open your eyes and adjust to your surroundings . .

094 Prescript.   NAIL BITING – OVERCOME
(Follow Relaxation)

The reason we are here today is because . . you have made a firm decision to stop biting your fingernails . . You want to let your fingernail grow long enough . . to care for them properly . . And permitting yourself to be hypnotized means you will be successful in eliminating this habit . .

Biting your fingernails is a habit you have learned over a period of time . . But it's an easy habit to get rid of because . . biting your fingernails fails to serve any purpose in your life . .

You know you have the ability to move your hands any time you want to move them . . It's easy for you to put your hands any place you want to put them . . All you need to do is decide where you want to put them . . and you can do it . . You can put them on top of your head . . or you can put them on your knee by merely making the conscious decision . . to move your hand to that spot . . From now on . . if your hand starts moving towards your mouth . . you will be aware of what is happening and you will realize that you can stop it . . And you will stop it . . and you will move it somewhere else . .

Your subconscious mind is increasing your will power and self-control . . and is making it easy for you to be free from the habit of biting your fingernails . . You have decided to stop biting your fingernails because you want them to grow . . And they will continue growing longer and stronger because you will not bite them any more . .

Now, from this moment on . . you are going to be very, very proud . . You are going to be very proud of the fingernails that you have . . You have beautiful fingernails and they are growing to exactly the desired length . . And you are going to take care of them, keeping them exactly the way they should be . . And from this moment on . . you are through biting your fingernails altogether . .

You can keep your nails neat and trim with an emery board and with a nail clipper . . You can carry these tools with you, if you like . . You can carry a nail file . . You can clip off the cuticle . . You can do anything with them that you like . . But not bite them . . You are through putting your fingers in your mouth altogether . . Should you make that mistake at any time . . they will taste very, very bitter . . As bitter as the most bitter substance you have ever tasted . . So that should a finger ever find its way into your mouth, you would immediately be aware because of the bitter taste . . You will bring it to your attention at once and quickly remove the finger from your mouth before any biting or disfiguration has taken place . . You are through disfiguring yourself in any way . .

This hypnotic session is a way of opening discussion of your problem with your subconscious mind . . You are allowing your subconscious mind to know that you wish to break the habit you have developed . . of biting your fingernails . . And that you want to replace that old habit with a new habit . . And that is . . caring for you hands . . You can even become compulsive about the care of your fingernails and hands . . in order to keep them looking nice . . You're through hiding your hands . . You're through shoving them into your pockets or folding them under your arms in order to keep them from being seen . . You are going to want them to be seen now . . because you're going to be extremely proud of the way you care for your hands, fingers and fingernails . .

Now, all of these suggestions take complete and thorough effect upon your mind, body and spirit . . and seal themselves into the deepest part of your subconscious mind . . And they reinforce themselves over and over again, becoming stronger and stronger with every breath you take . . Now you can sink deeper and deeper into relaxation . . as you let these suggestions take complete and thorough effect upon you . . The habit of biting your fingernails is broken . . The habit of taking good care of your fingernails is instilled . . The urge to put your fingers in your mouth, for any reason, is gone . . And as you relax now . . you are confident in the knowledge that you have conquered this problem . . All of these suggestions are the absolute truth to you and take complete and thorough effect . . upon your mind, body and spirit . .

EMERG

I want you to use your imagination now . . I want you to visualize yourself
. . slowly moving towards the beach . . You may be driving or flying . .
It doesn't matter . . But you are moving nearer . . very slowly . . It's a
beautiful day and you can hear soft, soothing sounds in the background . .

The sun will soon be setting and you are getting closer . . to the beach . .
You will be getting there in time to see the sun setting on the horizon . .

You have arrived at the beach . . You are sitting there, watching the bright
red sun as it slowly goes down over the horizon . . Notice the colors as
they begin changing from orange to crimson . . And as it continues
descending . . it becomes a deep, dark red-orange . . As the sun gets
nearer to the water . . you notice that it actually appears to be two suns . .
One in the sky and one in the water . .

You are continuing to feel more calm and peaceful . . as you notice how
the sun seemingly disappears . . into the water . . The colors continue
changing from orange-red to lavender and then to a purple-blue . . And
you continue to feel more relaxed and more at ease . . Everything around
you keeps becoming more calm . . and more still . . The water seems so
peaceful and smooth . . almost like glass . . reflecting a tranquil beauty
. . The ocean sounds seem to travel on forever and ever . .

You are hardly noticing, as you keep feeling more comfortable and tranquil
. . that you are also feeling more safe and secure . . Your entire body is
responding to the idea of complete relaxation . . And you are realizing that
. . this calmness and peacefulness are available to you at all times . .
Every time you look at water, your mind responds to that signal . . and
causes you to become calm and relaxed . . and feel very peaceful and at
ease . . Every time you look at water, your nerves become very relaxed
and at ease . .

I am also telling you of another signal you can use . . to experience
immediate relaxation any time you choose . . All you need to do is bring
your thumb and index finger together . . and that will cause you to become
calm and relaxed . . You will immediately experience a feeling of peace
and tranquility . . just by touching your thumb and finger together . .

Continue relaxing, calmly and peacefully now . . In just a moment I will talk to you again . . and give you some additional suggestions that will be helpful . .

(Give building self-confidence or self-acceptance or some other positive suggestions.)

NOTE :   PREPARE 'HEALING HANDS' BY CREATING PRESSURE BETWEEN THE PALMS (CHACRA'S). THIS IS ACCOMPLISHED BY 'ALMOST' TOUCHING FINGERTIPS TOGETHER AND GENTLY PUSHING THE PALMS TOWARD EACH OTHER, UNTIL A PRESSURE (ENERGY) IS FELT. IF PAINFUL AREA IS AVAILABLE TO TOUCH, PLACE BOTH HANDS ON OPPOSITE SIDES OF PAINFUL AREA . IT IS NOT NECESSARY TO TOUCH THE FLESH BUT CONTINUE TO FEEL THE ENERGY FLOW BY PUSHING THE CHACRA'S (fingertips and palms) TOWARDS EACH OTHER. GIVE THE FOLLOWING SUGGESTIONS :

You are beginning to feel a healing warmth flowing through the tissues of your skin . . The healing processes of your body are working in unison and you are beginning to feel more comfortable . . more at ease and more calm . . Your entire body is becoming more relaxed as the energy penetrates . .

All pain, all discomfort and all swelling are diminishing . . flowing out from your body, easily and naturally . . as if they were being drawn out with a magnet . .

The healing processes of your body are functioning properly now . . and will continue working properly . . And are healing your body completely and perfectly . .

Your muscles, nerves, tendons and ligaments are relaxing more and more . .

Swelling is decreasing and all of your joints are becoming normal in size . .

You are continuing to feel more comfortable as all pain and discomfort are leaving your body . . And your body is healing perfectly and completely . .

When the healing has been completed . . you will be able to do everything in a relaxed way . .

Your muscles are becoming stronger, yet they are loose and flexible . . and are functioning easily and comfortably . .

Notice, as I hold my hands in this position, that you are feeling more comfortable and more at ease . . You are feeling emotionally calm and serene . . It is such a peaceful and relaxing feeling . . You are beginning to experience wonderful sensations all through your body . .
(pause and hold the area for several minutes.)

NOTE : ENERGY INDUCEMENTS INTO VARIOUS BODY PARTS REQUIRES ABOUT 20 TO 30 MINUTES. GENTLY REMOVE HANDS WHEN COMPLETE AND CONTINUE WITH SUGGESTIONS.

Even after I remove my hands, you will continue feeling wonderful . . You will keep improving more each day . . And you will be very happy to realize the progress you are making . .

When you awaken from the hypnotic state . . you will feel much better than you did before we began this session . . You will feel calm and peaceful . . relaxed and comfortable . . rested and refreshed . .

The processes of your body are functioning properly now and are healing your body perfectly . . Your body is responding to its own natural healing energies . . to provide you with a well balanced, healthy condition . . (pause)

You have made great accomplishments today and it is time now to end this session . . In just a moment I will begin my count from one to five . . And when you hear the count of FIVE . . you will open your eyes, feeling wide awake, alert and ready for a new challenge . . I will begin . .

ONE   . . Rising up now . . Gently arising . .
TWO   . . Moving up slowly . . Waking more and more . .
THREE . . Your body wants to stir a little . . move your muscles now . .
FOUR   . . Let your arms and legs gain more strength now as you awaken.
FIVE   . . Open your eyes now and adjust to your surroundings . .

A person can learn a lot by watching construction workers build a house . .
I don't know everything involved in building a house . . However, I do
know that they are constructed differently in various parts of the country . .
Most homes that are built in hurricane areas are constructed with steel beams
in the frame . . to make them stronger and capable of withstanding a
hurricane force wind . . In northern parts of the country, most homes are
built with a basement . . They dig the foundation deep in the soil . . by
pouring in truckloads of cement for the basement floor and walls . . Some
of the walls are reinforced with steel bars . . to prevent cracking or
crumbling . . Many parts of the country have water so close to ground level
. . that they merely pour slabs . . and build the homes on the slabs . . Or
they have the ground floor of the home built up . . two, three or sometimes
ten feet above ground level . . to keep water out when water level is high . .

As you are continuing to drift into a more peaceful, more relaxed state of
hypnosis . . your mind is realizing that the male penis is comparable to a
home . . in that, each person's penis is different from all the others . .
Some penises are short and thick . . Some are long and slender . . Some
are short and slender . . while some are long and thick . . And regardless
of the size of all the penises in the world . . most men feel that their penis
is . . too small . . Most men have not seen the penis of very many other
men, or they have not observed other penises closely . . Yet they still feel
that their penis is too small . .

Possibly as a child, they saw their father's penis . . and it seemed so large
to them because they were comparing it to their own . . which, of course,
at that time, had not reached full growth . . However, since you feel that
you would like your penis to be larger . . you have the right to make that
decision . . and the subconscious levels of your mind knows what to do . .
to cause your penis to grow larger . .

First of all, an important key is for you to decide . . how large you want
your penis to be . . So decide now whether you want it to be one, two or
three inches longer than it is now . . And decide whether you want it to be
a half inch thicker or a full inch thicker . . Concentrate on your penis as
you are making these decisions . .

I want you to use your imagination now and think of your penis as being just
the way you want it to be . . Concentrate on that as I am talking to you . .

There may be times when I am talking and it may seem like my voice is a long distance away . . There may be other times when I am talking and you may not even be aware of my voice . . That is okay because your subconscious mind will hear and receive everything I say . . and will cause it to happen in an easy, natural way . .

You have probably heard the story of Alice in Wonderland . . And you may remember that when she saw the bottle with the label that said, Drink Me, she did drink . . and she got larger . . then smaller . . And you will find it interesting to notice that as you continue to relax . . things are beginning to change for you as well . . You will probably notice that your left arm is beginning to feel heavier than ever before . . And your right arm is feeling so light, it feels like it wants to lift up towards the ceiling . . Notice that your left arm is continuing to feel heavier . . And without even noticing it . . your right arm is feeling lighter than a feather and is beginning to lift up towards the ceiling . .

As that continues, I want you to notice your right foot . . Notice the feeling of your shoe on your right foot . . It may seem that your right foot is getting bigger and bigger as your left foot begins feeling smaller and smaller . . Be aware of the changes you are experiencing in both of your feet . . as your right hand and arm keep lifting up towards the ceiling . .

Things are changing . . readjusting . . Similar to the way trees keep adjusting . . Many trees shed their leaves during the fall and winter months . . only to have them bloom again in the spring and summer . . and the trees continue growing . . And without noticing it . . your penis is beginning to renew its growth pattern . . and is becoming exactly the way you want it to be . . Each night, just before you go to sleep . . I want you to close your eyes and visualize your penis . . exactly the way you want it to be . . All levels of your subconscious mind will receive this image and will cause it to happen . . just that easily . . And just as surely as your inner mind causes your hand to become numb . . when I put that suggestion into your mind . .

In just a moment I am going to count from one to five for you to awaken from the hypnotic state . . You will come up to a wide awake, fully alert state, a little more, each time I say a number . .

And when you hear me say the number FIVE . . you will be back in a fully alert state . . Your left hand and arm will be back to their normal feeling and size . . Your right hand and arm will be back to their normal feeling and size . . And both your right foot and your left foot will be back to their normal feeling and size . .

I will begin my count now . .

EMERG

(NOTE)   IN ADDITIONAL SESSIONS, YOU CAN USE PRESCRIPTIONS FOR 'ENLARGING BREASTS'. JUST CHANGE BREAST TO PENIS.

PHOBIA TREATMENT - CHILDREN

(Metaphor)

At this point you are completely . . and deeply relaxed . . Very deep now . . Completely relaxed . .

There was a little boy who was very rich . . He was so rich that he had a big, huge, special room . . just for his toys and treasures . . And he would go to that special room, every day . .

You would think that he would be a very happy little boy . . having so many wonderful toys and treasures . . But actually, the boy was very sad because . . even though he had many beautiful toys and many treasures . . there seemed to be one thing that ruined everything for him . .

Sitting over in the corner of the room . . behind all the toys and treasures . . so it could barely be seen . . sat a large, green dragon . . And that dragon seemed to be watching the little boy . . all the time . . It never took its eyes off the little boy . . And that would spoil all of his fun . . Because . . he was so afraid of the dragon . .

He would even have dreams about the dragon . . rushing up to him and throwing him down the stairs and . . trying to kill him . . And every night he would wake up screaming . .

He never could explain to anyone about his nightmares because . . he was afraid that the green dragon would get him, if he told . . And the little boy kept feeling more unhappy . . In fact, he became so unhappy that . . sometimes he would dance around and play very hard . . He would laugh loudly and talk, and talk, and talk . . thinking it would make him forget about the dragon in the corner . . But, no matter how loud he laughed . . how hard he played or how much he talked . . whenever he stopped he would look in the corner and there would be the green dragon . . Still staring at him . . The little boy just kept feeling dejected . . and fearful . .

This problem continued for a very long time . . Each day, the little boy would start out by playing with his toys . . Trying to enjoy himself and trying not to think about the green dragon . . And each day, he would end up, sitting there, feeling sad . . with tears running down his face . .

One day, a friend came to visit him . . The friend was another boy, his same age and size . . The visitor looked around the room . . really amazed at all the wonderful toys and treasures . . He ran around, picking up one toy after another . . Overjoyed at all of the toys to play with . .

But the little rich boy felt anxious and worried . . He kept looking over at the green dragon . . He didn't join his friend in his fun and enthusiasm . .

Suddenly, his friend ran over to the green dragon to sit on it . . Like sitting on a rocking horse . . And the rich little boy yelled, fearfully, "NO, NO, DON'T DO THAT" . . Of course, the friend asked, "Why not?" And the little rich boy replied, "Because he is a fierce and wicked dragon . . He will try to harm you because he is so evil . . I know, because, he tries to harm me . . I'm terribly afraid of him" . .

His friend laughed and said, "Look at this." . . He turned the dragon so the little rich boy could see the back of it . . And there, on the back of the terrible dragon was . . a long, shiny, black zipper . .

The little boy didn't know what to think of that . . He looked more closely . . still trembling with fear . . And his friend asked, "Don't you want to see what's inside?" . . And the little rich boy stammered, "Uh, I'm not sure" . . And his friend laughed as he unzipped the back of the dragon . .

The dragon's green suit fell away and . . guess what was in there ? . . Another little boy . . And the little boy who came out of the dragon's suit just laughed, and said . . "I really enjoyed being a dragon, until I was discovered . . I knew you were afraid . . All this time I just sat here, making you fearful . . And the little rich boy said, "That was very mean of you! Why did you do that"? "Oh," answered the new little boy . . I did it because I knew it would be fun . . And besides, you have so many toys and treasures . . If you hadn't had the dragon, you might never have known how lucky you are" . .

Then the three boys became good friends and . . began laughing and playing together . . And guess what they did? They began taking turns, zipping themselves up in the dragon suit . . and, playfully, trying to scare each other . . Then they pretended to be afraid of the dragon . . And they were all laughing and having a lot of fun . .

The little rich boy clapped his hands and said, "Now we can lots of fun and play with all of my toys and treasures" . . And so, they did . . But the thing they enjoyed most was, playing Dragon . .

Now, the little rich boy was finally happy . . No longer afraid for no reason . . And he enjoyed playing with all of his toys and treasures . . And Soon, word spread around the neighborhood . . and more little boys and girls came to play . . with all the wonderful toys and treasures . . Oh, yes . . and even the dragon was there . .   EMERG

Your body has been created in such a way . . that it is capable of healing itself perfectly . . If you cut your skin . . the healing processes of your body . . cause the tissues of your skin . . to heal . . You may wash the cut to cleanse it . . or if it is a severe cut . . you may have the doctor put stitches in it . . But, it is still the natural healing processes of your body . . that causes the skin to mend . .

If you should, somehow, break a bone . . you may have a doctor set the bone . . But, it is still the natural healing processes of the body . . that causes the bone to grow back together . .

The same processes that heal scratches . . cuts and broken bones . . can heal other blemishes on your skin . . And can restore your skin perfectly . .

The processes of your body are also designed . . to cleanse unneeded waste material . . out of your body . . through your elimination system . . Some of this 'waste matter' is cleansed out of your body . . through the pores of your skin . . as you perspire and sweat . . Sometimes, the pores become clogged . . for a number of reasons . . and waste matter is held in, beneath the clogged pores . . And that is what causes blemishes . . or pimples . . to form on the skin . .

It has been found that . . clogged pores . . are easy to overcome . . And that pimples on your skin . . are equally as easy . . to cure . . In fact, even now, the processes of your body are functioning properly . . to eliminate all waste matter . . And in the future . . the pores of your skin will be open . . and your skin will keep becoming more smooth and more healthy . .

Your heart is pumping blood through your circulatory system . . carrying with it . . the new cells and nutrients needed . . to renew your skin . . While at the same time . . it is carrying the impurities . . out of your body . .

By having this hypnotic session . . your subconscious mind is being made aware . . of your desire to renew and refresh . . the skin on your body . . From now on . . your subconscious mind is causing your body processes . . to function more effectively . . and cleanse more of the waste matter out of your body . . through your kidneys and your bowels . . And the pores of your skin will continue . . becoming more open and dryer from secretion . .

Your elimination system will keep functioning more perfectly . . and will cleanse all waste materials . . and impurities . . out of your body, in an easy, natural way . .

Your subconscious mind is also controlling your appetite . . And will cause you to desire . . and choose to eat . . only the foods that your body needs . . to keep you healthy and strong . .

You will eat and drink only non-fattening foods and liquids . . that are good for your body . . And you will eat and drink . . only when your body needs food or liquids . . And after you have eaten . . the small amount of food your body actually needs . . to keep you strong and healthy . . you will feel perfectly content and satisfied . . And you will stop eating . . when you know you should eat no more . .

You will wash your skin regularly, and use a towel to pat it dry . . after rinsing thoroughly . . In a short time, your skin will be flawless and healthy . . You will be happy to notice the improvements . . as your skin keeps becoming more smooth . . more clear . . Healthier and more attractive, each and every day . .

EMERGE

PREMENSTRUAL SYNDROME - OVERCOME
(Follow Relaxation)

As you are continuing to relax . . I want you to open your eyes and look . . at the back of your RIGHT hand . . As you do this . . a feeling of heaviness will develop . . in your RIGHT hand . . As you notice that feeling of heaviness . . I want you to lift up your LEFT hand and keep it up . . until I tell it . . to go back down . . (Pause until LEFT hand lifts)

Good . . Your LEFT hand can go back down now . . As you continue concentrating on your RIGHT hand . . I will begin stroking your LEFT hand . . And I want you to notice all the feelings you are experiencing . . in your RIGHT hand . . as your LEFT hand becomes completely numb . . (COMMENCE STROKING LEFT HAND AND PROCEED WITH SUGGESTIONS.)

Notice any feelings you are experiencing in your RIGHT hand . . Your RIGHT hand may begin feeling heavier . . You may notice a feeling of warmth . . coming into your RIGHT hand . . Or it may begin tingling . . Notice everything you are experiencing . . in your RIGHT hand . . as your LEFT hand becomes completely numb . .

Are you aware of the feelings you are experiencing in your RIGHT hand ? . . (Wait for Response)

Now . . I'd like for you to notice that your LEFT hand is feeling very numb . . You are experiencing numbness in your fingers . . In the palm of your hand . . The back of your hand . . and, all through the entire hand . . (Pause) Notice that the numbness is increasing even more now . . And as it does . . it's such a pleasant feeling . . that it feels as though it's too much trouble . . to even move a finger . . It feels as though it is going to sleep . . Almost as though it is no longer a part of you . . And as you become aware of that . . you will nod your head, YES . . (Pause, until client nods.)

AFTER CLIENT NODS, YES, PICK UP HAND BETWEEN FINGERNAILS OF THE THUMB AND MIDDLE FINGER AND ASK CLIENT, "What does it seem like I am doing now" ? . . (Wait for Response.) If client says, "It feels like you are pinching me" . . Reply, "Do you mean, you can feel the pressure of the skin between my fingers?" If client says, "Yes" . . Reply, "You don't feel any pain at all, do you ? (Wait for Response) If client says, "I feel some pain" . . Continue holding hand by fingernails, and Reply, "The hand is continuing to feel more numb . . Tell me when you feel nothing but the pressure of the skin between my fingers" . . (Wait for Response)

(When you are confident the client has numbness in the hand. continue as follows:)

You are responding well to my suggestions . . In just a moment . . I'm going to have you open your eyes . . And even with your eyes open . . you will remain in a hypnotic state . . You will be able to keep your eyes open . . until I tell you to close them again . . When I tell you to close your eyes . . you will close them and immediately drift into a much DEEPER hypnotic state . . And you will continue responding to the suggestions I give you . . Okay, Open your eyes now . . Look and see what I am doing to your hand . . Now, you realize that your subconscious mind caused changes . . so that only your LEFT hand became numb . . Your RIGHT hand has all the normal feelings . . Your LEFT arm has all of its normal feelings . . I'm going to pinch your LEFT arm, lightly . . so you will notice it has all of its feelings . . (Pinch arm lightly, and ask) "Can you feel that?" (Then pinch back of RIGHT hand, and ask) "You notice a little pain in your RIGHT hand, don't you?" (Wait for Response, then say) Now you realize that your subconscious mind causes changes, without any conscious effort by you . . I put the suggestion into your mind . . that your LEFT hand would become numb . . Then I told you a signal I would use . . The signal was . . stroking your LEFT hand . . And it kept becoming more and more numb, each time I stroked it . .

Your mind has learned to respond to signals . . Everything we do . . is in response to signals . . Whatever we do . . we are responding to signals . . When you make a decision to brush your teeth . . you send a signal to your subconscious mind, which in turn . . causes you to make all the correct movements . . To open the toothpaste tube . . squeeze some onto your toothbrush . . Put the brush against your teeth and move your hand in the proper way . . And you make all of these movements, without even thinking about them . . It's that way with everything we do . . When we make the decision to do something . . that is a signal we send to our subconscious mind . . And the subconscious mind responds . . by causing our body to make all of the necessary movements . .

Sometimes, things happen in your body . . that need adjusting . . and you feel pain or discomfort . . Your body continues to function normally . . Still, you are aware of the pain and discomfort . . consciously . . but your subconscious mind needs to be made aware . . that you are not pleased . . with what is happening to your body . . And you want to make changes . . That is why you are here now . .

Now, your subconscious mind is understanding . . that having a brief menstruation period each month, is normal and natural . . For that is a part of the normal preparation of the body . . to enable it to become pregnant . . You were created with the ability . . to have a perfectly normal, functioning body . . Your body knows how to function . . in an easy, natural way . . Enabling you to experience your menstrual period, comfortably . .

I want your subconscious mind to review . . what is happening . . to cause you to experience such discomfort . . during your menstrual period . . and work out the solution . . to resolve that problem completely . . Your subconscious mind is reviewing, examining and exploring . . the causes and effects of that problem . . And your mind is understanding it . . from a more adult . . more mature, point of view . . Realizing that menstruation is a normal activity . . and should be experienced easily, calmly and comfortably . . It should be just as normal and natural as urinating or . . having a bowel movement . .

Your subconscious mind is reviewing and imprints, impressions, thoughts and ideas . . that have gone into your mind . . that may have been causing that problem . . Your mind is assessing that information . . and understanding it from a different point of view . . And understanding, that it is okay now . . to resolve that problem completely . .

You are continuing to relax . . calmly and comfortably . . All levels of your mind are cooperating . . Working out a very pleasant solution . . to that problem . . Continue relaxing another moment . .

When your mind knows it is okay for that problem to be resolved . . and that changes have begun . . and you are getting rid of that problem . . easily and comfortably . . one of your fingers will lift up . . towards the ceiling . . And your finger will remain up . . until I tell it to go back down . .

NOTE : IF CLIENT'S FINGER DID NOT LIFT TO INDICATE CHANGES HAVE STARTED , GO TO, "THERAPY BETWEEN SESSIONS". GIVE THOSE SUGGESTIONS BEFORE AWAKENING CLIENT .

You are doing very well . . It feels so good . . just to continue relaxing . . You are doing just fine . . Later on, when you awaken from the hypnotic state . . your whole body will feel good . . From the top of your head all the way down . . to the bottom of your feet . .

Your subconscious mind is very sensitive to everything I say . . And so, I will remind your subconscious mind that . . even after you awaken from the hypnotic state . . and at all times during your daily life . . these suggestions will continue to influence you . . Just as strongly . . just as surely and . . just as powerfully . . as they do while you are hypnotized . . You will be pleased with the improvements in your life . . Each day, the improvements will keep increasing . . And you can you awaken, each morning . .

Your self-confidence will continue increasing more each day . . And you will be attracting the attention of people . . who will recognize you . . as being one who is capable of achieving . . outstanding accomplishments . . People will be noticing that you are a real achiever . . And that will bring you new opportunities . . for personal advancement and prosperity . .

Remember that you attract to yourself . . what you think and what you believe . . So, always endeavor to keep your thoughts . . on the goals you want to achieve . . And on other, positive, ideas . . that are beneficial to you . . as well as to others . . Do not carry negative thoughts . . or you will bring back negative actions onto yourself . . Always maintain positive thoughts and actions . . And that will bring you your greatest happiness, joy and prosperity . .

One of the most important goals in life . . is to keep becoming a better person . . And you can do that, by being the positive . . self-confident and self-assured person . . you are capable of being . .

You will continue becoming more successful . . because you deserve to be successful . . You are a good person . . You are a very important person . . You are a powerful person . . These are all true statements about you . . And you know it . . Your subconscious mind knows it . . God knows it . . And, therefore, it is a fact . .

You know that achieving success is not merely a matter of chance . . or luck . . When we study about successful people . . we learn that they have taken the actions necessary . . to produce their own success . .

Whether it has been success in marriage, in high grades at school . . success in business . . or in their spiritual growth . .

Success begins in the mind . . You develop an idea of what you want to accomplish . . And you keep repeating that idea, over and over, in your mind . . Especially, just before you go to sleep at night . . When you keep doing that . . you become aware of . . other ideas . . of how to take the necessary actions . . to put your ideas to work . . And then, you keep working on it until you achieve your goals . .

To simplify your key to success, this is what you do . . ONE - Develop your idea or inspiration . . of what you want to accomplish . . TWO - Keep thinking about that idea, several times, every day . . THREE - Write plans of what needs to be done, to make your idea successful . . FOUR - Take the actions needed to put your plan to work . . and FIVE – Always . . be positive . .

It is your birthright to be a happy, healthy and successful person . . you were created by the same creator . . who created every you awaken, each morning . . be sure it is permanent and lasting . .

Being hypnotized is always a wonderful, relaxing experience . . And you will become more aware of the benefits . . you are to experience from it . . each time I hypnotize you . .

You realize that your subconscious mind . . caused the changes in your body . . without any conscious effort by you . . to make your hand numb . . And now, your mind is causing you to experience pleasant changes . . that will enable you to have an easy, comfortable menstrual period . . for a short time each month . . Your menstrual period will be experienced in an easy, natural way . . As a normal cleansing process of your body . .

The healing processes of your body are working properly . . because you want them to work . . Your subconscious mind is obeying your thoughts and desires . . for you, to experience a comfortable menstrual period each month . . Your body is responding . . And you will be very happy as you notice the continuous progress you achieve . . Continue to relax . . .
(Pause)

In just a moment, I will be counting from ONE to FIVE, for you to awaken from the hypnotic state . . And when you awaken . . all the normal feelings will be back in both of your hands . . Your whole body will feel relaxed and comfortable . . Your mind will be alert and you will feel peaceful and calm . . I will begin my count now . .

ONE . . You are aware that soon you will awaken . . You are coming up . .

TWO . . Coming up a little higher now . . and your mind is waking . .

THREE . . Feeling good now . . Feeling wonderful, all over . .

FOUR . . Coming up faster now . . Breath in deeply . . and

FIVE . . Feeling relaxed and wonderful . . You may Open Your Eyes . .

383

As you continue drifting into a DEEPER and DEEPER hypnotic state . . I want you to imagine that you are walking along a path . . through the woods . . that leads up onto a beautiful mountain . .

As you are walking, very casually . . allow your comfort level to increase . . And without even noticing . . you will continue moving into a deeper and deeper relaxed state . . Relax deeper now . . DEEPER . .

As you walk along this path, through the woods . . you will be aware of a variety of trees . . Some large . . Some small . . And by looking upward . . through the trees . . you will see a beautiful, blue sky . . with fluffy, white clouds, drifting high above you . . Soon you will notice the trickling stream . . coming down from the mountain . . And you will see several waterfalls . . as you continue your journey, up onto the mountain . .

As you walk . . just take your time and appreciate things along the way, that interest you . . Many people enjoy the sounds of nature . . such as the different kinds of birds, singing . . The sound of the wind through the trees . . Frogs croaking . . Sometimes they even hear crickets . .

Seeing and hearing the wonders of nature . . really reminds us that . . we could never put a price on the beautiful lakes and streams . . or the beautiful sunsets . . or the wonders of the flowers and the trees . . and animals . .

As you continue your stroll, up into the mountains . . I want you to notice that you are also carrying a pack on your back . . Feel the weight of the pack that you are carrying on your back . . And become more aware that it keeps feeling heavier . . with each step you take . . That pack is filled with all of the things that have been causing your problems . . It is filled with things like . . anger, bitterness, resentment . . jealously . . rejection . . contempt . . And everything that has been causing the problems of _____ .

You sense that it is only a short distance now, to the top of the mountain . . In fact, you are so close to the top . . that you can see it, just ahead . . the path you are taking . . leads to a large, open meadow . . with beautiful green grass and many kinds of wild flowers . . And now, you are walking into that meadow . . noticing all of the colors of the flowers . . and their natural beauty . .

In the center of the meadow, you can is a large open space . . Walk out into the open space . . Take the pack off your back and lay it on the ground . . You are ready now . . to get rid of all those heavy burdens, you have carried for so long . . Along with the feelings of guilt and remorse . . that have heaped themselves . . on top of those problems you have been experiencing . . You have been carrying all of this around with you for so long . . And now, you are ready to get rid of it all . . In just a moment . . I am going to ask you to open that pack . . and pull out the anger . . the bitterness . . the feelings of rejection . . the jealousy . . the contempt . . And all the other items that have been weighing you down . . Keeping your spirit from progressing . . Unhook the snaps on the top of the pack now . . and open it up . . And as you pull those objects out . . one at a time . . Stack them in a pile beside you and . . write their name on a label . . and attach that label to each one . . naming, what they are . . (Wait for Response)

Now, if your pack is empty . . I'd like you to look in the bottom of that empty pack . . You will find a box of matches . . I want you to build a fire with those matches . . a BIG fire . . in that open space, on top of the mountain . . Now, pick up all those objects you pulled out of the pack . . and, one at a time . . toss them into the fire . . And as you do this . . read the label on each one . . so you will fully understand . . later on . . .

You're going to be pleased to notice that . . with each object you toss on that fire . . your feelings of calmness and serenity will increase . . You will feel a very large load being lifted from you . . And you will continue feeling more at ease . . It will give you a strong feeling of relief . . You are feeling yourself being cleansed . . of all those excessive feelings . . from your system . . And noticing your feelings of peace and comfort increasing, with each object you throw into that fire . . Pick them up now . . One at a time . . Read their label and . . toss them onto the fire . . (Pause) By the time you are rid of all those objects . . you will be pleasantly surprised to notice . . how peaceful you feel . . within yourself . .

When you have thrown all of those objects into the fire . . and have seen them burn up . . And go up in smoke . . Your subconscious mind will cause one of your fingers to lift up . . And it will remain up until I tell it to go back down . . (Wait for response, with encouragement)

Okay, your finger can go down . . And now . . just lay back on the soft, comfortable grass . . And watch all of those problems going up in smoke

. . Getting rid of everything that has been causing any kind of difficulty . . And as you watch the smoke gently rising up into the sky . . you can feel all of your problems quickly dissolving . . You feel a great sense of relief . . and release . . You are getting rid of all those problems . . Watch closely . . as the gentle breeze carries them farther . . and farther away from you . . You can breath deeply . . and exhale slowly . . a few times . . and really enjoy the freedom . . the relief . . the calmness and the peacefulness, flowing all through you . .

Those feelings of comfort and serenity . . will remain with you . . even after you awaken from the hypnotic state . . You have rid yourself of those terrible burdens . . They will bother you no more . . You are free . .

Your subconscious mind is working out the best solution . . and is releasing you from the control of any . . unpleasant experiences from the past . . Your mind realizes that the past is gone . .

Nothing is of the past . . but memories . . and that is not where you are . . You are living today . . for tomorrow . . Your mind refuses to recognize past memories . . as a way of life for you, today . . And your mind refuses to let those past memories . . cause you difficulties now . . in your present life . . You are becoming more free and complete with each passing day . .

Every part of your body . . All organs, glands, muscles, nerves and tissues . . your entire circulatory system . . your metabolism . . your intestines and elimination system . . Every system of your body, mind and spirit are working well . . in accordance with God's Laws of health, strength and vitality . . Peace, poise and confidence are growing stronger within you . . You are becoming stronger, healthier and more secure each day . . and you will continue to be amazed and pleased . . with your improvements . . Prepare yourself for your new life . .

Continue to relax a few moments longer . . then, I will begin my count . . from one to five . . When you hear the number five . . you'll be wide awake, feeling refreshed and relaxed . . (Pause briefly)

EMERG

(Follow Relaxation)

I understand you may be having a little difficulty in getting things done . . Maybe you're procrastinating . . Maybe you're rationalizing . . Not taking action . . Maybe all you have to do . . to resolve your difficulty . . is to make a phone call . . or write a letter . . or go to see someone . . But you keep putting it off . .

First of all, let's realize that you are attempting great things in your life . . Right ?   And greatness does not come easy . . You have set your goals . . You are trying to establish your destiny . . But you are stifled by a barricade you have yet to overcome . . And if you don't . . Well, that is why there is so much mediocrity around . . But you are a star . . You are above the average . . You are a rhinoceros ! You are a success . . And all you have to do . . is the one thing that you are putting off . . And you will rise above that mediocrity . .

Now, I know that you don't want to do it . . You could just as easily forget about it . . and not worry about ever doing it . . Just like so many other failures out there . . It's easy to quit, isn't it ? . .

To take the easy way out? . . and just give up without ever knowing you gave it your best effort . . That spells automatic failure . . And you are not built that way, are you ? . . You're a star . . and if you don't do what needs to be done . . it's going to eat at you, inside . . You would be frustrated for the rest of your life . . Because you would never know what the result might have been . . It could have been the turning point of a fabulous success story . .

Do you know what success is ? . . Success is simply . . a series of doing things that failures will not do . . And when you're up there, telling your success story . . it will be the result of what you are going to do, right now . . This one little thing you're going to do . . is the key to your success . . It's the key to your Rolls Royce . . To your appearance on the Jay Leno show . . Your travels, around the world . . Your dream home on the hill . . Your peace of mind . . while knowing that others will keep the ball rolling for you . . And your helping others to achieve success . . For their success, depends on your success . . All things hinge on what you are going to do . . Right Now !

Okay, first, Let's set the proper attitude . . And that attitude, simply, is that . . life is a jungle . . And that is exciting because . . You are a Rhinoceros . . You're free to roam wherever you want . .

You're free to accomplish anything you want to . . Yes, the jungle can be very exciting . . if YOU make it exciting . . You know that there are a lot of wild animals out there . . But you are bigger than any of them . . Right ?

Just let me remind you of what the alternative, to the jungle, is . . The alternative is . . the pasture . . And you know what they keep in the pasture . . Cows . . Dirty, old, fat, lazy, disgusting cows . . And talk about Boring . . All the cows do is wander the boundaries of the pasture . . Following each others tails . . Eating all day . . Getting fatter and fatter . . and FATTER . . And then, one day, the farmer opens the gate . . And they are led off . . one by one . . to slaughter . . That is your alternative . . So, let's keep away from the pasture . . Let's get back into the jungle . .

Right Now . . The jungle is where your opportunities are . . And it's where you'll find the rewards . . The risks . . The excitement and the challenges . . And, best of all . . the other Rhinos . . You would be pretty lonely, as a charging Rhino . . in a pasture full of cows . . So, the jungle is characterized by action . . And now that you've put yourself back into that jungle . . that's what you are going to do . . Take action . .

Let's get back to the task at hand . . that you are going to do right now . . This one, perhaps, uncomfortable task . . that is the key to your entire future . . It is what you're going to take care of, right now . . You may have to eat a little dirt . . but you're not going to sit around, like a cow . . waiting for slaughter . . Because you're in the jungle now . . And if you don't move to action . . you'll go down in quicksand . . Where the bugs will torment you . . The sun will boil your flesh and you will rot, right where you stand . . Get charging !!! You're a success . . You're a Rhinoceros !!! Go do it now . . Make those good things happen . . You can do it . . Only you can do it . .

You're a fabulous star with a fantastic future . . You're in control of your destiny . . And we want you . . to do the one thing you need to do . . so you can be with us . . Go do it, right now . . Don't put it off any longer . . You're a superstar winner . . because you take action . .

Exciting things are right around the corner . . but you've got to walk around the corner to know what's there . . Go do it right now . .

388

You are rising up . . Rising up higher . . and higher . . Above the crowd . . Above all of that mediocrity . . Above the pasture . . Like a rising star, in the morning light . . Rising higher . . and higher . .

You're taking action now . . You are going to change your life . . to the way it was meant to be . . Yes, You're ready now . . to do the one thing that will make everything real . . And you're charging on . . like a Rhinoceros . .

I will begin my count now . . from ONE to FIVE . . And when you hear the number FIVE . . you will be wide awake . . feeling good . . Feeling refreshed and ready to commit yourself to accomplishing the one thing you need to do . . to reach the goals you have set for yourself . .

I am counting now . . from one to five . . You will become a little more awake . . with each number you hear . .

1, 2, 3, 4 and 5 . . Open your eyes . .

You showed up for your appointment today . . and that is a big step
. . toward overcoming your problem of procrastination . . You are
relaxing deeper now . . DEEPER . . and DEEPER . . Just continue
relaxing . . And as you continue moving, into a deeper . . and
DEEPER . . hypnotic state . .

I'll be giving you suggestions . . that will cause you to do the
various things you need to do . . when they are suppose to be done . .
In fact, you will enjoy getting at the things you have to do . . and
getting them done . . To the extent that . . you will soon be getting
your work . . and many other tasks, completed . . More and more
rapidly . . It will give you a great feeling of pride and accomplishment . .
to get your work . . and other tasks completed . . ahead of time . .

Each day, you keep realizing . . more and more . . the importance of
finishing your work . . And your other projects . . that you have
agreed to complete . . And you will find it enjoyable . . to get them
done on time . . And in many instances . . ahead of time . .

You are experiencing more pride in your daily activities . . and in
your work . . and in your special projects . . You are setting priorities
and realizing the importance . . of getting them done, on time . .
And in many instances, ahead of time . .

Your creative abilities . . keep emerging more and more each day . .
Causing you to develop unique and creative ways . . of handling your
responsibilities . . You identify the projects that are important . . And
you devote the amount of time needed . . to get them done . . as
rapidly and efficiently as possible . . From now on, you set goals for
yourself to accomplish . . And your creative mind enables you to develop
effective ways . . to achieve those goals, successfully . .

As you complete each task . . you continue learning from your
success . . And that increases your confidence in achieving the next
task . . You are able to make decisions wisely . . And you have
confidence in your decisions . . It keeps becoming easier for you . .
to make decisions . . You have confidence in your ability . . to make the
right decision, at the right time . .

You keep feeling a greater sense of accomplishment . . and a sense of well being . . By completing your work and your other projects, on time . . You are experiencing a greater feeling of pride . . in doing things that need to be done . . And getting them done rapidly . . When you have work to do . . or a project to complete . . you get at it . . And you get it done in a sufficient amount of time . .

Your friends, family and associates . . notice your new attitude . . your ambition . . and your desire for accomplishment . . And they respect your sense of pride . . And sense that pride as well . .

Your abilities to be successful are increasing rapidly . . You look forward to beginning . . and completing . . new projects . . You look forward to making decisions . . You look forward to the many rewards . . of completing a task or project . . in a sufficient period of time . . You look forward to . . getting your work, your tasks and your projects, completed . . And, on time . .

Your self-confidence . . self-reliance and self-sufficiency . . keep increasing more each day . . And you continue becoming more proud . . of your accomplishments . .

You have done very well, my friend . . Continue to relax a few moments longer . . as your subconscious mind absorbs everything we have talked about . . (Pause)

I will begin my counting now . . from ONE to FIVE . . When you hear the number FIVE . . you will open your eyes . . You will wake a little more with each number you hear . .

1 . . 2 . . 3 . . 4 . . and . . 5 . .

You are now in a deep hypnotic state of relaxation . . And you can continue moving into an even deeper state . . as you listen to my words . . And let yourself go, completely . . Just let yourself go now . . Relax . . You don't need to think about anything at all . . Just continue relaxing . . And your subconscious mind will enable you . . to respond to all of the suggestions and instructions I give you . . You are emptying your mind of any thoughts . . And your awareness is narrowing down . . as you continue moving into . . a deeper . . drowsier state . . that is closely related to . . a dreaming state . . You are becoming drowsier . . and more relaxed . . as you respond to the suggestions and instructions I give you . . And you will always be aware of my voice . . when I speak to you . . And you will automatically respond to my directions . . You are feeling more calm . . and more at ease . . as you follow my instructions . .

In just a moment, when I tell you to begin . . I want you to start counting backwards . . from one hundred . . Slowly, like this . . one hundred . . ninety nine . . ninety eight . . ninety seven . . And you will continue, slowly counting on down . . as far as you can . . As you count slowly backwards . . beginning at one hundred . . somewhere along the way . . you will lose count . . Perhaps in the lower eighties or seventies . . It doesn't matter when the numbers disappear . . because with each number you think . . your mind and body will keep relaxing more . . each time you say a number . . And I want you to try to count at least, to eighty . .

You are not trying to think of anything . . You are merely continuing to relax . . while you are counting . . And moving into a deeper . . more comfortable state of relaxation . . Other sounds keep fading away . . more and more . . And as you are counting backwards in your mind . . you can experience a deep, soothing drowsiness coming over your entire body . . You can reach a deep, dreaming state . . And at the same time, you will always hear my voice . . when I talk to you . .

As you continue counting backwards . . the numbers keep fading away . . fading away . . And when you lose count . . you will be in a deeper hypnotic state . . than you have ever been in before . . As soon as that happens . . you will see a large screen television set in front of you . . It will have a remote control to operate it . . And the remote control will be in your hand . .

You can continue counting backwards from one hundred . . until the numbers disappear . . or you lose count . . And as soon as the numbers disappear, or you lose count . . you will see a large screen television set with remote controls . . And the control will be in your hand . .

You will use the control to turn on the television set . . And as the set warms up . . you will be wondering what you will see . . When the picture becomes clear . . you will notice that it is showing some scene from your own life . . Perhaps it will be a personal news flash . . Or it may be a review of your early school days . . Or a glimpse into your family life or . . it may show something of your work . . Or you, being with your friends or family members . .

You don't know what you will be seeing on the screen . . But I want you to notice everything that is happening . . and I want you to tell me what you are seeing . . Regardless of what you are seeing . . you will remain relaxed and calm . . And you will tell me as much about it as you are willing for me to know . . You will be able to change the channel or turn off the set . . any time you want to . . And that is why your subconscious mind will permit you . . to see what will be the most helpful to you . . in overcoming that problem . .

Just continue counting back from one hundred now . . When the numbers disappear or you lose count . . you will see the television set . . And you will turn it on . .

(proceed)

A short time ago . . I used a series of numbers . . to help you to relax . . Now we will go through another set of numbers . . that you are familiar with . . which will bring your forgotten memories . . into sharper focus for you . .

You are comfortable . . and your mind is completely relaxed . . You have complete faith and trust . . And you are confident . . that no harm can come to you . . And everything you say . . is confidential . . You are safe . . You are secure . . And you are not alone . . I am with you at all times . .

When I tell you to begin . . I want you to count back . . slowly . . from your present age . . until you are back at the age of . . six . . (tentative age)

As you say each number . . beginning with your present age . . you will feel yourself becoming younger . . And when you reach your teenage years . . you will notice yourself becoming smaller . .

As you count back slowly . . you can easily forget the experiences that happened, after . . the age each number represents . . And you will be happy to find that . . as you forget those years . . and the experiences of those years . . your memory of earlier ages in your life . . will increase . .

When you reach the number, six . . you will be back at the age of six . . When you get to the age of six . . you will be able to remember and recall . . everything . . that happened at the age of six . .

And you will recall and relive your life . . just as you lived it then . .

You will feel the same feelings . . and think the same thoughts . . as you did at the age of six . . And you will experience the same actions . . and reactions . . as you had at the age of six . .

You are going back now . . Back in time . . Easily and comfortably . . as you deeply relax . .

When you arrive at the age of six . . you will find it is your sixth birthday . . If you had a birthday party . . at the age of six . . you will be at your birthday party . .

I am going with you . . And you will be able to hear my voice . . any time I talk to you . . And you will verbally respond to all suggestions or instructions . . I give you . .

You will relive and recall . . real experiences . . just the way they happened . . when you were six years of age . .

If I suggest that you, physically, do something . . that is happening at that time . . you will do it, only . . as you did it, at that time . .

As soon as you are six years of age . . you will tell me . . out loud . . everything that is happening . .

If I tell you to open your eyes . . when you are six . . you will open your eyes . . And you will see only what you saw . . at that age . . And you will remain in a DEEP hypnotic state . . even with your eyes open . .

If I tell you to go to some other period of time . . you will become the age . . that I suggest . . and will go, at once, to the period of time . . that I suggest . .

As you are reliving those experiences . . you will be unaware of your present location . . and will know only what is happening at that age . . And you will always hear my voice . . as I talk to you . . And you will always respond . . in describing your experiences . .

After you have finished . . reliving your experiences from the past . . I will ask you to come back to your present age level . . And you will easily come back to the present time . . And, you will easily awaken . . when I suggest you awaken . . from the hypnotic state . . After you awaken from this hypnotic session . . you will easily recall, with complete accuracy . . everything that was said or done . . or that you experienced . . in your earlier life . .

During the time you are reliving those experiences . . from your past . . you will be unaware of your present age . . and your present time . . You will know only what is happening . . at the age level of six . . or other age levels that I suggest you go to . . You will always hear my voice clearly . . And you will always respond . . and follow my instructions . . whenever I talk to you . .

Okay, if you are ready now . . I want you to begin counting backwards . . slowly . . from your present age . . Soon, you will notice yourself becoming smaller and smaller . .

How old are you now ? . . And the next number is . .

(NOTE : KEEP MENTIONING THAT THE CLIENT IS BECOMING YOUNGER . AND WHEN THE CLIENT GETS DOWN TO ABOUT FIFTEEN, MENTION THAT HE OR SHE IS GETTING, PHYSICALLY, SMALLER.)

WHEN CLIENT REACHES AGE, SIX, CONTINUE WITH . .

Now, you are six years of age . . And you are at your birthday party . . Look around you and tell me what you see . .

What kind of clothes are you wearing ? . . Look in a mirror and tell me what you look like . .

What are you doing, right now ? . .

Who is there with you ? . .

(Discuss the purpose client had for regressing.)

NOTE : AFTER ESTABLISHING THAT THE CLIENT HAS REGRESSED TO AGE OF SIX, YOU CAN CONTINUE BY HAVING CLIENT GO TO EARLIER - OR LATER - AGES . . OR TO A PREVIOUS INCARNATION, AS DESIRED.)

EMERGE as required

REGRESSION TO A PREVIOUS LIFE
(Follow RELAXATION - Deep)

CONTINUE THIS SESSION FOLLOWING "REGRESSION TECHNIQUE", WITH CHANGES, AS FOLLOWS :

You will use the controls to turn on the television set . .   As the set warms up, you will have your choice of several channels . . Each channel will be showing a time . . when your soul was in another body . .   It will be showing a previous . . or a future . . incarnation . . of your experience . . You may appear to look the same as you do now . .   Or you may be of the opposite sex . .

When the set warms up . . you will be seeing yourself during a lifetime either before . . or after . . your present lifetime experience . . It is your choice whether you want to go into the future or past . .

CLARIFY THIS POINT WITH CLIENT BEFORE PROCEEDING.

The picture will become very clear and vivid . .   It will be showing scenes from a different incarnation . .   And as soon as you notice what is happening on the screen . . I want you to describe what you are seeing . . What is familiar to you ? . .   Do you recognize anyone with you ? . . Et cetera.

NOTE : KEEP REPEATING SUGGESTIONS ABOUT SEEING A PREVIOUS INCARNATION UNTIL CLIENT BEGINS DESCRIBING WHAT HE OR SHE IS SEEING.   CLIENT MAY WISH TO GO INTO A FUTURE INCARNATION BUT SHOULD HAVE A PREVIOUS LIFETIME REGRESSION EXPERIENCE BEFORE HAND.

TIME ALLOWABLE MAY BE SEVERAL HOURS.

You are doing very well . . You are relaxing . . and your mind is peaceful . . You are open to awareness . . and to understanding . . You are becoming more aware . . of the spiritual power within you . . The power that enables you to overcome obstacles . . and improve the direction of your life . . And to experience your God-given birthright . . of health . . happiness and success . .

While you are here on Earth . . you can experience a wonderful Human life cycle . . You have as much right to happiness, joy, love and prosperity . . as any other person in the world . .

You may not be aware of it yet but . . you are a very important part of creation . . You came here from the same creator . . that every other person came from . . And you are here for a purpose . .

You are here because you are very special . . And because you are very special . . you do not need to 'measure up' . . to any other person's expectations of you . . You are not here, to be what someone else expects you to be . . You are YOU . . and you are unique . . You are here to work on your own spiritual plan . . and to fulfill God's plan . . in your own special way . .

You do not owe it to any other person . . to be the way he . . or she . . thinks you should be . . You are to be . . the way you want yourself to be . . You are in control . . of your own life . .

Each day, your self-confidence continues growing stronger . . Your self-acceptance and self-reliance continue increasing . . And you keep enjoying your life . . more fully . .

You always do your best to be a thoughtful, loving and understanding person . . You have the ability to use good judgment . . to make wise decisions . . and to achieve great goals in your life . .

You have within you . . the qualifications to handle every situation or circumstance . . that comes up in your life . . You possess the knowledge and ability . . to overcome every obstacle you face . . And you are developing the habit of being successful . . That habit is the product of . . repeatedly directing yourself . . to a specific action . . And you are developing the habit . . of performing the actions . . that will lead you to happiness . . and success . . Knowing that once you establish those habits . . they continue working for you . . automatically . .

Every challenge you encounter . . you will meet with confidence, sureness and with power . . Because you will keep all of your thoughts, positive . . And that will attract happy, positive conditions to you . .

Each of us possesses between twenty and thirty times more physical . . and mental . . abilities . . than we ever use . . So, the success we attain . . is determined by how much we use the abilities . . that we have . .

Each day, you become more determined . . to put your talents and abilities . . into action . . And you realize that . . no one . . can keep you from being successful . . You were born with the ability . . and the power . . to achieve any goal that you want to attain . .

You continue becoming more optimistic . . in your personal view of life . . And you are rewarded by your ability to recognize . . new opportunities and great possibilities . . opening up to you . .

As you continue drifting . . into a deeper and DEEPER . . more peaceful, hypnotic state of relaxation . . your subconscious mind is receiving the imprints I am presenting . . And is causing them to be a strong influence on your personality . . and on your daily performance . .

Your faith, courage and determination . . are becoming stronger . . and you continue to expand your personal view of yourself . . Recognizing your abilities and making good use of . . your God-given talents . .

You are encouraged by your development of . . a greater attitude . . of love and understanding . .

You want to be loving and kind . . in all of your responses and actions . . towards others . .

You know that if you make a mistake . . you want others to be understanding towards you . . And the same is true of your feelings toward them . . They are human . . and they make mistakes . . like all humans do . . By being a loving and kind . . and forgiving person . . you produce an atmosphere . . an aura . . of happiness and harmony around you . . You create your own, beautiful world . . in which to live . .

If you ever feel mistreated by someone . . ask yourself if you have done something to deserve such mistreatment . . If you feel you do not deserve their mistreatment . . then realize that it is the other persons mistake . . Therefore, there is no reason for you to feel badly . . or for it to hurt you, in any way . . You are understanding . . of the person who mistreats you . .

Think to yourself . . "That person is a human . . and is still evolving . . to develop his or her own . . self-acceptance" . .

Learn from that persons conduct . . Be determined to be more loving . . and more kind to yourself . .

Always remember that you grow stronger . . by learning from situations that are difficult . . They will keep your confidence increasing . . and improving . . And will enable you to handle any situation that comes up in your life . .

Never allow yourself to become unhappy . . because of what other people do . . You can't control the actions of another person . . However, you can control the way you let their actions affect you . .

There is an old proverb, which says . . "Let everyone sweep his own doorstep . . and all the doorsteps will be clean" . . That is what you are doing . . right now . . You are sweeping your own doorstep . . You know how to be a good, loving person . . You know how to keep improving yourself . . And you know you are worthy . . of happiness and success . . And from now on . . you will anticipate happiness and joy in your life . . And you will expect to gain good experiences . .

Right now, you are feeling an inner renewal . . taking place within you . . You continue developing more zest and enthusiasm for life . . and for living . . Each day, you keep feeling more alive . . more energetic . . more enthusiastic . . and more powerful . . You are YOU . . and you are good . .

I want your subconscious mind to absorb everything we have talked about . . as you continue to relax . . for a little longer . . In a moment I will bring you back to a normal state of being . . Rest a little longer . . (pause)

I am going to begin my count now . . from One up to Five . . And when you hear my count out the number, Five . . you will become awake, alert and aware of your surroundings . .

ONE . . TWO . . THREE . . FOUR . . and . . FIVE . .

You may open your eyes now . .

I want you to continue relaxing now . . It is not important for you . . to consciously listen to my words . . from this point on . . In fact, you don't need to consciously pay any attention to what I am saying . . because your subconscious mind . . and all other levels of your inner mind . . is absorbing everything I say . . and can enable you to put everything I say to you . . into your own actions . . Without any conscious effort from you . .

Even though you presently have . . the power and the ability . . to achieve any goal you want to achieve . . there are certain actions that you can take . . that will enable you to progress more easily . . and more rapidly . .

You are already taking one of the most important actions you can take . . to increase your self-confidence . . Permitting yourself to be hypnotized . . is one of the most helpful . . and most beneficial actions you can do . . for increasing your self-confidence . . And for helping yourself . . in all other areas of your life . .

In the past . . you may have been timid about doing certain things . . that would enable you to achieve greater success and happiness . . But now, your confidence is increasing rapidly . . And you are acquiring the confidence you need . . to handle every situation or circumstance . . that comes up in your life . .

Your confidence is increasing more each day . . And you believe in yourself . . as being a person who possesses the knowledge . . the wisdom and the ability . . to achieve the goals you want to achieve . .

In the past . . you may have had some doubts . . But those doubts are fading away rapidly . . And all of your doubts . . will be gone completely . . by the time you awaken from this hypnotic state . . Those doubts are being replaced . . by a strong sense of confidence . . A confidence in your own abilities . . And you are developing a greater realization . . of your own importance . .

You are . . a very special person . . You have . . special talents and capabilities . . that no other person in the world has . . in the same way that you do . . And each day, you continue developing . . a greater realization of your own special capabilities . .

You can help yourself to progress even more rapidly . . by using a technique . . that will keep reinforcing and strengthening your concept of

401

yourself . . This technique will increase your self-awareness . . your self-confidence . . your self-acceptance . . and your self-reliance . .

You are a good person . . You were created . . by the same creator . . that created every other human being on this planet . . And you have within you . . the potential to be an outstanding success . . Most people never become aware of the potential within them . . as you are becoming aware . . through hypnosis . .

You have outstanding capabilities . . And you possess a tremendous power . . that you can use to be . . an outstanding success . . That power . . is the power of your own mind . . You can use your own mind . . to help yourself to attain even greater success . .

I want you to repeat this statement, silently, to yourself . . Repeat this several times to yourself . . and remember it . . "Each day, I use the power of my mind . . to attain greater success" . . Repeat that . . over again, in your mind . . "Each day, I use the power of my mind . . to attain greater success" . .

After you leave here and go home . . I want you to write that statement down . . You will find that . . the more you look at that statement . . and repeat it to yourself . . the more your confidence will increase . . And you will continue attaining greater success . .

You can do anything you make up your mind to do . . You can achieve any goal you decide to attain . . By using your mind . . in a positive way . . you draw to yourself . . everything that benefits you . . in a positive way . .

Think these words in your mind now . . "I believe in myself . . I believe I can achieve any goal . . that I decide to attain" . . I'll repeat that . . "I believe in myself . . I believe I can achieve any goal . . that I decide to attain" . .

You will find it to be very beneficial . . to continue repeating these statements . . over to yourself . . several times, each day . . Especially, just before you go to sleep . . And the first thing when you get opposition from other people in the world . . You have as much right to good health . . happiness, joy and prosperity . . as any other person in the world . . And you have a good mind . . as well as the freedom to use your mind . . to achieve any goal you want to achieve . .

402

Each day, your realization of these true facts . . will keep becoming stronger in your mind . . You continue becoming stronger . . and more courageous . . Your self-confidence keeps increasing more each day . .

You have outstanding capabilities . . You have within you . . tremendous mental and creative powers . . So your motivation to be successful is increasing . . Your confidence is increasing . . And you have the courage you need . . to keep achieving even greater happiness . . greater joy . . and all of the many riches of life . . that you deserve . .

Another key to maintaining your self-confidence . . is your ability to relax . . and to remain calm at all times . . You will remain calm . . and relaxed . . whether you are at work or doing something for recreation and fun . . That will cause your body processes to function harmoniously . . And will enable you to do everything in an efficient and effective manner . .

Each day, you keep improving, physically, mentally, emotionally and spiritually . . You have a greater sense of personal well-being . . A greater sense of personal safety . . and you keep feeling more secure . . You enjoy life more, each day . . Your happiness keeps increasing . . And you become . . more enthusiastic and more optimistic . . each day . .

As you continue improving . . you will notice how you are becoming . . more able to depend upon yourself . . You will have increased confidence . . in your own judgments, your own opinions and in your own points of view . . Your self-confidence, self-reliance, self-acceptance and self-esteem . . keep growing stronger . . And you continue to be more successful in everything you do . . Everything I have told you is already happening to you . . because everything I have said is true . . You want to be successful . . Therefore, your desire and determination to be successful . . is being fulfilled . .

Your subconscious mind has accepted . . all of the suggestions I have given you . . and is causing you to progressively advance . . in all areas of your life . . Your life, therefore, keeps becoming more productive . . more useful . . Your body . . keeps becoming more healthy . . Your mind is also healthier . . happier . . and more at ease . . And you have postured yourself . . for even greater spiritual growth . .

In just a moment, I will begin my count . . from ONE to FIVE . . When you hear the number . . FIVE . . you will open your eyes and be wide awake and alert . . If you are ready now, I will begin . . ONE TWO THREE FOUR FIVE . . Open your eyes now . .

(Follow Relaxation)

Continue to let yourself relax . . Just as you are . . And as you relax . . I am going to give you some suggestions . . on self-discipline and self-persistence . . In fact, you will find yourself welcoming these suggestions . . and making them a permanent part of your psyche . . Because you realize that they are important to you . . And you realize that they are helpful in maintaining the success that you want to instill as a permanent part of your subconscious mind . . You also realize that your immediate success is going to be maintained . . through self-discipline and persistence . .

With discipline . . and persistence . . you are going to be able to convert . . your greatest weakness . . That thing you believe to be your greatest weakness, whatever it is . . It doesn't make any difference what it is . . You are going to be able to convert that 'weakness' . . into a strength . . And you are going to convert it to a strength . . through self-discipline and self-persistence . .

Now you may have heard of, Norman Vincent Peale, who said . . "You can become strongest in your weakest point" . . In fact, he was so convinced of that . . that he related a story about a man named, Glen Cunningham . . Glen Cunningham was that fellow whose legs were so badly burned, as a child . . that he was told he would never walk again . . But the young boy rejected that idea . . and through self-discipline and persistence . . became one of the fastest Olympic milers in history . .

I am going to give you a few examples . . so that you realize . . you can . . convert your weakest point . . into your greatest strength . . There was a fellow named, Paul Henderson . . He was a sickly, puny, weakling . . and he was beaten many times . . But he refused to accept defeat . .

Through self-discipline and self-persistence . . he constructed a home built weight lifting outfit . . And he transformed himself into the strongest man in the world . . Literally, breaking records that stood for many years . .

We have often said, "Oh, if only I had had the patience to wait it out" . . And that's what you have been asking for . . The patience to wait it out . . The persistence to keep plugging away . . The persistence to keep going forward . . and keep striving for the mark, again and again . . and again . . Regardless of failures . .

Because we know the system works . . We know that positive suggestions DO have their cumulative effect . . And we know that when we tell ourselves . . we're going to succeed . . we ARE going to succeed . .

You are much better off by persisting . . than by giving up . . And you are much better off by disciplining yourself . . than by being in a position where others . . must discipline you . .

You need self-discipline and self-persistence . . And those are going to be yours today . . Because you realize that, through self-discipline . . And you realize that, through persistence . . you can transform yourself from, whatever you are, right now . . into a completely and totally successful person . . beginning right now . .

You may have heard . . that Abraham Lincoln was a failure . . Yes, he was . . a lifelong failure . . up to the age of fifty . . But through self-discipline and persistence . . he transformed himself into the greatest, most humane . . most sympathetic and understanding . . of all of our Presidents . .

There are many success stories of people . . who have overcome great obstacles . . before finding success . . You will hear about them . . or read about them . . as time goes by . . But yours . . is the success story I am interested in . . Your self-discipline and persistence . . will make it happen . .

So, I would like to ask you . . right now . . What is your main weakness? . . Think about that for a moment . . What is your main weakness ? . . Well, you say . . It might be any number of things; Fear . . Loss of temper . . Lack of confidence . . Alcohol . . Excessive eating . . Sexual frustrations . . Inhibitions . . Over spending ? . . Only you can recognize your main weakness . . Whether it be Selfishness or Depression . . or any of the other things I've mentioned to you . . Realize that, weakness is only a weakness . . because you focus your attention on all the little focal points around it . . but never directly on it . . Even though you are quite aware of it . . You intentionally avoid that one focal point . . or weakness . . And you spend a great deal of effort . . suggesting to yourself that . . because of this weakness . . which you have failed to recognize in the past . . Because of this weakness, you can't succeed . . You can't improve . . You can't get better . . You've labeled yourself, "Can't" . . Yes, you've exhibited a great deal of effort . . convincing yourself that because of your weakness . . you can't succeed . . You can't get any better than you are . .

Now, we need to look for a solution to this dilemma . . And that's what we are going to do, right now . . Look for a solution . . But you are not alone . . I am here with you . . To assist and guide you through this . . Together, we will find it . .

You know, when you dwell upon a problem . . the only thing on your mind is . . a problem . . But when you concentrate on a solution . . you come up with a solution . . once you get the problem out of the way of your thinking . . So you are going to eliminate concentrating on your problems . . And you're going to start concentrating on solutions . . right now . . Because the solution of the problem should be resolved . . right now . . And when you resolve it . . that will prove to yourself that you are, indeed, successful . . Right now, you are going to prove to yourself . . literally, beyond any doubt . . that you can do what others have done . . I only gave you examples of well known people . . because they are people . . just like you . . They each, found success . . and you can do it, too . . And you're going to do it by transforming your greatest weakness . . into your most prized asset . . You choose what your weakness is . . You know it better than anybody else . . And, right now, you're going to transform that weakness . . into an asset . . by using self- discipline . . and through your own persistence . .

And when you transform your greatest weakness into a great strength . . what more proof of success can you have, than that ? . . What could be better proof to you, than that ? . . You can do it today . . You can do it, right now . . You can turn your greatest weakness . . into your greatest strength . . by listening carefully to the following suggestions . .

After you leave here today . . I want you to find a quiet place, where you can be alone . . for some quiet reflection . . I want you to go over your life . . over your actions . . or lack of actions . . And I want you to consider . . your greatest weakness . . What are you not doing . . that you should be doing . . And what excuse do you give yourself . . for your lack of action . . Realize . . that that excuse is . . your weakness . . I want you to write it down . . Write down . . your greatest Weakness . . Literally STOP and DO IT . . And I am giving you the suggestion that you will stop . . you will take the time . . you will think about it . . and you will write it down . .

And I suggest you write down any number of other weaknesses you think you have . . And after you write them down . . study each one of them and tell yourself . . as you contemplate that list of weaknesses . ."I am going to transform each one of these weaknesses into strengths . . beginning with my greatest weakness . . and I am going to begin my transformation, today" . . (Repeat)

Then you'll begin . . Then you'll start making those changes . . And that is what's important to you . . No procrastination here . . DO what you just told yourself you are going to do . . You have already seen that, by saying what you are going to do . . and then doing it . . you'll begin to develop a new habit that will counter the old one . . You'll begin to condition yourself to perform . . And successfully perform . . Now, that's self-discipline . . That's persistence . . And together, they will put you on the road to success . . Transform this weakness, that you think you have . . into the strength . . that you will have . . Because it's true . . that the biggest battle for success . . is to conquer yourself . . The biggest battle . . is conquering one's self . . and you have resolved, right now . . to conquer yourself . .

You are resolving, right now, to perform the way you ought to perform . . And you'll perform that way, without fail . . because you're resolved that you're going to perform that way . . This kind of resolution . . once it becomes a habit . . will stick with you forever . . So you're going to resolve to make these changes . . And you'll continue with these changes . . until they become such habits . . that they will stay with you all the time . .

In the beginning, you'll recall . . you took the easiest way . . And you have been following that way . . out of habit . . Allowing yourself to hold onto the very thing . . that is making you ill, emotionally . . And that is the reason success has evaded you . .

You're going to begin by conquering your greatest weakness, first . . To prove to yourself that everything is possible . . And then, you'll gain the confidence to be successful . . in every other endeavor that you choose . . And you realize, right now . . that the battle against yourself . . begins with the resolution that you're going to make the change . . And it only ends after self-discipline has become engraved in your mind . . It only ends after self-discipline has become so engraved . . and so conditioned . . into your subconscious mind . . that success is an automatic habit that you simply cannot break . .

You're beginning to think 'success' right now, aren't you . . So much so that you're even willing to allow those thoughts . . to become habits with you . . Just think . . A habit that you cannot break, no matter how hard you try . . How wonderful it is, to begin to think 'success' . . It's really wonderful, to decide you really are going to be persistent . . in overcoming your problem . . And you realize that persistence . . is the direct result of habit . . And you are habitually persistent . . when you condition yourself to be . .

You understand that . . when you condition yourself to be a failure . . you'll wind up as a failure . . And when you condition yourself to be a coward . . you'll run away . . And you'll end up, running away from life . . Another shortcut to failure . . But realize this . . If you condition yourself to meet life, head on . . If you condition yourself to persist . . over and over, over and over . . and over again . . you will, in fact . . condition yourself to enjoy persisting . . Yes, enjoy it . . even in the face of failure . . Even in the face of depression . . That is when you've conditioned yourself to be persistent . . And that persistence will pay off for you . . You're conditioning yourself to be self-disciplined . . You're conditioning yourself to live . . and live abundantly . . And you're conditioning yourself to change those old habits . . into new ones . . The ones that will put you right onto the pathway of success . .

There are always choices to make . . In this world, we either discipline ourselves so that we can handle each situation . . or we discipline ourselves so that we cannot handle them . . You know what your choice is . . And you know you want to be persistent . . in reaching your goals . . And you know . . you want the discipline in your life . . to cause you to be persistent . . To be successful, in every way . . The quickest, safest and surest way . . is to turn your greatest weakness into your greatest strength . . And you'll do this through self-discipline and persistence . . and the resolution, that you are going to change . . You are going to make your start, as soon as you can, by writing your list of weaknesses . . Then begin converting them into your greatest strengths . .

Now, I am going to give you a moment of silence . . And during this moment of silence . . I want you to visualize yourself . . resolving those weaknesses and converting them for the better, right now . . Begin by selecting your main weakness and resolve to change that one first . .

That moment of silence begins now . .

EMERGE

I want you to continue relaxing now . . just as you are . . I am going to give you a few suggestions and instructions . . that will help you to feel differently . . about yourself . . and where you are going in this life . .

Many times, people notice . . how talented another person is . . in painting or singing . . playing tennis or working on computers . . or in giving a speech or, even . . telling jokes . . And because you feel you are not as good as that person . . in the one talent you are noticing . . you fail to take into consideration . . the fact that you are even more talented . . in many other categories . . than the person you are noticing . .

It is time for you to start seeing things . . from a new perspective . . And realize that if other people looked at you . . the way you look at others . . they would probably feel inferior . . by noticing those things which you do, better than they do . .

Instead of noticing the talents that others have . . that you don't have . . start noticing all of the talents you do have . . that others do not have . . You may have a tendency to start feeling a little superior to most of those people . . However, you can give yourself permission to understand that, just as you are here . . by the grace of the creator . . all other people were created by that same creator . . None of us have any right or reason to feel inferior . . or superior . . to anyone else . .

You have many reasons to feel good about yourself . . And realize that you have capabilities . . far beyond what you have been consciously aware of knowing . . And you have the ability to keep improving . . your talents, your skills and abilities, more each day . .

From now on . . you are understanding that it is okay . . to feel proud of yourself . . by putting forth your best effort . . in using the talents, skills and abilities that need to be used . . to accomplish the goals you want and need to achieve . . You can do it now . . today . . And you can do it tomorrow . . And you can continue doing it, from now on . . for the rest of your life . .

You can understand all of this, quite clearly . . And you are feeling more and more comfortable about it . . Your confidence is increasing rapidly . . Your self-acceptance is getting stronger . . And you are feeling more and more secure . . within yourself . .

You understand that you become . . what you think . . So you are thinking, only good, positive thoughts . . about yourself . . This new way of thinking and feeling . . is increasing rapidly . . because it is true . . You are a good person . . You are a talented person . . You are just as good and just as capable of being successful . . as every other person on this Earth . . You are feeling happy about that realization . . Notice now, that you feel confident . . and pleased . . Your subconscious mind understands this . . even if you are still unsure . . of how much of it you are really aware of . . consciously . . Still, you will notice . . that your thoughts . . about yourself . . are changing quite rapidly . . And you will continue to become more and more proud . . of your accomplishments, each day . .

Continue to relax . . as your subconscious mind absorbs . . everything we are discussing . .

You know what to do now . . And you know what needs to be done . . So, from now on . . whatever needs to be done . . you will DO IT . . And as you are doing it . . always put your very best effort into it . . You will find, your creative abilities emerging more each day . . Your hidden talents . . Your secret knowledge . . will keep emerging . . And you will keep becoming more and more aware . . that in your mind, are memories . . and learning's . . and experiences . . The many things you know . . And the many things . . you can do . . All those things are going to come out . .

As you continue relaxing now . . your subconscious mind is, automatically, providing the awareness you need . . to put these suggestions . . into your own actions . . as you go about your daily activities . . And you will continue progressing . . in all areas of your life . . physically . . mentally . . emotionally . . and spiritually . .

You have done very well . . Relax, as you are . . for another moment . . Then I will bring you back . . by counting from ONE to FIVE . . When you hear me say the number FIVE . . you will open your eyes . . and you will be wide awake . . But, for now . . continue to relax . .   (Pause)

Now . . I will begin the count . .

ONE   TWO   THREE   FOUR   FIVE

As you continue relaxing . . you find yourself going . . a little deeper and , , DEEPER . . until, finally . . you are deep enough . . to step out onto the pathway in front of you . . It is an easy little path to follow . . leading down a winding trail . . into a beautiful forest . . The sun is shining . . and you can hear the birds singing . . There is a very pleasant little stream, flowing close to the pathway . . And you notice a very pleasant aroma in the air . .

As you are strolling along . . you suddenly notice a large mound . . of freshly dug dirt on the right side of the pathway . . You look closer . . and notice a wooden door . . that leads into the underground . . And it is open . . You step through the doorway and you enter a tunnel . . which is somewhat dark . . However, there is a glimmer of light . . coming from the other end of the tunnel . .

You begin walking . . towards the light . . You continue moving into a deeper . . and DEEPER . . state of hypnosis . . It is more peaceful now . . as you continue walking . . into the light . . Moving closer . . It gives you such a warm, peaceful feeling . . as the light seems to get brighter . . and larger . . as you get nearer and nearer . . to the light . . You keep walking . . Finally . . you reach the far end of the tunnel . . And as you step out of the tunnel . . into the light . . Your eyes begin to focus . . And you realize . . that you are in the middle of a beautiful garden . . There are trees . . and hanging vines . . like a tropical forest . . And there is laughter . . You hear some very cheerful laughter . . coming from just around the curve in the pathway . . through the garden . . You follow the path, around the curve . . and move towards the sound of the laughter . . It sounds so delightfully happy . . At last you meet a happy smiling person . . in the middle of the path . . who introduces (Him / Her self) as, Universal Wisdom . . The owner of the garden . . You are invited to walk . . in any parts of the garden you wish to . . and explore anything you desire to see . .

The first thing you notice is a pool, filled with water . . The water is so clear that . . as you look down into it . . you see the reflection of yourself . . And you are amazed because . . you look exactly the way you want your body to be . . Slim . . Trim . . And your entire body is perfectly proportioned . .

You look around and you notice that the person called . . Universal Wisdom . . is still with you . . He / She motions you to come closer because He / She has a message for you . . Quietly, He / She speaks to you . . with information about yourself . . that you had been previously unaware of . . You ponder on this information for a moment . . (Pause) After you have absorbed this information . . I want you to tell me as much about it . . as you are willing to share . .

WAIT FOR RESPONSE. IF APPROPRIATE, FURTHER DISCUSSION WITH "UNIVERSAL WISDOM" MAY BE SUGGESTED.

After gathering all the information you need . . for now . . you continue walking through the garden . . The winding path leads to many interesting wonders of the garden . . Suddenly, on the path before you . . is a young child . . The child is smiling, as you bend down nearer to him / her . . and he / she whispers something in your ear . . You realize that he / she is telling you something about yourself . . that you had forgotten, years ago . . He / She tells you about an incident from your own childhood . . Something that you need to remember now . . to help you enjoy your life more fully . . Would you like to share with me, what the child talked to you about ? . .

You look at Universal Wisdom . . as you leave the child . . and continue to walk . . And you wonder, how that child knew . . the information he / she had whispered in your ear . .

Universal Wisdom, seems to sense what you are wondering . . and reminds you . . that we all possess a tremendous amount of knowledge . . that we are not consciously aware of . . And when we become more and more attuned . . to the knowledge within us . . we, then, begin experiencing . . perfect peace . . And we feel truly overjoyed . . to be alive . . And we realize that we can achieve any goal . . we set our mind to . .

You continue on your way . . and you arrive at a small clearing . . where three, small butterflies are fluttering . . joyfully . . above the flower garden . . Their wings seem to hum a lilting melody . . about the beautiful day . . and they stir up the exciting, joyous feelings of happiness that you are having . . You pause for a moment . . listening to the beautiful melody . . And you want to take that melody with you . . Then you resume your walk . . down the pathway . .

You are coming to the end of the garden now . . Universal Wisdom, is still with you . . reminding you of all of the great insights you will experience

412

. . as a result of your journey through the garden . . He / She points the way to the opening of the tunnel . . by which you will leave . . "But this is not the end", you are reminded . . "This is but the beginning . . I will tell you something now", Universal Wisdom says to you . . "which will be very important for your future" . .

(Therapist) Now . . I want you to concentrate on this information . . from Universal Wisdom . . and allow it to become absorbed . . into your subconscious mind . . Relax your mind . . Relax . . And absorb the information . . the Universal Mind . . speaks to you now . . (Pause, 1 to 2 minutes)

You have completed your journey . . through the garden of Universal Wisdom . . You are stepping back into the tunnel . . making your way back through it . . The light is at the far end . . It looks small, at first . . but as you get nearer and nearer to it . . it becomes larger . . and brighter . . You are at the end of the tunnel now . . and you can step up, into the light once more . . You will soon be returning to the activities of your daily life . . And you will carry with you . . the tremendous amount of wisdom . . you have within you . . It may take a little time . . but you are determined to put that wisdom into action . . Knowing that you will keep becoming more knowledgeable . . and more successful . . in all areas of your life . .

I am going to count now, from 1 to 5 now . . And on the count of 5, you will open your eyes to an alert waking state . . feeling clear of mind . . relaxed . . and wonderful . . I will begin . .

One - You will remember everything you have experienced today . . with understanding and clarity . .

TWO - You are now connected to your inner strength and higher power . . supporting your good . . You will carry that inner strength with you throughout your day . . every day . .

Three - Everything I have told you is true and is already happening . . and you are already successful in manifesting the positive suggestions that I have given you . . into your daily life and consciousness . .

Four - You are beginning to be more aware of your body as it fully awakens and wants to stir . .

Five - As you open your eyes now, you are feeling clear, rested and wonderful . . For you are a wonderful person . .

413

There was a gardener . . who wanted to make a flower garden in her yard . . She looked through a seed catalogue . . picking out by color, whatever looked good . . from all the beautiful pictures that she saw . . She chose yellow marigolds, white chrysanthemums, blue larkspur, purple delphiniums . . and a mix of colors in morning glories, asters, lilies and roses . .

After selecting the many, many different seeds she wanted to plant . . she sent off her order . . so she would have the seeds back in plenty of time . . for the spring planting . . She waited patiently for the seeds to arrive . . Finally, a large package was delivered to her mailbox . . She opened them hurriedly . . and found dozens of packages of seeds inside . . She became quite excited . . and began planting them immediately . .

She planted row after row . . making lovely beds in her back yard . . And in the front of the house, she planted them around her porch and along the walkways . . Then along the sides of the house . . and the walls . . and around all the trees . .

As the days passed, she watered them and weeded them . . and watched them closely . . getting quite excited each time a green shoot began . . showing through the warm, damp earth . . And each day, she watched her plants proudly . .

Some were growing tall . . Some, medium in height and some, quite short . . Some bushed out . . Some stayed slender . . And some had many leaves while others had only a few leaves . .

Each morning she jumped out of bed, excited about seeing the changes that had taken place during the night . . And each day, she was rewarded . . seeing new leaves and new growth . .

The day came when she began finding new buds on many of the plants . . And she felt concern because . . some were fat and some were so little and hard . . And others were long and squat . . And she worried as she weeded . . Yet continued to watch and work them each day . .

When it didn't rain, she watered them carefully . . And she loosened the earth around each stem . . And all the time . . she worried . . secretly . . Because some were so very different . . from the others . . And she was not sure the plants were doing what they should be doing . .

So she watched . . She waited and she worried . . And continued working the beds until . . one day . . she saw a flower . . And in the days that followed . . she saw hundreds of flowers . . All different colors, different shapes and different heights . . And she realized that, even though they were different . . they were, each, lovely and perfect . . in their own way . .

She saw that the round and squat buds became lovely round flowers . . And the long, skinny buds became beautiful slender flowers . . And the little hard, shiny buds . . became little clusters of flowers . . And she really enjoyed all of them because they were all so unique . .

She understood that it was all right for them to be different . . And so, she was filled with joy and happiness . . as each day . . she saw more flowers blooming in many different sizes, shapes and colors . . And her garden was lovely because there were so many beautiful flowers in it . . All them of seemed to belong together . . even though they were all so different from each other . .

And she felt very proud of her little garden . . as people came from all over to enjoy seeing it . . Everyone talked about the ones they liked best . . But the gardener only smiled because she knew . . they were all good . . very good . . Each one, in its own special way . .

EMERGE

SEXUAL ADJUSTMENT

I want you to continue relaxing now . . just as you are . . I am going to give you a few suggestions and instructions . . that will help you to attain your goals . . The suggestions and instructions I will give you . . are going directly into the storehouse of your subconscious mind . . And they will begin working immediately . . to enable you to make the adjustments needed . . to achieve your maximum, enjoyable, sexual satisfaction . .

Each day, these suggestions have a stronger influence on you . . Causing you to experience a happy, well adjusted sex life . .

Your entire organism . . of your body . . is cooperating with these suggestions . . causing your body processes . . to function more perfectly and naturally, each day . .

Your subconscious mind understands . . that the sex urges you have . . are normal and natural . . It is the way nature has provided . . to enable you to give and receive love and affection . .

You will continue developing a greater understanding . . of the natural urges of your body . . And that will cause you to experience . . greater happiness and fulfillment . . in a love-sex relationship . . with the partner of your choice . .

I want you to use your imagination now . . I want you to imagine yourself . . making love with your chosen partner . . Get that impression in your mind, clearly . . Think of yourself, in bed . . naked . . with your chosen partner . . Submerge yourself in these enjoyable feelings . . as you caress each other . . (Pause)

See . . and smell . . and feel yourself . . in sexual intercourse . . with your chosen partner . . Hear the words you are saying to each other . . and the sounds you are making . .

Now, make the picture brighter . . and bring it closer to you . . Make everything come alive . .

Make it more real . . and notice the wonderful feelings you are experiencing . . See yourself . . and feel yourself . . experiencing sexual fulfillment . . Notice the odors . . and taste . . the aromatic flavors that come . . with sexual fulfillment . . (Pause)

416

You are realizing that sex is a wonderful . . body-soul expression . . of love and affection . . It's a wonderful way of uniting your body and soul . . with the body and soul of another . . And your sexual relationship, with the partner of your choice . . keeps becoming more and more enjoyable . . each time you make love . .

You will be calm and at ease . . when you are having sexual relations . . And you will feel confident and secure . . as you unite your body . . with the body of your chosen partner . . You will be able to express your affection . . which makes the relationship more compatible . . You will find that a mutually satisfying sexual relationship . . will increase your happiness . . And will also instill a greater feeling of happiness and security . . in your chosen partner . .

You will read good books and articles . . about sex . . to increase your knowledge . . about the normal and natural sexual responses . . of your partner . .

Each day, you will experience an increased level . . of self-confidence, self-reliance and self-acceptance . . That will automatically cause you . . to be more successful . . in all other areas of your life . .

You now have a more relaxed attitude about sex . . And you continue developing . . a more wholesome, more mature attitude . . that causes you . . and your partner . . to experience a happier, more fulfilling, sexual adjustment . . with each other . .

Sex is normal and natural . . And you each have a right to experience . . sexual fulfillment . . All inhibitions, fears or feelings of guilt . . are gradually fading away . . And you will notice your sexual experiences . . continuing to become more enjoyable . . and more satisfying . .

The thought of having sexual relations with your chosen partner . . will be so stimulating for you . . that you will easily become sexually aroused . . And you will calmly anticipate . . a very enjoyable, fulfilling experience . .

Each of you . . will be a co-participant in your sexual relationship . . by taking an active role . . in the sexual experience . . Actively participating, each time you are together . .

You continue developing more enthusiasm . . about your sexual relationship . . And you keep experiencing even greater pleasure from having sex . . than ever before . .

You will always use considerate and loving techniques . . that will assure you and your partner . . the most satisfaction in your sexual achievements . . And you will do your best . . to keep yourself physically attractive . . to your chosen partner . .

Mentally and emotionally . . it keeps becoming easier to discuss various ways . . to increase sexual happiness and enjoyment . . for you and . . for your chosen partner . .

Each day, your self-confidence keeps increasing . . enabling you to give . . and to receive . . love . . in a normal, natural way . .

You continue developing greater love and understanding . . for each other . . and for others . . The more love and understanding you project to others . . the more you'll find love and understanding . . flowing back to you . . Your life will be filled with . . a wonderful feeling of complete compatibility and love . .

You look forward . . each day . . with confidence and anticipation . . Knowing that each day . . will be filled with radiance, joy, love and happiness . . And you arise each morning . . filled with enthusiasm, energy and vitality . .

Continue to relax a moment longer . . as your subconscious mind absorbs everything we have talked about . . Enjoy the comfort of hypnosis . . as you always do . . each time I hypnotize you . . (pause)

In a moment, I will begin my count . . from One down to Five . . And when you hear me count out the number Five . . you will open your eyes, feeling awake, alert and alive . . And ready to take on the rest of your day . .

EMERGE

As you are continuing to relax . . I want you to open your eyes and look . . at the back of your RIGHT hand . . As you do this . . a feeling of heaviness will develop . . in your RIGHT hand . . As you notice that feeling of heaviness . . I want you to lift up your LEFT hand and keep it up . . until I tell it . . to go back down . . (Pause until LEFT hand lifts)

Good . . Your LEFT hand can go back down now . . As you continue concentrating on your RIGHT hand . . I will begin stroking your LEFT hand . . And I want you to notice all the feelings you are experiencing . . in your RIGHT hand . . as your LEFT hand becomes completely numb . . (COMMENCE STROKING LEFT HAND AND PROCEED WITH SUGGESTIONS.)

Notice any feelings you are experiencing in your RIGHT hand . . Your RIGHT hand may begin feeling heavier . . You may notice a feeling of warmth . . coming into your RIGHT hand . . Or it may begin tingling . . Notice everything you are experiencing . . in your RIGHT hand . . as your LEFT hand becomes completely numb . . Are you aware of the feelings you are experiencing in your RIGHT hand ? . . (Wait for Response)

Now . . I'd like for you to notice that your LEFT hand is feeling very numb . . You are experiencing numbness in your fingers . . In the palm of your hand . . The back of your hand . . And, all through the entire hand . . (Pause) Notice that the numbness is increasing even more now . . And as it does . . it's such a pleasant feeling . . that it feels as though it's too much trouble . . to even move a finger . . It feels as though it is going to sleep . . Almost as though it is no longer a part of you . . And as you become aware of that . . you will nod your head, YES . . (Pause, until client nods.)

AFTER CLIENT NODS, YES, PICK UP HAND BETWEEN FINGERNAILS OF THE THUMB AND MIDDLE FINGER AND ASK CLIENT,
"What does it seem like I am doing now" ? . . (Wait for Response.)

If client says, "It feels like you are pinching me" . . Reply, "Do you mean, you can feel the pressure of the skin between my fingers?" If client says, "Yes" . . Reply, "You don't feel any pain at all, do you ? . . (Wait for Response) If client says, "I feel some pain" . . Continue holding hand by fingernails and Reply, "The hand is continuing to feel more numb . .

419

Tell me when you feel nothing but the pressure of the skin between my fingers" . . (Wait for Response.)

(When you are confident the client has numbness in the hand, continue as follows:)

You are responding well to my suggestions . . In just a moment . . I'm going to have you open your eyes . . And even with your eyes open . . you will remain in a hypnotic state . . You will be able to keep your eyes open . . until I tell you to close them again . . When I tell you to close your eyes . . you will close them and immediately drift into a much DEEPER hypnotic state . . And you will continue responding to the suggestions I give you . . Okay, Open your eyes now . . Look and see what I am doing to your hand . . Now, you realize that your subconscious mind caused changes . . so that only your LEFT hand became numb . . Your RIGHT hand has all the normal feelings . . Your LEFT arm has all of its normal feelings . . I'm going to pinch your LEFT arm, lightly . . so you will notice it has all of its feelings . . (Pinch arm lightly, and ask) "Can you feel that?" (Then pinch back of RIGHT hand, and ask) "You notice a little pain in your RIGHT hand, don't you?" (Wait for Response, then say) Now you realize that your subconscious mind causes changes, without any conscious effort by you . . I put the suggestion into your mind . . that your LEFT hand would become numb . . Then I told you a signal I would use . . The signal was . . stroking your LEFT hand . . And it kept becoming more and more numb, each time I stroked it . .

Your mind has learned to respond to signals . . Everything we do . . is in response to signals . . Whatever we do . . we are responding to signals . . When you make a decision to brush your teeth . . you send a signal to your subconscious mind, which in turn . . causes you to make all the correct movements . . To open the toothpaste tube . . squeeze some onto your toothbrush . . Put the brush against your teeth and move your hand in the proper way . . And you make all of these movements, without even thinking about them . . It's that way with everything we do . . When we make the decision to do something . . that is a signal we send to our subconscious mind . . And the subconscious mind responds . . by causing our body to make all of the necessary movements . .

Sometimes, things happen in your body, or your mind . . that need adjusting . . and it causes you to feel excitement in your stomach and in your penis . . Your body continues to function normally . .

420

Still, you are aware of the excitement and the pleasure you know it will cause . . consciously . . But your subconscious mind needs to be made aware . . that you are not pleased . . with the destructive consequences you bring to your mind . . and to your body . . And you want to make changes . . That is why you are here now . .

Now, your subconscious mind is understanding . . that having a brief desire for sex . . is normal and natural . . For that is a part of the normal functioning of the body . . to enable your sexual partner to become pregnant . . You were created with the ability . . to have a perfectly normal, functioning body . . Your body knows how to function . . in an easy, natural way . . But it does not know how to react . . when your conscious mind directs it to perform anal sex . . or ejaculate into the mouth of another man . . Or he, to ejaculate into your mouth . . These are very negative acts . . against the natural doctrines of nature . . And negative acts create negative consequences . . .

I want your subconscious mind to review what is happening . . to cause you to experience such discomfort . . in your conscious thinking . . and work out the solution . . to resolve that problem completely . . Your subconscious mind is reviewing, examining and exploring . . the causes and affects of that problem . . And your mind is understanding it . . from a more adult . . more mature, point of view . . Realizing that masturbation is a normal activity . . and should be experienced easily, calmly and comfortably . . It should be just as normal and natural as urinating or . . having a bowel movement . . It is also implanting in your conscious awareness . . the grave consequences of your behavior . .

By allowing yourself to be hypnotized . . and to express your desire to be free from this problem . . you are activating your subconscious mind to review any imprints, impressions, thoughts and ideas . . that have gone into your mind . . that may have been causing that problem . . Your mind is assessing that information . . and understanding it from a different, more adult point of view . . And, understanding, that it is okay now . . to resolve that problem completely . .

You are continuing to relax . . calmly and comfortably . . All levels of your mind are cooperating . . Working out a very pleasant solution . . to that problem . . Continue relaxing another moment . .

When your mind knows it is okay for that problem to be resolved . . and that changes have begun . . and you are getting rid of that problem . . easily and comfortably . . one of your fingers will lift up . . towards the ceiling . . And your finger will remain up . . until I tell it to go back down . .

NOTE : IF CLIENT'S FINGER DID NOT LIFT TO INDICATE CHANGES HAVE STARTED, GO TO, "THERAPY BETWEEN SESSIONS". GIVE THOSE SUGGESTIONS BEFORE AWAKENING CLIENT.

You are doing very well . . It feels so good . . just to continue relaxing . . You are doing just fine . . Later on, when you awaken from the hypnotic state . . your whole body will feel good . . From the top of your head, all the way down . . to the bottom of your feet . .

Your subconscious mind is very sensitive to everything I say . . And so, I will remind your subconscious mind that . . even after you awaken from the hypnotic state . . and at all times during your daily life . . these suggestions will continue to influence you . . Just as strongly . . just as surely and . . just as powerfully . . as they do while you are hypnotized . .

You will make the necessary changes in your life . . .whatever is required . . A new environment . . new friends . . Perhaps a new job . . Acquaint yourself more strongly with the opposite sex . .

Study and understand their needs and desires . . You have expressed your need for self-satisfaction . . Now, it is time to consider others . . Your real friends and family . . You will be pleased with the improvements in your life . . Each day, the improvements will keep increasing . . And you can be sure it is permanent and lasting . .

Being hypnotized is always a wonderful, relaxing experience . . And you will become more aware of the benefits . . you are to experience from it . . each time I hypnotize you . .

You realize that your subconscious mind . . caused the changes in your body . . without any conscious effort by you . . to make your hand numb . . And now, your mind is causing you to experience pleasant changes . . that will enable you to have an exciting masturbation . . each time you do it . . by yourself . . And it will be experienced in an easy, natural way . . As a normal cleansing process of your body . . It is understood that you must excrete semen from your body, periodically . .

In time . . perhaps at church or at a mall . . or grocery store . . you will meet a lady . . who will make your life comfortable . . Until then . . you will be content with self-masturbation . .

The healing processes of your mind are working properly . . because you want them to work . . Your subconscious mind is obeying your thoughts and desires . . for you, to experience a comfortable transcending of your mind . . Your body is responding . . And you will be very happy as you notice the continuous progress you achieve . . Continue to relax a while longer . . (Pause)

In just a moment, I will be counting from ONE to FIVE, for you to awaken from the hypnotic state . . And when you awaken . . all the normal feelings will be back in both of your hands . . Your whole body will feel relaxed and comfortable . . Your mind will be alert and you will feel peaceful and calm . .

I will begin my count now . .

ONE . . You are aware that soon you will awaken . . You are coming up now . .

TWO . . Coming up a little higher now . . and your mind is waking a little more . .

THREE . . Feeling good now . . Feeling wonderful, all over . . For you are a wonderful person . .

FOUR . . Coming up faster now . . Refreshed and alive . . Breath in deeply . . and

FIVE . . Feeling relaxed and wonderful . . You may Open Your Eyes now and breath deeply . .

As you continue relaxing . . you go a little deeper . . and a little DEEPER . . until, finally . . you are deep enough . . to completely enjoy . . the fully relaxing sensations of this experience . .

Notice the pleasant sounds in the background . . Perhaps you hear birds singing . . as the wind rustles the leaves in the trees . . And you notice a very pleasant aroma in the air . .

I want you to continue relaxing now . . just as you are . . I am going to give you a few suggestions and instructions . . that will help you to attain your goals . .

There was a neighbor . . who wanted to plant a flower bed . . She looked through a seed catalogue, picking out, by color . . whatever looked good . . from among all the beautiful pictures she saw there . . After selecting the many, many different seeds she wanted to plant . . she sent off her order . . so she would have the seeds back in plenty of time for the spring planting . .

She waited patiently for the seeds to arrive and finally . . in the mailbox one morning . . a large package was delivered . . She opened it hurriedly and found dozens of packages of seeds inside . . She was quite happy and excited . . and began planting them immediately . .

She planted rows and rows in lovely beds . . in the back yard . . And in the front of the house . . she planted them around the porch and around the trees . . And along the sidewalks . .

As the days passed, she watered them and weeded them and watched them closely . . Getting quite excited each time a little green shoot began showing its way . . through the warm, damp earth . .

And daily, she could see the plants growing . . With some growing tall; some were medium in height and some . . were quite short . . Some of them bushed out . . and some stayed slender . .

Some had many leaves, while other . . had only a few leaves . . She was surprised and delighted to see how different each plant was . . from the other plants . .

Each day she jumped out of bed, excited about seeing all of the changes that had taken place . . during the night . . And each day she was rewarded, with all sorts of new leaves and new growth . .

The day came when she began finding buds on many of the plants . . And she felt concern because . . some were fat and some were little and hard . . And some were long and squat looking . . And she worried as she continued weeding . . watching and waiting . . day by day . .

When it didn't rain, she watered them carefully . . And she loosened the earth around the stems . .

And all the while, she worried, secretly . . Because some were so different from the others . . And she was not sure the plants were doing what they should be doing . .

So she watched and waited . . and worried . . and continued to work in the beds until, one day . . she saw the first flower . . And in the days that followed, she saw hundreds of flowers . . All were different sizes . . different colors and different heights . . And she noticed . . even though they were each different . . each one was lovely . . in its own way . .

She noted that the round and squat buds became lovely, round flowers . . And the long, skinny buds turned into beautiful, slender flowers . . And the little hard, shiny buds became . . little clusters of flowers . . And she really felt proud of the way each one had turned out because . . they were all so uniquely different . . And each one was so beautiful . . in its own unique way . .

She told herself that it was all right for them to be different . . And so she was full of joy and happiness as each day . . she saw more flowers blooming . . in many different sizes, shapes and colors . . And her gardens were lovely because there were so many different flowers in them . . All of the flowers seemed to belong together, even though they were so different from each other . .

And she was very proud of her garden . . as people came from all over to enjoy it . . Everyone talked about the ones they liked the best . . But the gardener only smiled because she knew . . each one of them was good . . Each one, in its own, special way . . Continue to relax a bit now . . as your subconscious mind absorbs what we are discussing . . And then we will go on . . (pause)

I want to mention that . . I had recently hypnotized a young, married lady . . And while she was hypnotized . . relaxing . . I had mentioned the many improvements that she would be noticing . . Then, when she awakened from the hypnotic state . . it took her a minute or two to reorient herself . . So I had her remain in the recliner for a couple of minutes longer . . to be sure she was back in a wide awake, fully alert state . . before going out into the reception room . . where her husband was waiting to take her home . .

The following week, when she came in for another session . . she told me that . . as they were driving home . . she was thinking about the session we had completed, the week before . . and realized . . that she couldn't remember anything about it . . But she knew she had been hypnotized by me because . . she felt a hundred times better than when she came into my office . .

She said, as she was riding home in the car . . she was unaware of noticing any of the scenery . . And she seemed to be daydreaming about other things . . and not noticing where she was going at all . . with her husband driving . . It was an excellent time for her to have her own daydreams . .

I don't know exactly when the scene changed . . It may have been when the car entered the tunnel . . and she saw a face . . It impressed her strongly . . She was surprised as she realized how much she liked the look of that face . . And how relaxed and comfortable it made her feel . .

Whether it is something you notice by the smoothness of the facial muscles; or the relaxed fullness of the mouth, or the softness of the eyes . . or maybe, the comfortable breathing . . She was fascinated, just looking into that face . . and seeing herself . . And something else was there . . Something she couldn't quite recognize . . but she couldn't stop looking into that picture . . The more she looked at it the more she realized . . there was something very sexy . . about the way her eyes sparkled . . and her stomach muscles . . trembled . . as she looked into that scene . .

And as she was watching the face . . and memorizing those experiences . . she must have drifted back into a hypnotic state because . . the next thing she recalled . . was how the background had changed . . And she was seeing herself in a . . desirable situation . . with that face . . and that complete relaxation . . and that comfort . . And that powerful strength

426

. . Yes, she felt she was 'safely sexy' . . Interacting with the man whom she loved . . Interacting in a way that pleased her considerably . .

And you can be very pleased . . and excited . . watching yourself interacting . . in a way that you enjoy . . Doing something different . . Your conscious mind doesn't need to believe it's possible for you to actually . . act that way . . Provocative, perhaps . . Still, you can really enjoy the scene that your subconscious mind projects . . Or, more likely, you are consciously projecting the scene . . and your subconscious mind just keeps those feelings constant . . Just continue to relax and . . flow with it . . Enjoy this moment . . while you are immersed in this beautiful scenery of love . . (pause)

Then the car hit a bump in the road . . and the scene changed to reveal her . . interacting again . . This time, with some of the men at work . . You interact in different ways with different people . . And even though she kept the same qualities constant . . they were translated to a different situation . . And you can sense your sexuality when you are around other men . . It's still there . . but you only let it reveal itself in a more . . professional manner . . It may be only recognized in the pride you have in yourself . . The aroma of your well selected perfume . . or the way your body looks . . so good . . as you stand and talk with them . .

The car hit another bump and the scene changed again . . There she was, with some women who had caused her difficulty in the past . . It's not clear, why it had been difficult . . but she saw herself asking them for help . . She saw herself, down in a hole, holding her hands up towards them, saying . . "Could you please help me out of here?" . . She felt very safe, as they responded . .

Another jolt of the car . . and the scene changed again . .

Your conscious mind doesn't need the time to review . . because your subconscious mind is able to allow you to understand all of this . . Quite rapidly and clearly . .

To her, it must have seemed like hours, instead of minutes . . that she rode in the car . . Watching those interactions . . Memorizing some things with her conscious mind . . Experiencing other things, subconsciously . . And when she came out of the tunnel . . the shifting of lights disrupted the scene . . And she suddenly became aware of the fact that . . the car had never gone into . . any tunnel . .

427

She felt blessed, she thought . . as she became overjoyed with a sense of great comfort and security . . And then she realized that she had learned so much, simply from . . daydreaming . . Some things that would be very helpful to her . . and to her relationships . . When the car was parked, safely at home, in the driveway . . she got out of the car, laughing . . and feeling very happy to be home . .

You are continuing to relax even more now . . and your subconscious mind is accepting . . my suggestions . . and is improving your health . . and is enabling you to live your life in a more peaceful . . more calm, more relaxed way . .

Each day, these suggestions will become even more effective . . you are learning to use these principles of relaxation . . which you are now experiencing . . in all phases if your daily life . . and that will keep you calm and relaxed . . at all times . .

In every situation or circumstance . . that comes up in your life . . you will be calm and relaxed . . Your nerves will be relaxed and steady . . and you'll be able to do everything in a relaxed way . . You will be able to cope with . . every day changing circumstances . . in a loving, peaceful way . .

Now, I am going to count from 1 to 5 . . and on the count of 5 . . you will open your eyes . . to an alert, waking state . . feeling clear of mind, relaxed and wonderful . . for you are a wonderful and confident person . . I will begin . .

One.   You will soon be in a normal, conscious state of mind . .
Two.   You are now connected to your inner supporting strength . .
Three. Everything I have told you is true . . and is already happening . .

Four.   Beginning to be more aware of your body as it fully awakens and wants to stir . .
Five.   Let your hands and feet move . . Stir and stretch as you open your eyes, feeling clear, feeling rested and wonderful . .

You are very relaxed now, aren't you . . But I want you to go deeper now . . relax deeper . .

Listen only to the sound of my voice . . I am going to give you suggestions that will benefit you . .

As in most families . . each of us had a two wheeled bicycle . . when we were young children . . You probably had one . . As I recall, learning to ride that bicycle . . taught me a lot about myself . . Mostly, How to balance my body . . It also helped me develop good coordination . . In fact, learning to ride a bicycle, taught me a lot of things . . Things that I didn't even realize, as a child . .

Any parent who will not let their children learn to ride a bicycle . . is really doing a disservice to their child . . In riding a bicycle . . you learn something about motion . . balance, coordination . . rhythm and timing . . that becomes the foundation for further development . . later on, when we become adults . .

You may not remember every detail . . of what you did to learn how to ride that bicycle . . But you did learn . . And when you achieved that goal . . it increased the kind of confidence you needed to have . . Even in relationships with other people . .

It reminds me of a movie I saw, a long time ago . . in which Gene Wilder . . played the part of a man . . who was very shy and insecure . . He was obsessed with the belief that he was a failure . . with every woman he attempted to date . . He thought he had to perform, sexually . . and just knew she would be disappointed with his performance . . No matter who she was . . Finally, he met a woman . . who knew how to take things slow and easy . . And she enabled him to be very comfortable . . At first, he invited her to go out dancing . . And she reminded him of what every child knows . . about looking at the smile on the face of a special friend . . when you are enjoying each other . .

Disregarding the fast tempo of the music . . she just stopped, still, on the dance floor . . And held out her arms to him . . inviting him to dance slowly with her . . and hold her near to him . . The evening continued like that . . even when they got back to her apartment . . And she lit candles . . and began to . . slowly . . undress him . .

She released a clasp . . of her own clothing . . And then . . comfortably, looking at him, she sweetly said . . "You'll have to do the rest" . . As he looked at her beautiful naked body . . focusing on the pink nipples of her breasts . . she asked, "Did you think I would be bigger?" And he said, "I had no idea you would be so beautiful" . . Then she put on a record and they danced . . in the quiet intimacy of her candle lit bedroom . . before going out for a moonlight romp on the beach nearby . . Much later, when they were sitting in front of a fireplace . . holding each other tightly . . he placed his hand up against her heart . . Commenting on the fact that it was beating so rapidly . .

"Nervous?" he asked . . "What do you have to be nervous about?" She responded, simply, "I'm the one who has to do it . . Do you want to know what would make me feel good?" He responded, "If I could know that . . it would make me very happy." And very softly, she carefully explained that . . "While having you inside me would be very nice . . I don't want that now . . Right now, I just want you to touch me and kiss me . . But keep your eyes open and . . just look at me . . Soon, I will tell you more things, but first . . I need a little bit more confidence" . .

And then, she just looked at him . . all over . . And let herself be looked at . . And she smiled the most tender, beautiful, vulnerable, yet, trusting smile you could imagine . . Eyes wide open . . A delicate, innocent little smile . . Very still . . warm . . and wonderful . .

And then, through the magic of movies . . Blending with . . and superimposed . . in front of that young woman's face . . was the much younger little girl she had once been . . shining through . . Smiling that same smile . . with confidence, innocence and openness . . Playing in the front yard sprinkler, with a little boy . . And the little boy's face, of course . . temporarily replaced the face of the shy, young man . . And there was his innocence . . and trust . . and curiosity and love . . as he looked into the face of that smiling little girl . . Water was splashing on them both . . And they hugged . . as the drops rained down around them . .

The two adults, who were soon pressing their lips together . . tenderly . . then more passionately . . embracing . . had somehow, been able to reach into the storehouse of learning . . that only a child has . . and applied that sense of knowing . . how beautiful and precious you are . . to a current situation . . with someone you know

430

you can trust to recognize it too . . And that simple act of honesty . . Looking at each other . . touching each other . . embracing . . and kissing . . was far more intimate than whatever overt sexual contact followed . . For it is certainly the intimacy that lends a magic . . and a mystique . . to the, otherwise, expressive act . . of sexual intercourse . . (Pause)

I will leave you with these thoughts to guide you . . There is no reason to ever fear, for love . . as long as it is approached . . in a manner that is compatible . . to both of you . . Love is to share . . But first . . it is a bonding of trust . . and respect . . for each other . .

Take another moment to relax . . as your subconscious mind absorbs . . all that we have talked about . . (Pause)

In just a moment . . I will begin my count . . from ONE . . to FIVE . . When you hear the number FIVE . . you will open your eyes and be wide awake . .

I will begin my count now . .

ONE

TWO

THREE

FOUR

FIVE

You are very relaxed now, aren't you . . But I want you to go deeper . . Gently relax Deeper . . Listen only to the sound of my voice . . I am going to give you suggestions that will benefit you . .

You have probably heard the song, with the words . . "Old Man River . . He just keeps rolling along" . . Regardless of anything that happens . . the river keeps flowing . . headed somewhere . . And although there may be obstacles along the way . . It keeps moving along . . to its destination . .

As I talk to you . . your mind can remember that song . . And another song . . that talks about . . the perfect love . . or, a beautiful morning . . And another song . . And another . . Those songs may become so vivid in your mind . . that you may visualize the band playing . . and the singer . . singing, first, one song . . and then another . .

You may visualize the band . . and the singer . . And you may become even more involved in those songs . . as your memories of them project their beautiful melodies, back to you . . And it may seem like the vibrations of the music are flowing . . through every part of your body . .

There may be a little confusion in your mind . . as you try to project one singer over another . . or one band playing while you concentrate on another . . at the same time . . But you are capable of hearing both . . at the same time . . And your subconscious mind . . can still listen . . and receive everything I am saying . . because it is not important for you to, consciously, listen to what I am saying . . Your subconscious mind is free . . to absorb everything I tell you . . And you can be pleasantly surprised to find . . your subconscious mind, making true . . everything I say to you . .

You may find some confusion . . in knowing, whether you are listening . . to music with one ear and me . . with the other . . Or whether you are listening to one song with one ear . . and another song with the other ear . . And not paying attention to what I am saying at all . . And that's okay . .

It is beautiful music you are hearing in your mind . . isn't it . . You may be so interested in the music . . that you do not realize . . how easily your subconscious mind is receiving . . everything I say to you

432

. . And is causing everything I tell you . . to happen, automatically . . as you go about the activities of your daily life . .

There are many things you are consciously aware of . . And there are many things you are capable of doing . . which you are not consciously aware of . .

You can be in a comfortable position, in front of me . . And you can adjust your legs to a more comfortable position, if you like . . And I can hold a slip of paper, with printing on it . . toward you . . and you would be able to read it . . even if I had it turned upside down . . That is something you know you can do . . And you can feel pleased to know you can do that . . as you continue to adjust yourself . . to a more comfortable position . .

We could both do it at the same time . . And we can both feel pleased . . You can do it in your way . . And I can do it in my way . . And even though we may differ . . in the way we do it . . We both can find a lot of satisfaction . . in doing it . . And there are many other things you can do . . just as easily . . without thinking about it, consciously . . You can begin experiencing a very pleasant, very enjoyable sensation . . starting in your feet . . and gradually moving up, into your calves . . A tingling . . soothing sensation . . Rising up above your knees now . . coming higher . . and higher . . Such a pleasant sensation . . soothing to you . .

As soon as you begin feeling that wonderful, tingling sensation . . moving up into your thighs . . and into your stomach . . with a warm, tingling sensation . . one of the fingers on your right hand will raise up . . and will remain up . . until I tell it to go back down . . (Pause for response) You're responding very well . . You're doing everything that comes naturally . .

It reminds me of a poem I read . . "And when thyself shall pass . . to relax upon the grass . . It shall, as a soothing drink . . fill an empty glass . .

It is natural . . It's like filling a long empty void . . Or massaging . . the right spot . . It feels so good . . to let yourself go . . You have free access to everything your conscious mind knows . . about your body . . But does not know, that it knows . . And what your body knows freely . . and wants to bare . . and wants to release . . it can release . .

Your subconscious mind has an amazing ability . . to learn rapidly . . and is learning rapidly . .

You are learning to use, quite well . . all knowledge that you have . . Body and mind language . . Body and mind knowledge . . And using all of it well . . You are learning to experience . . and enjoy . . the natural feelings . . and sensations . . of your own body . .

What does your body know . . which you know . . and know well . . both consciously and subconsciously ? . . It knows how to keep you breathing . . It knows how to keep your heart pumping the blood . . through your circulatory system . . And it knows how to cause you to experience enjoyable feelings and sensations . . in your sensual organs . . In your genitals . . And it knows how to automatically cause . . your soft nipples . . to stand right out . . Your mind and body know . . that you have soft tissues that can become erect . .

You also have other knowledge . . that you may not have used for a long time . . But you do have the knowledge . . and you can begin using that knowledge now . .

When your body was developing . . you had the knowledge . . to connect your toe-bone . . to your foot bone . . and your heel-bone to your ankle bone . . And you knew how to make all the other connections . .

As further example . . your external genitals are connected to your internal genitals . . And your internal genitals are connected to . . your ovaries . . To your adrenals . . And all of the connections continue, on and on . . All of the connections have been completed, perfectly . . And you know how to use them all . . automatically . . without any need to, consciously, think about anything . .

All of the connections have been made properly . . And your endocrinal gland system is overflowing . . with vibrating, sexual feelings . . And all of your sexual feelings . . are connected with your nervous system . . and with your body functions . . and with your other feelings . . And you can prove it to yourself . . by putting my suggestions . . along with your feelings . . into your own actions . .

You will discover a magical transformation taking place . . when someone gently massages . . the nipples of your breasts . . with their hand or with their lips . . And you will be pleased . . and perhaps, amazed . . at how wonderful it makes you feel . . as your chakra's light up . . with exciting sensations . .

You will automatically experience wonderful, sexual feelings . . in every part of your body . . And you will know that every word I say is true . . In fact, I'm quite sure you already know it is true . .

You will be happy to enjoy it . . You will find it to be like, when you see a small baby . . and you have the uncontrollable urge to stop and pick it up . . And you know, that is what you will do . . So does the baby . . You can't keep from it . . You really enjoy it . . and it comes so naturally . .

If you were having doubts about yourself in the past . . You will realize . . those doubts are wrong . . They will fade away rapidly . . Your body knows . . Your conscious mind knows . . And your subconscious mind knows . . Only you . . the person . . does not know . . So I will tell you . . The tender kiss . . The sweet caress . . The gentle cupping of your breasts . . The chills of excitement . . and the enjoyable sensations . . running all through your body . . The tickling, tingling in your stomach as your aching loins long to press hard . . against another being . . is the normal, natural yearning, you are experiencing in your body . . And one that needs to be fulfilled . .

You are blessed to be a woman . . because women have been blessed by God . . Men have only one place to express an orgasm . . but women have many . .

You are feeling very enthusiastic about it, aren't you . . You are happy . . .and excited about it . . You are already feeling a sense of satisfaction . . by organizing what I am saying, into your own actions . . And it will be for your own benefit . . for your pleasure and satisfaction . . And that has been so long in coming . . You know that the more you caress him . . the more you will enjoy the wonderful . . sensations . . you are feeling . . You are anticipating it . . and looking forward to it . . Culminating in the most orgasmic climax . . of your life . . And you will be so thrilled . . and so pleased . . to experience . . and to share . . such joy and happiness . .

Relax, in a moment of silence now . . as your subconscious mind absorbs . . what we have discussed here today . . (Pause)

In just a moment . . I will begin my count . . from ONE . . to FIVE . . When you hear me say the number, FIVE . . you will open your eyes and be wide awake . . I will begin my count now . .
ONE   TWO   THREE   FOUR   FIVE

(Follow Relaxation)   COURAGE TO REVEAL

You are very relaxed now, aren't you . . But I want you to go deeper . . Gently relax, Deeper . . Listen only to the sound of my voice . . I am going to give you some information . . that will help you with the problem . . you are experiencing . .

This is about two young boys named Bob, and his friend, Jim . . Like all boys do, they were out in the yard playing one day . . They were building a fort, with scraps of wood they had found . . Bob suggested they should put the boards straight up . . for the walls . . But Jim thought they would be better if they were on their sides . . So, they compromised . . They agreed to have two walls, with boards straight up . . and the other sides would have boards lengthwise . . so they could add a window and a door . . It was going to be a good fort . .

After they got the boards standing upright . . Bob began nailing them in place . . Jim was handing him the nails . . Then Bob noticed that Jim kept rubbing his pants . . He didn't think any more about it . . until he noticed he was doing it more and more . . Jim went to get more nails . . and when he came back . . they kept working until they had the walls nailed in place . .

As they stood there . . looking at the fort . . Bob noticed Jim, rubbing himself again . . and he asked . . "Hey, Jim, What are you doing?" . . Jim turned RED . . He was very embarrassed . . and he asked Bob if he could keep a secret . . Bob said, "YES." . . Jim asked him, "Are you sure ? Do you promise?" . . And Bob promised that he wouldn't tell anyone . .

You may not even be able to guess . . what Jim told Bob . . He told Bob that he, and his uncle . . would wrestle together, quite a lot . . He didn't want to . . but his uncle would shame him into it . . calling him a sissy, if he didn't . . And he said, "Sometimes my uncle grabs me . . and touches me . . And I don't like the way he touches me . . It gets me thinking things . . that I know I shouldn't be thinking about" . . Bob replied, "Hey, He shouldn't be doing that . . It isn't right . . We should go tell somebody" . . And Jim said, "NO ! You promised to keep it a secret" . . Bob objected "You've got to tell your Mother or your Father . . or some adult . . because he may not ever stop doing it" . .

Bob had seen a movie at school . . about what to do when someone touches you . . or tries to hurt you . . And he explained to Jim how important it is . . for him to go and tell somebody . . Anybody . . Jim said he had tried but they wouldn't believe him . . He had tried to tell his parents . . what his uncle was doing . . But they just wouldn't believe him . . And his uncle told him that if he told anybody else . . it would get his uncle in trouble, big time . . and it would be Jim's fault . . He didn't know what to do . . Bob suggested that maybe he should tell someone at school . . Jim said he would be too embarrassed . . But Bob insisted that it was important . . and that he should keep telling . . until somebody listened . .

Jim felt confused . . He didn't know what he should do . . He knew he didn't like what his uncle was doing . . But he also knew . . he had to tell someone who could do something . . to make his uncle stop . .

Both boys decided to stop working on the fort for the day and go home . .

Jim said, "I know my uncle will be at my house, when I get there . . He'll be there 'til late tonight . . Do you think I could stay overnight at your house?" . . "Sure," Jim replied . . "Come on in. I'll talk to my Mom" . .

The next morning, they both went to school . . then went to their separate classes . . Jim took a deep breath . . he could feel his heart pounding in his chest . . because he knew he had to do something . . that would take a lot of courage to do . . And he didn't know how it was going to turn out . . He just knew it had to be done . .

Finally, he decided to go ahead and just do it . . He headed towards the counselor's office . . He got right to the door, but then, remembered . . the counselor was a woman . . He stopped and thought about it . . She was the only one he could think of to tell . . Getting his courage up again . . he walked into the counselor's office . . and asked to speak with her about . . something very important . .

She could see right away, that he was very scared . . And she asked him to sit down . . Then she asked him to close his eyes . . and to breathe deeply . . and then to exhale, slowly . . five or six times . . She said, that would relax his whole body . . She was very understanding . . So, Jim did as she asked . . And after doing that . . he opened his eyes and felt very relaxed . .

Finally, he felt at ease enough to start talking . . And told her the whole story . . about his uncle . . touching him . . on his private parts . . and how he felt about it . . How it hurt him . . kind of, inside . . and got him so confused . . And how he felt guilty . . like it was his fault . . And, if anything happened to his uncle . . that would be his fault, too . .

The counselor complimented Jim . . for having the courage to come forward and tell . . what his uncle had been doing to him . . And she assured him that . . none of it had been his fault . . And that he should not feel guilty for something, someone else had done . . He was a victim . . He was not to blame . . And he was right . . to tell someone who cared . . and could help . .

Then she began asking him questions . . And the more she asked . . the easier it was for Jim to talk to her . . And he knew they would figure out a way . . to get his parents to help him, too . . And, somehow, they would get his uncle to stop . .

When he left the counselor's office . . he felt so much better . . And he felt proud of himself . . for having the courage to tell someone . . who was able to help him . . That's what the counselor is there for . . To help kids with problems . . (like yours . .)

I'd like you to take another moment . . just to relax . . as your subconscious mind absorbs . . all that we have talked about . . And after you awaken . . if you have any questions . . or if you want to talk to me . . about anything . . I want you to know that I am your friend . . and you can trust me . . I want to help you in any way that I can . . Just relax now . . Relax . .   (Pause)

In just a moment . . I will begin my count . . from ONE . . to FIVE . . When you hear the number FIVE . . you will open your eyes and be wide awake . . I will begin my count now . .

ONE TWO THREE FOUR FIVE

You are responding very well to everything I am saying . . And now you are ready for your inner mind . . to begin making the proper adjustments in your body . . providing for yourself, far greater pleasure and enjoyment . . than you have ever experienced before . .

Permitting yourself to be hypnotized lets your subconscious mind know . . that you sincerely want every part of your body to function properly . . so you will be healthy and strong . . And will be able to experience . . true, sexual satisfaction . . with your chosen partner . .

You have made a wise decision . . And you will be pleased and very happy . . that you have asked me to help you overcome . . this frustrating, sexual problem . .

You realize that the subconscious level of your mind controls all of the functions and activities of your body . . So the conscious level of your mind can continue relaxing . . as your subconscious mind responds . . to everything I tell you . .

Listen to the soothing sounds . . coming from the tape recorder (Air Conditioner) . . You don't need to make any effort to listen to my words . . because your subconscious mind will hear everything I say . . And will cause you to automatically respond . . to everything . . I tell you . .

You know what it's like to daydream about something . . and not really be looking at anything . . And not really listening to anything . . And as you are daydreaming . . someone in the room may be talking . . but you don't notice what is being said . . Just as easily . . you can enjoy the comfort of being . . in a deep hypnotic state . . And later on, when you awaken . . you don't need to remember anything that happened . . while you were hypnotized . . And so, you will not . . remember anything that happened . . while you were hypnotized . .

Relax deeper now . . DEEPER . . Relax . . DEEPER and DEEPER . . Listen, easily, to the soothing sounds . . coming from the tape player . . And you can experience the feeling of drifting away . . Much like when you drift into a natural state of sleep . . Your subconscious mind will be hearing each word I say . . as your conscious mind relaxes . . enjoying the restful . . peaceful feeling . . of drifting . . floating your body . . just above your chair . . Just relax . . RELAX . .

439

There may be some sounds that you are not familiar with . . but you will find yourself enjoying it fully . . and more fully . .

It feels good . . to let yourself go completely . . Gently and easily . . you continue drifting into a deeper . . and DEEPER . . more comfortable state . . The music continues to play in the far background . . and an enchanting aroma . . comes to your senses . . Breath in that pleasant aroma . . It is so sensual . . so pleasing . . As you hear one part of the music . . another piece may come to mind . . A piece . . that you can enjoy, over and over again . .

You don't need to pay attention to me . . Just give your attention to the enchanting aroma . . and the beautiful music . . in the background . . And you will begin to notice the wonderful sensations, pulsing all through your body . . It will seem like it is caressing . . every part of your body . . And it keeps becoming more enjoyable . . more pleasurable . .

Just relax . . because your subconscious mind understands everything I say . . Even things that you don't understand . . Just relax and go with it . . Your subconscious mind is going to give you some really wonderful . . sensual vibrations . . and sensations . . all over your body . . (pause)

Your entire body and organism is cooperating . . with everything I tell you . . Your subconscious mind understands . . that sexual urges and desires . . are normal and natural . . It is one of the ways God has provided for you . . to experience a union of oneness . . and express yourself . . through love and affection . .

You will be pleased . . as the natural urges of your body keep increasing . . and you will continue enjoying these sensations . . and a greater love-sex relationship . . with your chosen partner . .

Your conscious mind is very busy . . listening to the sounds of the music . . And your subconscious mind is listening . . to everything . . that I say . . And everything I say is very meaningful to your subconscious mind . . (pause) Your conscious mind is hearing only the music . . and your subconscious mind is free . . to limit itself . . to everything that I say . .

You will always enjoy having me hypnotize you . . Every time I hypnotize you . . you will enjoy it even more . . You will enjoy the wonderful, sensuous feelings of comfort . . peacefulness . . tenderness and love . .

Your subconscious mind is really taking over control now . . And what you experience . . will be very pleasing to you . . And now, you are beginning to feel a sense of confidence . . and a sense of competence . . and sureness . . with sensations that you haven't had for a long time . . You are feeling very strong and . . excited . . about it . . And you will be pleased that it will continue . . even after you awaken from the hypnotic state . .

Every time you are with the partner of your choice . . those wonderful feelings and sensations . . will keep growing stronger . . And you will realize that they are normal and natural . .

You understand that your sexual urges are normal . . Having sexual relations with your chosen partner . . is a body-soul expression . . of love and affection . . It is one of the ways God has made available . . for the uniting of your body and soul . . with the body and soul of your chosen partner . .

Even after you awaken from the hypnotic state . . you will continue experiencing these wonderful feelings and sensations . . as your body is responding, normally and naturally . .

The cells of your body are alive . . and they know how to function properly . . The cells of your body know how . . to conduct their activities, normally . . and restore every part of your body to normal functioning . . The cells of your body are continuing . . to work in more perfect harmony . . Causing your metabolism . . your hormones . . and all of your glands and organs . . to function harmoniously . .

You will continue experiencing . . pleasant sensations . . flowing through the tissues . . of your skin . . Restoring, rejuvenating and revitalizing . . every part of your body . .

You want your body to function properly . . You want to enjoy, normal and natural, sexual stimulation . . You want to enjoy . . sexual satisfaction and fulfillment . . And your subconscious mind is cooperating . . with your wants and desires . . And is causing you to experience . . arousing changes . . that are increasing your pleasure and enjoyment . . of sexual relations . . with the partner of your choice . .

As the sexual parts of your body become more responsive . . and stronger . . this will cause all other parts of your body . . to keep becoming healthier . . and continue functioning, more perfectly . .   EMERGE

(Follow Relaxation)

You are doing quite well . . Just continue to relax . . as I present you with information that will be of great help to you . .

It has been found that each cell of your body . . performs functions that no one . . has ever duplicated . . Those processes occur . . by receiving directions from your subconscious mind . . And your subconscious mind functions . . by receiving directions from your experiences . . and through information you have received . . from things you see, hear, touch . . or anything that makes an impression in your mind . . Even though you are not consciously aware of it . . your subconscious mind is continuously receiving . . imprints and impressions . . from everything that you experience . .

And your subconscious mind keeps the healing processes of your body . . working, at all times . . The healing processes of your body . . are continuously keeping your body temperature stabilized . . They are continuously nourishing tissues . . strengthening muscles, ligaments and tendons . . They are constantly repairing damaged skin, healing wounds, keeping your hair and fingernails growing . . And keeping your digestive system and your elimination system functioning . .

Those processes and activities of your body are normal and natural . . and they continue working twenty four hours a day . . Causing your metabolism, your organs, your glands . . and all other parts of your body . . to do their work perfectly . .

It is amazing, the way the human body has been created . . with billions of cells, muscles, nerves, glands, various organs . . blood, pulsating in a circulatory system . . And there are many other parts . . All functioning in perfect harmony . . to keep your body healthy, strong and in perfect physical condition . .

The only time the processes of the body . . do not perform perfectly . . is when some thoughts or ideas, have gone into the mind . . and are causing interference . . But, when that happens . . it can be corrected easily . . by getting your mind to review the imprints and impressions . . And understand them, from a more adult . . more mature point of view . .

Even the Bible says, "You can be transformed by the renewing of your mind" . . And that's what we are doing now . . And your mind will soon be causing . . all of your body processes . . to function harmoniously again . . by reprogramming your mind . . with proper thoughts and ideas . . your subconscious mind then causes your bodily processes to function properly . . To rebuild and strengthen your body . . cell by cell . . And heal any damage or disease , completely and perfectly . .

By making your subconscious mind aware of your need for improvement . . you will notice pleasant changes taking place . . as your skin is healing . . and becoming healthier and more smooth . .

Scientists tell us, the body is more than 80 % liquid . . Even your bones are soft and porous . . and are filled with a fluid substance . . Your bones are penetrated by capillaries of blood . .

Your subconscious mind can send energy vibrations into every cell of your body . . and can cause pleasant changes to take place . . and heal your skin completely and perfectly . .

The strongest force of energy in your body . . comes from your subconscious mind . . Your body is changeable . . It can be shaped and renewed . . by thoughts that go into your mind . . Your subconscious mind is now aware of your wants and desires . . and is directing the cells of your body . . to energize every fiber of your skin . . And is causing your skin to keep becoming more moist and smooth . . more flawless . . and healthier . .

DEMONSTRATE THE POWER OF THE IMAGINATION BY HAVING THE CLIENT HOLD BOTH ARMS OUT IN FRONT OF HIS/HER BODY AND IMAGINE A BUCKET, HANGING ON THE LEFT HAND, WITH THE HAND, PALM UPWARD . . AND STRINGS TIED AROUND THE RIGHT WRIST WITH HUGE BALLOONS TIED TO THE STRINGS, FLOATING UP TOWARDS THE CEILING, LIFTING THE RIGHT HAND AND ARM. COUNT TO TEN, SAYING YOU ARE POURING TEN POUNDS OF SAND INTO THE BUCKET, WITH EACH NUMBER YOU SAY. COUNT SLOWLY, ALLOWING TIME FOR THE SUBCONSCIOUS MIND TO CAUSE THE LEFT HAND TO DROP . . AND THE RIGHT HAND AND ARM TO FEEL LIGHTER, AND LIFT UPWARD.

AFTER COMPLETING THE ABOVE DEMONSTRATION, HAVE THE CLIENT GET THE NORMAL FEELING BACK IN BOTH HANDS AND ARMS, AND THEN, CONTINUE AS FOLLOWS :

Now, you realize that when you imagine something . . your subconscious mind causes your body to respond . . to what you imagine . . So now, I want you to use your imagination again . . And this time . . I want you to visualize your skin . . as being smooth and flawless . . soft and supple . . exactly the way you want your skin to be . . Think of yourself as having skin that is smooth, healthy, beautiful . . like a baby's skin . . flawless and perfect, in every way . . Get that image in your mind and hold it there . . (Pause)

Your subconscious mind is responding to that image . . of your perfect, healthy skin . . and is causing the processes of your body to function perfectly . . Cleansing all impurities, out of your body . . through the natural processes of your elimination system . . Your skin is gradually changing . . and is becoming smooth . . and flawless . . and perfect . . Exactly as you want it to be . .

Each night, just before you go to sleep . . close your eyes for a couple of minutes . . and visualize your skin, the way you want it to be . . Smooth, firm, healthy and flawless . . As you continue to visualize your skin, the way you want it to be . . your subconscious mind will cause your body processes to function perfectly . . and heal your skin . . and will keep it smooth and beautiful . .

Each time you wash your skin . . you wash away old cells and molecules, that are no longer needed . . They are replaced with new, fresh, healthy cells, that keep your skin young and vibrant . .

Your metabolism and elimination system will continue functioning properly . . cleansing the inside of your body . . Your entire organism is constantly cleansing and renewing itself . . And your skin keeps becoming more smooth . . more flawless . . and healthier, each day . . The circulation of your blood is improving . . and is carrying the nourishment's and energies needed . . to the tissues of your skin . .

At times, you may feel a slight increase of warmth . . And perhaps, a mild tingling sensation on your skin . . as the healing processes are working . . to provide extra nourishment to those areas where healing is most needed . .

Each day, your health will continue improving . . Every cell, atom and molecule of your body is functioning harmoniously . . to produce perfect health and beautiful, smooth skin . . Your subconscious mind has accepted the suggestions I have given you . . You will be noticing improvements as you continue experiencing the healing processes flowing through every part of your body . . Cleansing, purifying, rejuvenating and restoring the tissues of your skin . . perfectly . .

EMERGE

SKIN RASH - OVERCOME

(Follow Relaxation)

You are doing very well . . Just continue to relax . . as I present you with suggestions . . that will help to resolve the problem you are having . .

Permitting yourself to be hypnotized lets your subconscious mind know . . that you sincerely want every part of your body to function properly . . so you will be healthy and vibrant . . And will be able to experience . . social interactions, without feeling self-conscious . . about your appearance . .

You have made a wise decision . . And you will be very pleased and happy . . that you have asked me to help you overcome this skin rash problem . .

As a result of you permitting yourself to be hypnotized . . your skin is going to begin healing . . And the healing will continue . . until your skin becomes smooth and flawless . . and perfect . .

Your skin . . and your whole body . . is becoming stronger, healthier and more vibrant . . Your circulation is improving . . Especially the circulation of the little blood vessels . . that supply nutrients and new cells to the skin . .

Your heart is pumping blood through your circulatory system . . and that is causing more nourishment to be carried to the skin . . This will cause your skin to become healthier, more normal in texture and more youthful . . Your skin is becoming more healthy in every way . .

As your circulation continues to improve . . your nerves become stronger and steadier . . You'll find that you are able to respond to every situation or circumstance . . in a peaceful, loving way . .

I want you to use your imagination now . . I want you to visualize yourself . . sitting there, comfortably . . feeling strong, peaceful, relaxed, calm and comfortable . . See yourself ONLY . . as a loving, kind and considerate person . . who is compassionate, caring and intelligent . . Think of yourself as being capable of making decisions, wisely . . and feeling confident in the decisions that you make . . You are wise . . and strong . . and well loved and respected . . by everyone . .

Now, look closely at your skin . . Magnify it, in your mind . . You can see the changes taking place . . You can see it becoming smoother . . silkier . . and more flawless and perfect . . Envision the skin rash, leaving your body . . It is falling off . . and floating away . . toward outer space . . Floating out so far that it is disappearing completely . .

Now, you have a genuine feeling of confidence, coming over you . . . It feels good, doesn't it . . Notice the sense of sureness . . and the sense of knowing . . that your skin is healing perfectly . . and permanently . . Hold that vision, firmly, in your mind . . (Pause) You will remain peaceful and calm at all times . . as you go about the activities of your daily life . .

You desire and select to eat . . only foods that are healthy for your body . . You eat foods and drink liquids . . that strengthen your muscles and bones . . and cause your skin to become perfect . . Every day, your muscles, your bones . . your skin . . and all other parts of your body . . keep becoming healthier and more perfect . .

As a result of this experience . . you are feeling more confident . . You are feeling better, mentally and physically . . You are experiencing a strong sense of sureness . . in knowing . . that the rash will disappear . . as your skin continues to heal . . through hypnosis . .

EMERGE

I want you to sit back and feel comfortable . . Just relax and close your eyes . . . just for a little while . . You have decided to quit smoking . . This is your own decision . . You are doing this for your own benefit and . . for your own well being . . This means that it will be easy for you to get rid of the smoking habit completely . . And you will be surprised at how easy it will be for you . . to get rid of the smoking habit . . through hypnosis . .

In fact, you have already stopped smoking . . because you are realizing how calm and relaxed you are . . right now . . even though you don't have a cigarette in your hand . . or in your mouth . . and you don't have one burning in an ashtray . .

This relaxation you are experiencing . . is a very peaceful and calming state . . which you have produced yourself . . I didn't ask you to relax . . I merely gave you suggestions and you relaxed yourself . . And you can automatically relax yourself . . just the way you are now . . every time you look at water . . Looking at water is a signal to you . . and your subconscious mind will respond to that signal from now on . . and for the rest of your life . . Causing you to become relaxed, calm and peaceful . . for at least six hours . . every time you look at water . .

So, you have already stopped smoking . . And you will never smoke again . . unless you have a strong psychological reason that you need to appease . .

You know your body needs water . . to keep your body processes functioning properly . . You also know you need food . . to provide the proper amounts of nourishment your body needs . . And you also know that there is nothing in cigarettes . . that provides anything your body needs . .

So, you will never smoke a cigarette again . . unless you feel you must smoke or die . . Of course, you realize too, that you do not need to smoke to stay alive . . In fact, your health will keep improving . . now that you have quit smoking . . You will feel so much better because . . eliminating the smoking habit will prolong your life . . So, you know you will never need . . and never want . . to smoke again . .

Today you have stopped smoking completely . . and your subconscious mind is causing your body processes . . to function properly, to cleanse out all nicotine, tar . . and other impurities, from your body . . through the normal processes of your elimination system . .

As each hour passes, you have less desire to smoke . . Two hours from now, you will have even less desire to smoke . . And in a short time . . all desire to smoke will leave your mind and body completely . .

Your will power . . and your self control . . are becoming stronger every hour . . enabling you to be completely free . . from the smoking habit . .

You will be calm and relaxed at all times . . even when you are around people who are smoking . . You will remain calm and relaxed . . even when you see ashtrays with cigarettes in them . . Any time you see people smoking . . you will feel excited and . . much happier . . now that you have quit smoking . . You'll be proud of the fact that you are no longer a smoker . .

Tobacco has no appeal to you . . You cannot enjoy the smell of tobacco . . even when someone else is smoking . . Because now, you can proudly say . . you are a nonsmoker . . You have quit smoking completely . .

You have completely released yourself from the smoking habit . . And you feel like that big load . . has finally been lifted from you . . You are excited and happy to feel the freedom you now enjoy . . All desire for smoking has been cleansed out of your mind and body . . With each hour that passes, you feel healthier, stronger and more clean than ever before . .

Complete relaxation will be yours . . whenever you look at water . . That is your signal to relax . . as well as your reminder that you . . are a nonsmoker . . from now on . .

While you are relaxing . . your subconscious mind is absorbing everything that is happening . . within your body and your mind . . Right now, you are undergoing a complete cleansing . . physically, mentally and spiritually . . Continue to relax a moment longer . . (pause)

Now, I want you to breath deeply . . through your nose . . Hold it a moment, then . . slowly . . exhale . . out through your mouth . . Do that again . . Inhale deeply . . through your nose . . Hold it . . And exhale . . out through your mouth . . Very good . .

Now you can open your eyes . .

SMOKING - ELIMINATE THE HABIT

(Follow Relaxation)

You are continuing to relax deeper now . . Deeply relaxed . . Going deeper into relaxation . .

You are going to be very happy that you decided to let me hypnotize you . . Permitting yourself to be hypnotized . . lets your subconscious mind know . . you have a strong determination to stop smoking . . In making the decision to be hypnotized . . to eliminate the smoking habit . . it shows that you have accepted the responsibility . . for your own body . . And are making a commitment to treat your body well . . From now on . . you will always treat your body well . . and will do what is healthy for your body . .

In this state of hypnotic relaxation . . you can concentrate on the feeling of floating . . as though you are floating away . . on a fluffy, white cloud . . Floating out . . beyond space and time . .

At the same time . . your subconscious mind can concentrate on . . these three important reasons . . for why you have stopped smoking . .

1. First, you have quit smoking . . because you do not like the effect . . that smoking has on your body . . You need your body to live . . And you want to live for the rest of your life . . in a healthy body . . and so, you have stopped smoking . .

2. A second reason you have stopped smoking is because . . you have learned to respect your body . . And from now on . . you are determined to treat your body well . .

3. A third reason you have stopped smoking is because . . your body is the one important physical structure . . through which you experience life . . And you want to experience the rest of your life . . in a strong, healthy body . . Because your body is also . . the structure which carries around, your brain, from place to place . . And your brain controls all of your senses . . Your vision, your hearing . . your sense of taste and smell . . Your sense of perception and understanding . . and many other remarkable features . . Without a strong body to carry your mind . . to other places . . your life experiences would be greatly diminished . .

You have accepted the responsibility . . as your body's keeper . . You realize that you are responsible for your own body . . And by making this commitment . . to treat your body well . . and take care of your body . . it also gives you the power . . to be completely free from smoking . .

Notice that you are now thinking about what you are FOR . . rather than what you are against . .

Of course, you are against smoking . . because you know that smoking is an undesirable habit . . but your emphasis is now focused on your commitment . . to respect and take care of your body . .

Because of your commitment to respect and take good care of your body . . it is fitting and natural for you to protect your body . . against the harmful effects of tobacco . .

By making this commitment to protect and respect your body . . you have not only stopped smoking . . you will also be careful to eat and drink only . . foods and liquids that are beneficial . . to your body . .

You now have a disciplined concern . . that causes you to protect your body . . You select only foods and liquids . . that are beneficial for your body . . You eat only foods that keep your body slim, trim and healthy . . while protecting your body from the harmful habit of smoking . .

Think of these words in your mind now . . "I need my body to live . . I owe my body the respect and protection it needs . . to be healthy and strong . . I have stopped smoking . . completely and permanently . . I have stopped smoking . . completely and permanently" . .

In just a moment, I want you to think of the numbers . . 6, 5, 4, 3, 2 and 1 . . in your mind . . and keep relaxing more with each number that you think of . .

From now on . . each of those numbers takes on a new meaning . . And each time you think, hear, see or say . . one of those numbers . . your subconscious mind causes the meaning . . for that number . . to keep working more . . automatically . . in your life . .

SIX, means you are relaxing peacefully and calmly . . Every time you think, hear, see or say . . the number, SIX . . your subconscious mind causes you to relax . . more peacefully and calmly . .

FIVE, means that all impurities are cleansed out of your body . . through the natural processes of your elimination system . .

FOUR, means that your health keeps improving . . and your life continues to become happier . . and more enjoyable . .

THREE, means that your self-confidence, self-acceptance, self-reliance and self-esteem . . are growing stronger . .

TWO, means you are peaceful, calm and confident . . in every situation or circumstance . . in which you find yourself . . Whether you are alone or with others . .

ONE, means that you are completely free from the smoking habit . . And all desire for smoking is gone away completely . . Remember that YOU are number ONE . . and you feel great about your accomplishments . .

Continue relaxing now . . as you think of the numbers, 6, 5, 4, 3, 2 and 1 . . in your mind . .

There is nothing in cigarettes that provides anything your body needs . . so there is no reason to ever smoke again . . And now, you are feeling happy and proud of the fact . . that you have eliminated the smoking habit from your life . . Getting rid of the smoking habit . . causes you to have a strong sense of accomplishment . . and a strong feeling of satisfaction . .

Being free from the smoking habit is important to you . . and it will be helpful to other people . . who will be aware of what you have accomplished . .

When you awaken from the hypnotic state . . you will feel confident and happy about your achievement . .

Anytime you are around people who are smoking . . you will be relaxed and calm . . And when you see people smoking . . or see ash trays holding cigarettes . . it will remind you of how good it is . . to be free from the smoking habit . .

Tobacco has no appeal to you . . You can enjoy the smell of tobacco . . when someone else is smoking . . but you remain, always . . a nonsmoker . . And when you see other people smoking . . it will cause you to feel even happier . . that you have eliminated the smoking habit from your life . . Because of your own commitment . . and determination . . you are completely released from the smoking habit . .

Now you feel like that big load has been lifted from you . . As each day passes, you keep feeling cleaner and healthier . .

All of the nicotine . . the tar . . and the other impurities . . are being cleansed out from your sinuses . . out of your throat . . out of your lungs and out of your entire body . . through the normal processes of your elimination system . . And all desire for smoking is gone . .

You will never smoke again . .

Each day, these suggestions will become even more effective . . you are learning to use these principles of relaxation . . which you are now experiencing . . in all phases if your daily life . . and that will keep you calm and relaxed . . at all times . .

In every situation or circumstance . . that comes up in your life . . you will be calm and relaxed . . Your nerves will be relaxed and steady . . and you'll be able to do everything in a relaxed manner . . You will be able to cope with . . everyday changing circumstances . . in a loving, peaceful way . .

Regardless of what comes up in your life . . you will be in control of your emotions and feelings . . That is what will cause success to be yours . . more and more . . and soon you will have all that you want in your life . .

Now, I am going to count from 1 to 5 . . and on the count of 5 . . you will open your eyes . . to an alert, waking state . . feeling clear of mind, relaxed and wonderful . . for you are a wonderful and confident person . .

I will begin . .

One.   You will remember everything you have experienced today with complete understanding . .

Two. You are now connected to your spiritual, inner supporting strength . .

Three. Everything I have told you is true . . and is already happening . .

Four.   Beginning to be more aware of your body as it fully awakens and wants to stir . .

Five.   Let your hands and feet move . . Stir and stretch as you open your eyes, feeling clear, rested and wonderful . .

(Follow Relaxation)

You are continuing to relax deeper now . . Deeply relaxed . . Going deeper into relaxation . .

You have decided to get rid of the habit of smoking . . and you will be very pleased . . that you made that decision . . Because eliminating the smoking habit will cause your health to improve . .

It will also increase your energy level . . your strength and your vitality . .

Permitting yourself to be hypnotized . . enables you to stop smoking completely . . And you'll be pleasantly surprised at how easily . . you get rid of the smoking habit . . and the desire to smoke . .

You may notice that you are really calm and relaxed now . . even though you are not smoking . . And you will continue experiencing . . the same feeling of calmness and relaxation . . as you go about the activities of your daily life . .

I want you to relax even deeper now . . Deeper . . Go down deeper . . and relax . . Deeper, deeper . . and relax . . You are doing very well . . as you relax . . deeper . . Just . . relax . . (pause)

I want to ask you some questions now . . that can be answered with a simple yes . . or no . . Questions that your subconscious mind will answer . . Your subconscious mind can review, examine and explore . . the information in the storehouse of your mind . . and can give the correct answer . . to each question I ask . .

Your subconscious mind will answer each question . . by causing the index finger on your left hand to lift up . . That will be a YES answer . . The little finger on your left hand will lift up . . if the answer is NO . . If the correct answer is yes, your mind will cause your YES finger to lift up . . That is your index finger . . If the correct answer is NO . . your mind will cause your little finger to lift up . . That is your NO finger . .

Now . . we need to get to the underlying cause for your smoking at such an early age . . Did both of your parents smoke ?. . Only your Mother ? . . Were you left on your own a lot ? . . Did you have to work at an early age ? . . Did your friends at school smoke ? . . Was smoking a social custom with your peers ? . . Did anyone ever try to get you to stop ? . . Did you ever want to stop? . .

You have been smoking for a very long time now . . and you may need to have help . . from somewhere else . . The best help you can have is from within you . . And so, I want to ask your subconscious mind for a promise . . I want to ask your subconscious mind to make a promise . . to help you to give up smoking . . Please answer, YES or NO . . Will you make that promise ? . .

Wait for YES answer. If answer is NO, continue talking to subconscious to convince it. If answer remains NO, bring up client and ask if he would like a reschedule or 'give up'.

Be sure that you have used finger-response, or other technique, to have client released from the underlying cause of smoking. Also ask the subconscious mind to promise to help the client quit.

Every time you look at water . . you become relaxed, calm and peaceful . . and you remain that way . . for at least, six hours . . every time you look at water . . That will be your signal . . to take control of your desires and emotions . . Think, see or say the word, water, and you will immediately become calm and relaxed . . and your cravings will cease at once . . Think WATER . .

Your subconscious mind has promised to help you . . stop smoking completely . . Your mind is increasing your will power and self-control . . and is enabling you to be totally free . . from the smoking habit . .

You can enjoy the smell of smoke . . when someone else is smoking . . but you have quit smoking . . You have given it up completely . . and will never smoke again . . Your subconscious mind has promised to help you . . And now, you must make the same promise . . to help your body to become healthy once again . .

You have many good reasons . . for getting rid of the smoking habit . . It will improve your health . . It will strengthen your heart . . It will cleanse your sinuses, your throat . . and your lungs . . enabling you to breath more easily and freely . . And it will save you the expense of buying the cigarettes . . as well as the added expenses from burning holes in your clothing and furniture . . It gets rid of the tobacco smell on your clothing and your breath . . and it causes your nerves to be more relaxed and steady . .

You are beginning to realize that it is really good to be free . . from the smoking habit . . You are happy that you decided to allow me to hypnotize you . . to eliminate all desire for cigarettes . .

Your entire organism and body are cooperating . . to cleanse all desire for cigarettes . . out of your body, quickly . . After this session is over . . your mind will be on other, more important things . . And you will be pleased to know that you are smoke-free . .

There is nothing in cigarettes that provides anything your body needs . . so there is no reason for you to ever smoke again . . You have quit smoking completely . . And you are really feeling proud of your accomplishment . .

Your will power and self-control keep increasing every minute . . and you are free from being controlled . . by the smoking habit . . You have stopped smoking . . and you are happy to feel the freedom . . you now enjoy . .

Your health will keep improving . . You will have more energy, strength and vitality . . And you will be amazed at how much better you keep feeling . . as each day goes by . .

Regardless of what comes up in your life . . you will be in control of your emotions and feelings . . That is what will cause success to be yours . . more and more . . And soon you will have all that you want in your life . .

Now, I am going to count from 1 to 5 . . and on the count of 5 . . you will open your eyes. . . to an alert, waking state . . feeling clear of mind, relaxed and wonderful . . For you are a wonderful and confident person . . I will begin . .

One. You will remember everything you have experienced today with complete understanding . .

Two. You are now connected to your spiritual, inner supporting strength.

Three. Everything I have told you is true . . and is already happening . .

Four. Beginning to be more aware of your body as it fully awakens and wants to stir . .

Five. Let your hands and feet move . . Stir and stretch as you open your eyes, feeling clear, rested and wonderful . .

(Follow Relaxation)

You are continuing to relax deeper now . . Deeply relaxed . . Going deeper into relaxation . . In this state of hypnotic relaxation . . you can release yourself . . with a feeling of floating . . As though you are floating away on a soft, billowy cloud . . Floating out beyond . . space and time . .

You are responding very well to the suggestions . . directions and instructions . . I am giving you . . And now you are ready . . for your subconscious mind . . to make some pleasant changes . . that cause all nicotine, tar and other impurities . . brought from smoking . . to be eliminated from your sinuses . . From your throat . . From your lungs and from the rest of your body . . rapidly and completely . . Though the normal processes of your elimination system . .

Permitting yourself to be hypnotized . . lets your subconscious mind know . . that you are determined to never smoke again . .

You have accepted the responsibility . . for taking care of your own body . . and by having this session . . you have made a commitment to protect your body . . from now on . .

You have made a wise decision . . You have stopped smoking because . . you are dissatisfied with the way it affects you . . You need your body to live . . and you want to live, the rest of your life, in a healthy body . . So you are determined that you have stopped smoking . .

And now that you have quit smoking . . you know your body will be healthier and stronger . . And you'll find that you feel much better . . Now that you have discontinued the smoking habit . .

You can feel proud that it is your own decision . . You have ceased smoking for your own benefit . . For your own personal well being . . And for your own better health . .

You will be happy to notice . . how much better you feel . . now that you have stopped smoking . . And you will be surprised at how easily . . you have been able to eliminate the smoking habit . . through hypnosis . . And you can be sure it is permanent . .

Your subconscious mind knows exactly how to cause the activities of your body . . to rapidly cleanse all traces of nicotine, tar and other impurities . .

caused by smoking cigarettes . . out of your sinuses, out of your throat . . out of your lungs and the rest of your body . . And you will never smoke again . .

You will be happy to find that your subconscious mind . . has already started the process . . of cleansing the nicotine, tar and other impurities . . out of your body . . through the normal functions of your elimination system . .

All desire for smoking will be gone completely by the time you awaken from this hypnotic state . . And you will be pleased to find that your will power and self-control . . will keep increasing more with every hour . .

Every time you look at water . . Every time you think, see or say . . the word, WATER, it will make you feel calm . . and relaxed . . for at least, six hours . . Every time you look at water . . Every time you think, see or say . . the word, WATER, you will feel calm and completely at ease . .

You have stopped smoking already . . You realize that you are calm and peaceful now . . even though you don't have a cigarette . . in your hand or . . in your mouth . . And you don't have one . . burning in an ashtray . . And I have given you your signal . . which is water . . And that is keeping you calm and relaxed . . as you go about your daily activities . .

When you awaken from this hypnotic state . . you will know you are free . . from the smoking habit . . So, if you have cigarettes and a lighter with you . . you will leave them here . . on the desk . . before you leave this room . . And when you leave this room . . you will know you are free . . at last . . from the smoking habit . .

You are very calm and relaxed now . . And you understand that you become calm . . and relaxed . . every time you look at water . . Every time you look at water . . your nerves become more relaxed and steady . . And you continue to be more calm, emotionally . . Your subconscious mind is causing that signal to work automatically . . From now on and for the rest of your life . . keeping you calm and relaxed . . as you go about the activities of your daily life . .

In every situation or circumstance in which you are involved . . during your daily life . . you remain calm and relaxed . . whether you are alone or with others . .

So, you have already stopped smoking . . and you will never smoke again . . unless there is a strong psychological reason you need to smoke . . And it is very rare for a person . . to have a psychological reason for smoking . . So I am quite sure you have stopped smoking . . And you will find your health improving rapidly . . now that you have eliminated the smoking habit . .

You know that your body needs water . . Water is good for your body . . It helps to maintain a good fluid balance in your body . . It helps cleanse waste materials and impurities out of your body . . through the normal processes of your elimination system . . It keeps your kidneys healthy . . and keeps your urinary system clean . . It also eliminates the desire for snacks . . which enables your body to be slender and trim . . So you will enjoy drinking plenty of fresh water . .

Your body also needs proper foods to provide you with proteins, vitamins, minerals, fiber, potassium . . and other nutrients . . to keep your body slim, trim and healthy . . So you eat foods that are beneficial for your body . . You appreciate your body . . And from now on, you will always treat your body well . .

You know that your body needs water and food . . and you also know . . there is nothing in cigarettes that provide anything . . your body needs . . So there is no reason to ever smoke another cigarette . . You are happy to know that your smoking habit is gone forever . . You have eliminated the smoking habit for good . . and you are proud of your accomplishment . .

Getting rid of the smoking habit . . causes you to have a feeling of fulfillment . . and gives you a strong sense of satisfaction and pride . .

Permitting yourself to be hypnotized . . reveals that you have accepted . . the responsibility for your own body . . And you have made a commitment to always treat your body well . . It shows that you have taken the initiative . . and now you are putting everything I suggest to you . . into your own actions . .

You realize that getting rid of . . the smoking habit . . is very important to you . . It enables you to be an inspiration . . to a lot of other people . . when they become aware of what you have achieved . . And you will feel very proud . . to let them know . .

You are already feeling enthusiastic about it . . You are sensing a wonderful feeling of satisfaction . . from knowing you have stopped smoking . . And you will feel even better about it . . when you awaken from your hypnotic state . .

Tobacco has no appeal to you any longer . . You may enjoy the smell of smoke . . when someone else is smoking . . But when you see other people smoking . . it will cause you to be even more thankful . . that you have stopped smoking . . and that you are a successful . . nonsmoker . .

When you are around people who are smoking . . you will always feel calm and relaxed . . and will have no desire to smoke . . When you see other people smoking . . or see ash trays with cigarettes in them . . it will cause you to feel so happy that you stopped smoking . . When you see people smoking . . it will remind you of how good it is . . that you are free from the smoking habit . .

You are completely released now . . from the smoking habit . . You are happy to feel the freedom . . you now enjoy . . A big weight has been lifted from you . . and you keep feeling cleaner . . and healthier as each day passes . .

As each hour passes . . you have less and less desire . . for a cigarette . . Two hours from now . . you will experience even less desire . . to smoke . . And in a short time . . all desire to smoke . . will leave your mind and body completely . .

Your will power and self-control are becoming stronger . . with every hour . . enabling you to be completely free . . from the smoking habit . . From now on . . you are a proud, nonsmoker . . And you will never . . smoke another cigarette . . again . . (Pause)

I want you to continue relaxing for another moment or two . . in silence . . to allow your subconscious mind to absorb . . and resolve . . everything we have talked about today . . (pause)

You are now very comfortable, relaxed and totally at ease . . You are experiencing perfect peace of mind . . And in the future . . you can enjoy this same perfect calmness and respite . . any time you want it . . All you will need to do is to sit or lie down in a comfortable position . . close your eyes and imagine yourself in this . . comfortable state of mind . . Then count backward in your mind from TEN down to ONE . . By the time you reach number ONE . . you will be completely relaxed . . calm and at ease . . And you will know peace with the world . . And you can remain in that state for as long as you desire . . When you are ready to return to a wide-awake and alert state of mind . . you'll only need to open your eyes . . Whenever you do this . . you will always feel rested and refreshed . . full of energy, strength and vitality . . after relaxing this way, for only a few minutes . .

You will remember everything I have said to you today . . and you will greatly benefit from everything I have told you . . Continue now to relax, for just a little longer . . (Pause)

In just a moment we will be concluding this session . . I will be counting to FIVE for you to awaken . . You will come up to a wide-awake, fully alert state, when I say the number FIVE . .

ONE - Feeling so good . . feeling wonderful . . all over . .

TWO - your hands are tingling and your legs are feeling a bit numb yet . . Get the feelings back into your body . .

THREE - Coming up now . . More alert . . More aware . . Stirring into conscious awareness . .

FOUR - Gently inhale now . . Breathe out . . and . .

FIVE - Open your eyes now and focus on your surroundings . .

(Follow DEEP Relaxation)

You will continue drifting into a deeper, DEEPER . . more peaceful, hypnotic state . . of relaxation . . as I give you suggestions and instructions . . that will cause you to experience a continuous improvement of yourself . . physically . . mentally . . and spiritually . .

As you submerge yourself, going deeper . . and DEEPER . . You can notice how you are becoming . . even more relaxed and settled now . . Concentrate on that pleasant feeling of total relaxation . . Your mind and body are completely relaxing . . more and more . . relax . . All tension is leaving your body . . And all stresses and strains are moving out of your system . . as though they are being drawn out of your body . . by a powerful magnetic energy . .

You are learning to be relaxed and calm . . and will continue using these principles of relaxation . . during your daily life . . By learning to relax . . as you are doing now . . you will experience a happier, healthier, more enjoyable life . . A more productive life . . than ever before . .

You are beginning to notice a fresh feeling of energy and vitality . . flowing through your entire body . . Cleansing . . healing . . purifying and rejuvenating, as it moves all through your system . . Cleansing your entire body . . gradually and perfectly . .

We keep hearing on radio and television . . about 'Faith Healers' . . As though they are the chosen few . . who have been granted special powers from God . . to heal the sick and the handicapped . . But in reality . . we all have that 'special' power and energy within each of us . . That ability to be healed completely . . from any illness, disease or physical disturbance . . from within ourselves . . These are some words that are credited to Jesus Christ, by which he said . . "The Kingdom of God is within you" . .

Perhaps that gives us an explanation . . for the fact that we all have a power within us . . that is capable of cleansing, healing, purifying and restoring our body . . in a perfect way . .

The more research we do . . the more we find that it is our own mind . . that directs the healing energies of our body . . So, the important thing for you to realize is . . that you have a tremendous power within you . . that can renew, restore and heal your body . . completely and perfectly . . And those healing energies are all directed . . by your mind . . Your

461

subconscious mind has capabilities . . far beyond what you have been consciously aware of . . And your mind is remembering everything it needs to remember . . to cause the healing energies of your body to function as they are directed . . to heal your body completely . .

All limitations are being lifted . . And you are being revitalized with increased energy and inner strength . . Your body, mind and soul are continuing to function . . in a more harmonious way . .

Self-realization and understanding are opening up within you . . A feeling of peace is moving through every part of your being . . Instilling greater awareness of the power of God within you . .

You are letting go completely now . . And you are more aware of the feeling of peacefulness . . enshrouding your entire body . . A feeling of complete calm . . Like a blessing from God . . And that calmness and peacefulness will continue . . to enfold you . . during your daily life . . You have but one serious health issue . . that I am aware of . . that needs to be addressed . . And so, we will deal with that problem now . .

As you relax peacefully . . I want you to take a short journey . . deep within yourself . . Into the 'Human Chamber' that houses your very being . . It is said that the body is . . a temple . . Indeed, it is . . as you will discover . . The chambers of your temple hold many untold treasures . . fine tapestries and silks . . paintings that rival the Louve Museum . . From DeVinvi, there are marble statues . . All of the classical writings are in a huge library . . The floors are terrazzo and oak . . Marbled walls with fine standing fireplaces . . Everywhere you look there is finery and beauty . . As you wander the chambers and hallways, you notice photos and oils of your ancestors . . All of the family heirlooms you haven't seen since you were a child . . Many, of course, that you have never known to exist . . They are all breathtaking . . magnificent in their splendor . .

When you were born, all of these fabulous treasures were here . . in your temple . . to accompany you through life . . Later, after you had acquired a taste for a . . mature lifestyle . . you began to notice things becoming more 'dingy' . . taking on a rather worn and tattered appearance . .

Now . . even after the years of neglect and chaotic living . . the outside of your temple is still in good condition . . Firm and supple . . As you gaze into your mirror, you are pleased with what your eyes behold . .

462

A little grayer, perhaps, but over all . . not too different from your appearance as a child . . Surprisingly, your temple has held up quite well . . after all the storms and ravages of time . . Perhaps due to cosmetics and . . youth hormones . . Or simply, from good, healthful living . .

But now, we are going back . . Back down into the inner sanctum . . The chambers and hollows of your . . internal temple . . You noticed all of this . . when you were younger . . And you knew, even then, what was going to happen, didn't you . . if you were to neglect yourself . .

Look now, at your fine tapestries and wall hangings . . The oil painting . . the silks and the linens . . The statues and the oaken furnishings . . All of it now stands under layers of blackening soot . . Clouds of smoke hang in the air . . and great globs of ugly nicotine-stained tars streak down the walls and cover the flooring . . and the chandeliers . . Tar and nicotine . . ooze onto everything . . choking out the portals where fresh air once filtered in . . All is dark now . . Dismal and gloomy . . It is foul-smelling . . And the stench permeates everything . . It has been this way for so long now, you hardly notice . . Certainly not the way others notice . . The odors emanating from the bowels of your temple are . . deplorable . . But even worse, is the unhealthy condition of everything inside . . It is a blessing . . that no one can see . . the caked-on sludge encrusting your lungs . . choking out the very life from you . . Sealing you off from the very air you need . . to exist . . And it is clogging the flow of blood through your arteries . . The precious flow of blood that carries oxygen to your brain . . And vital nutrients, minerals and restorative energy, to all parts of your body . . Yes, this is your temple . . Your body . . Your very life . .

You are aware of the damage done . . inside of your temple, from years of smoking cigarettes . . But NOW . . is the time for change . . From the time you awaken, you will recall these scenes . . from the chambers of horror . . And you will have no craving . . and no need for cigarettes . . ever again . . (Pause) The restorative, healing processes of your body . . have now begun . .

You have seen healing powers at work . . The mysterious curing powers . . that heal cuts and broken bones . . So, you know that your body has the power to heal . . But more than just the obvious . . it can heal any damage, disease or sickness you ever experience . . And you are letting that healing

463

energy flow freely now . . Let it continue . . and you will be healed completely . . Breath deeply now . . Exhale . . and relax . . (Pause)

As you continue drifting . . into a DEEPER and DEEPER hypnotic state . . I want you to visualize yourself with a healthy, strong and beautiful body . . Exactly the way you want your body to be . . Inside and outside . . See yourself clearly . . and think of yourself with a perfect body . . Exactly the way you want your body to be, in every way . .

As you continue to think of yourself . . the way you want your body to be . . inside and outside . . your subconscious mind is accepting that image . . and is causing all of your body processes to function perfectly . . And is healing your body completely . . wherever the healing is needed . .

Each night, just before you go to sleep . . Close your eyes and think of yourself . . just the way you want yourself to be . . with a healthy, strong and perfect body . . with healthy lungs . . and a healthy heart . . As you continue to do that . . each night . . you keep reinforcing that image in your mind . . And your own mind causes you to develop . . your desired, perfectly healthy body . .

You will also find your self-confidence and self-acceptance . . growing stronger . . And you will continue improving in all areas of your life . . physically, mentally, emotionally and spiritually . .

You will have the knowledge to solve every problem that comes up in your life . . You will look forward to each day of your life with anticipation . . And you will find that each day will bring you greater happiness and joy . . You will arise each morning, feeling rested and refreshed . . And you'll continue having more energy, more ambition . . and more vitality . .

All of the suggestions and instructions I have given you . . are now in the storehouse of your mind . . And they are already working to keep improving your health . . and your way of life . . They are intended to influence your thoughts, your feelings and your actions . . in a positive, helpful way . . You will notice some very positive improvements . . And you will be very pleased . . with your continuous progress . .

In a moment, you will be, once again, in a normal state of mind . . Now, I am going to begin my count . . from ONE to FIVE . . and when you hear the number, FIVE . . you will open your eyes and be wide awake . . feeling refreshed and wonderful . . for you are . . a wonderful person . .

EMERG

You are doing very well . . as you continue to relax . . You are breathing easily . . and comfortably . .

I am going to give you some suggestions now . . that will help you with the problem . . you have been experiencing . .

A young man, I will call, John . . came to me, to be hypnotized . . He wanted me to help him 'build up' his body . . He was 23 years of age . . about 5 feet - 9 inches tall . . but weighed less than 120 pounds . . He was continually being picked on by others . . and he did not like losing all the time . .

In the first session, I gave him suggestions to get him started in . . a weight lifting program . . and I suggested he enroll in a karate class . .

John did both of his assignments, without question . . He began lifting weights . . and he enrolled in a karate class . . without any question . . After he had taken several of the karate classes . . he came back to see me . . I asked him . . if he didn't get tossed around a bit . . by some of the others in the class . . He said, "Yes, but that's different than getting beat up by some punk on the street" . . So, he felt that he had sufficient reason . . to continue studying karate . .

John was such a good student that . . within six months . . he had gained 25 pounds . . and was already taking part in karate matches . . And he had won three, of the four matches, he took part in . . He felt quite proud of himself, to be aware of his ability to do that . .

In a little more than six months . . he had gone from being . . a skinny young man . . who was constantly being pushed around . . to being a rather muscular man . . who was now confident of his abilities . . and who was capable of being in control of his life . .

Your subconscious mind understands that, in reality . . every person, actually is . . in control of himself or herself . . You were created by the same creator . . who created every other person on this Earth . . And you have been given the same freedom . . to make your own choices . . The same 'freedom of self-choice' . . that every other person . . has been granted . .

Many people do not agree with some of the things . . written in the Bible . . And, they have the freedom to accept or reject . . whatever they choose to 'accept or reject' . .

However, psychological research has proven . . that the following statements . . found in the Bible . . are true . . It says, "As a person thinks, in his own mind, so is he" . . It has been found that the thoughts in our mind . . cause us to become what we are . . And there is another statement . . found in Romans, Chapter 12, Verse 2, which says . . "You can be transformed, by the renewing of your mind" . . And that has also been proven to be true . . John . . whom I mentioned a few moments ago . . became transformed . . by renewing his mind . . And any time a person is experiencing any kind of problem . . that problem can be overcome . . by, simply, renewing the thoughts . . in the mind . .

You want to overcome the habit . . of snoring . . And the way to begin . . is by changing the thoughts . . in your mind . . Your subconscious mind understands . . that you can breath, just as easily . . just as smoothly . . and just as freely . . at night, while you are sleeping . . as you do, during the day . . when you are awake . .

I want to suggest . . that your inner mind . . begin to review . . what information has gone into it . . that caused you to begin snoring . . Your mind will assess that information . . evaluate it . . and determine whether there is a reason . . for you to continue the habit . . Your mind will work out the solution . . to resolve that problem . . rapidly and completely . .

When your subconscious mind fully understands the causes . . and has worked out the solution to that problem . . and knows that you have overcome the problem . . and will breathe easily and freely, at all times . . when you are sleeping . . one of the fingers on your left hand will lift up . . towards the ceiling . . and will remain lifted upward . . until I tell it to go back down . .

NOTE : ANYTIME FINGER LIFTS, TELL IT TO GO BACK DOWN. IF IT DOES NOT LIFT BY SESSION CONCLUSION, GO TO "THERAPY BETWEEN SESSIONS"

You are in a very deep . . very calm and comfortable state now . . Your entire body is relaxing peacefully . . and comfortably . . Your subconscious mind is very sensitive . . and receptive . . to everything I say . . and is hearing and receiving . . the suggestions I am giving you . . Causing each suggestion to begin working immediately . . And they will continue working automatically . . after you awaken from the hypnotic state . .

466

Without any conscious effort by you . . your subconscious mind keeps you breathing . . whether you are sleeping or awake . . Keeps your heart pumping blood through your circulatory system . . Causes your digestive system to continue functioning properly . . And causes every part of your body to respond to your conscious decisions . . Such as, causing your foot to lift up . . and step on the brake . . when you are driving your car . . and you need to stop . . Causing you to turn the wheel, automatically, when you come to a corner . . You do all those things, without consciously controlling what you are doing . . And just as easily . . you breathe smoothly, during the night . . while you are sleeping . . So, you will sleep easily and comfortably . . from now on . . Your subconscious mind understands . . There is no reason for you to snore . . when you are sleeping . .

The problem may be caused from a relaxed valve . . or a slack tendon . . or a need for muscle control . . Whatever the cause . . it will be discovered and rectified . . through your subconscious mind . .

Relax a moment longer as your subconscious mind absorbs . . what we have discussed here . . and resolves to make the necessary corrections . . to cure your problem . . (pause)

You are feeling confident and secure in the fact that . . you have overcome the habit of snoring . . completely and permanently . . And from now on . . you will sleep peacefully . . and quietly . . with no further disturbances . . for a restful, good nights sleep . .

In a moment I will begin my count, from One to Five . . And when you hear me count out the number Five . . you will open your eyes and be wide awake, alert and ready to continue with your usual activities . .

I will begin my count now . .

One   You are becoming more aware of your body . .
Two   You will remember everything you have experienced here today . .
Three Everything I have told you is true and is already happening . .
Four   Move your hands and feet a little . . Let them begin to stir . .
Five   You may open your eyes now . . how do you feel ?

SNORING - STOP

You are doing very well . . as you continue to relax . . You are breathing easily . . and comfortably . .

I am going to give you some suggestions now . . that will help you with the problem . . of snoring . .

Getting rid of that problem will satisfy you . . as a person . . The fact that you want to breathe easily and freely . . while you are sleeping . . is causing the subconscious level of your mind . . to review and examine . . what has been causing you to snore . . And it is working out the solution . . to help you get rid of that snoring problem . . quickly and permanently . .

The only thing I want you to do, consciously . . is to realize that you can . . go to sleep easily . . And you can sleep calmly and peacefully . . each time you go to bed . . for the purpose of sleeping . .

Even now, while you are in a hypnotic state . . you are continuing to breathe more easily . . And when you go to bed, for the purpose of sleeping . . you will automatically breathe easily and quietly . .

You are feeling confident in your ability . . and taking pride in your ability . . to sleep peacefully . . calmly and quietly . . until it is time for you to awaken . .

You've been experiencing that problem of snoring . . for some time now . . And consciously . . you haven't been able to get the problem resolved . . I don't know what you need to do . . to resolve the problem . . but there is a level of your mind . . that knows what has been causing the problem . . And knows exactly how to cause your system to adjust . . to get that problem corrected . . without any conscious effort by you . .

The level of your mind that knows how to correct the problem . . is working out the solution in a very pleasant way . . And when the problem has been resolved . . and your mind knows you will sleep easily, quietly and comfortably, each night . . one of the fingers on your left hand . . will lift up towards the ceiling . . and remain up, until I tell it to go back down . .

NOTE : ANYTIME FINGER LIFTS, TELL IT TO GO BACK DOWN. IF IT DOES NOT LIFT BY SESSION CONCLUSION, GO TO "THERAPY   BETWEEN SESSIONS"

Your mind is reviewing the information, thoroughly . . and is understanding that it is okay . . to resolve that problem, for now and forever . . And as your mind is working out the solution to that problem . . you are continuing to be more relaxed . . while moving into a more peaceful . . yet deeper . . and DEEPER . . state of hypnosis . . Calmly relax . . as you go deeper . . and DEEPER . . (Pause)

You are the only one . . who can help you to stop snoring . . And, right now, your mind is causing you to experience . . a very pleasant transformation . . And you will soon discover yourself . . going to sleep each night . . to sleep calmly and peacefully . . without snoring . . until it is time for you to awaken . . You will keep breathing easily and freely . . while you are sleeping . . And you will awaken each morning . . feeling rested and refreshed . .

So, when you awaken from this hypnotic state . . you will feel happy and confident . . Knowing that your own mind has worked out . . the solution to that problem . . And from now on . . you will be free from restless nights . . And the sounds of your snoring . . will no longer be a burden . .

Continue to relax now . . as your subconscious mind absorbs everything we have talked about . .

EMERGE

SPEAKING IN PUBLIC
Confidence Building

(Follows: Relaxation - Self Confidence)

This Prescription has helped many people overcome a fear of Public Speaking and to build confidence in their abilities with an audience.

You are doing well . . I want you to go a little deeper now . . Deeper . . (Pause)

In just a moment I am going to give you some suggestions . . which will help you with your problem . .

Repeat these words to yourself now . . "I can do anything I want to do . . I can achieve any goal I want to achieve . . I feel good, standing up and talking to people . . I am becoming an excellent public speaker" . . (repeat)

In the past you have experienced some emotions . . when you have tried to speak to an audience . . You are realizing that emotions can be a hindrance . . unless they are tethered . .

From now on, when you are in front of an audience . . or in a group . . and you are asked to speak . . you will be aware that the inner feelings . . that you experience . . are your own natural energy forces . . that are available for you to use . . That energy enables you to be calm and relaxed . . and to feel completely at ease . . in front of any audience . . or group of people . .

With that realization . . you can achieve any goal you wish to achieve . . You are becoming a successful public speaker . . You are permitting your own . . sensing ability . . to enable you to do the right thing . . at the right time . . And to say the right thing . . at the right time . .

At all times . . you speak clearly, firmly, positively, distinctly, calmly and effectively . . You always speak in a way that people enjoy . . And at all times . . you speak in a way that people can understand . .

When you are speaking to a group of people . . or in front of an audience . . you will always have your material prepared ahead of time . . and will go over it in your mind . . so that you are well prepared . . when you get up to speak . .

I want you to use your imagination now . . and imagine yourself getting up in front of an audience to speak . . See yourself, standing there calmly . . looking at your audience . . feeling that this is a wonderful . . and enjoyable experience . . See yourself talking calmly . . to the audience

. . Speaking clearly . . Getting each point across . . in a simple, direct way . . See yourself . . as you are speaking to the people . . loving them . . and really desiring to share with them . . what you have to say . . See yourself helping your audience to learn and to grow . .

Now, see yourself concluding your talk . . thanking the audience for the opportunity to share with them . . And picture yourself after the talk . . with everyone in the audience coming to you and thanking you . . Telling you how much they enjoyed and learned from you . .

As you see them shaking your hand . . you realize that you did an excellent job . . You are thankful for the opportunity to share with others . . and to help them by sharing your knowledge from your experience and research . . Sharing as you can by speaking to them . .

And you are realizing that you truly are a good speaker . . A very effective speaker . . Each day . . your self-confidence, self-reliance and self-acceptance keep increasing . . Each day you keep improving in your ability to easily and calmly speak . . to any group or audience . .

REF> SPEAKING IN PUBLIC - STAGE FRIGHT

EMERGE

You are very relaxed . . but I want you to go deeper now . . deeper relaxed . . Listen only to the sound of my voice . . I am going to give you suggestions now . . that will benefit you . .

You are afflicted with a problem . . as we discussed earlier . . That of, Speaking in Public . . For lack of a better term . . it is also akin to - Stage Fright . . Why is it called, 'Stage Fright' ? . .

Because it is a fright that is peculiar to being on the stage . . in front of a group of people . . The same as it is when speaking in public . . It is a common ailment . . Many people have suffered from it . . and many people have conquered it . . Fear of any kind is conquered . . not by force but by belief . . by faith . . and by conviction . . The fear of public speaking is no exception . . Once you are convinced that you are completely safe . . secure, self-confident, relaxed, and comfortable before your audience . . in front of a thousand people . . or only ten people . . then you will have completely conquered your public fear . . And this will be done in a very short time . .

As a matter of fact, you will be surprised and amazed at how rapidly . . you will gain the self confidence you seek . . Self confidence in any field . . is obtained by knowing . . that you know . . what you are doing in that field . . And that is accomplished, mainly, by constant practice . . After all, if you were doing a particular act . . which you have done a hundred time before . . or reciting a particular speech . . which you had recited a hundred times before . . then you certainly would have plenty of confidence . . regarding that performance . . or that particular speech . .

A doctor is at home in his hospital . . A lawyer is at home in the courtroom . . But the lawyer may not feel so secure in a hospital . . nor the doctor, at home, in a courtroom . . The doctor may wonder why people are afraid of a hospital . . And the lawyer, feeling quite at home in a courtroom, may wonder, why would anyone feel uncomfortable coming there . . Yet, to be on the witness stand . . may be a very frightening experience . . Especially if it is the first time . .

Furthermore . . if that first time in front of a group . . has been a traumatic experience . . as I suspect it may have been for you . . then each succeeding time carries with it . . that conditioning to fear . .

Fortunately, we know what causes the fear . . In public speaking, the fear is caused by a feeling of insecurity that we possess . . when we appear before a group . . The feeling that we may, in some way, embarrass ourselves . . either because of poor preparation . . or poor delivery . . That we will become embarrassed and be laughed at . . or in some way . . fail . . Therefore, the only way to get rid of this . . stage fright . . is to turn the tables on the audience . .

Winston Churchill once had stage fright . . So, what did he do ? . . He visualized his audience . . All sitting in their underwear ! What could be more ridiculous ? And what could be more embarrassing ? For the audience, that is . . to be clad only in their underwear . . So, instead of them laughing at him . . he laughed at them . . in his mind, of course . .

When you go up there to speak . . I would like you to visualize your audience as though they are all . . in their underwear . . Why ? Because it puts them on the defensive . . instead of you . . If anyone is going to do any laughing . . you will be laughing at them . . not the other way around . . And you make up your mind to do that, right now . .

So, that is your first suggestion . . Visualize your audience in their underwear . . Certainly they cannot be laughing at you . . if they are in their underwear . .

The second feature that make the stage a frightening place to be . . is the fact that you are so outnumbered . . There may be a thousand of them . . but there is only one of you . . A thousand in the audience and only one on the stage . . That can be a frightening thing . . to be outnumbered . . a thousand to one . . But you do have something that is far more advantageous . . You have the stage . . and you have the microphone . . the position you occupy is far more advantageous than all the positions in the audience . . For you have the attention of the audience . .

And so, you are going to remember . . that since you have the attention of the audience . . and they do not have the attention of each other . . whatever you say will effect them greatly . . And it is far more embarrassing for them . . to speak out against convention . . then it is for you to speak to them . . So the second point is . . You have the advantage of the attention of the audience . . because you occupy the stage . . The prominent position . . And you are going to remember that . .

Thirdly, there is not a bit of difference . . between talking to an audience of five thousand . . or to an audience of one . . Because in either case . . you address your remarks as though . . you are speaking to that particular person . . As you gaze out over your audience . . you pick out certain individuals and . . you ignore the rest . . You merely talk to those individuals . . As your gaze changes . . Look them right in the eyes . . And speak as if it is directed only at them . . And if your eyes pass over a few people . . don't worry about them . . You simply ignore them and pick up on someone else's eyes that are fixated on you . . or on your words . . You are very lucky to have the advantage of looking from where you are . . You have an entire group to select from . . certainly, you will find someone out there to direct your words to . .

Furthermore, you are fortunate in that you are the one . . who can change your vision direction . . at any time . . You can move from one person to another, at will . . and you will . . As you look from one person to another . . addressing your remarks to that particular individual . . you can change and begin talking to the entire group . . But, remember, that you are still only talking to one person at a time . .

It is true that if you have a larger group . . you may need to project your voice further . . You may need to slow down your rate of delivery . . Certainly a delivery in a stadium . . with a hundred thousand people . . and having speaker phones all over . . needs to be very slow . . and deliberate . . With many pauses . . While in a room filled with one to two hundred people . . you can go much faster . . But basically, it needs to be remembered . . that you are always . . only speaking to one person . . and the ratio is . . 1 to 1 . . One speaker on the stage . . One audience in the seats . . You are really only talking to one . . not to 5000 . . You have one audience and the ratio is . . one to one . .

Now by being completely prepared in every way . . so that you know what you are going to say . . what you are going to do . . and how things will be done . . And you have practiced and rehearsed until you are letter perfect with it . . Then you'll come to the stage with an air of confidence and self-assurance . . that no one in the audience could ever have . . After all, you know what you are going to say . . They do not . . You know what you are going to do . . They do not . . So, you are ahead of them all the time . . And you will stay ahead . . Completely and in every respect . .

Now I want to recapitulate exactly what I have suggested to you . . First of all . . Visualize the audience in their underwear . . You put them at a disadvantage . . Second, get the attention of the audience and keep it . . Thirdly, remember that it is one to one . . One of you and one audience . . and you'll speak to one person at a time . . Fourth and perhaps most important . . you'll have adequate preparation . . Once you do, you'll know exactly what you are going to do . . comfortably and confidently . . You'll be self-confident; you'll relax your body, concentrate your mind . . smile and speak . . Easily, comfortably and confidently . . That is exactly the way you will perform . . each and every time . . And you will be amazed at how wonderful you will do . .

EMERGE

You are doing very well . . And I want you to just continue to relax . . just as you are doing . . But I want you to go a little deeper now . . Continue to relax . . but go deeper . . DEEPER . . I would like you to take a few more minutes . . to increase your comfort level, even more . . You may continue becoming even more relaxed and comfortable . . by visualizing . . a time and a place . . a situation . . where you felt so comfortable . . that nothing else mattered . . except that comfort . .

Let your subconscious mind recall . . one of those situations . . in which you experienced a sense of total, blissful . . physical and mental comfort . . Let that complete feeling come over you . .

You can hear the pleasant, soothing sounds in the background . . as you re-experience . . all of the sensations, the feelings . . and the peacefulness . . that goes with the joy and comfort . . you are experiencing . . Notice the profound feeling of . . complete relaxation you have . . all over your body . . And you will notice that part of your body . . that really needed relaxation the most . . And you will notice that the nerves . . in that part of your body . . are no longer pulsating . . Every nerve in that part of your body is becoming relaxed . . and steady . . Calm and gentle . . Complete relaxation is now moving . . from your feet . . right up through your body . . And it is moving from the top of your head . . coming down through your body . . You are inside a cocoon of warmth and gentle comfort . . and you are feeling that comfort . . in every part of your entire body . . Wrapping you gently . . like a baby . .

As you experience that feeling of complete relaxation and comfort . . moving all through your body . . it can keep becoming more and more automatic . . so you won't even need to think about it, consciously, anymore . . You can just let yourself become a part of that relaxation . . Just as it becomes a natural part of you . . And you will be pleased to learn . . that you don't need to, consciously . . listen to me . . because your subconscious mind is hearing . . and absorbing . . everything I say to you . . And will respond in it's own comfortable way . . You can thoroughly enjoy . . whatever you are experiencing . . And your subconscious mind will cause you . . to go into the proper depth needed . . to accomplish whatever it feels is important for you . . to achieve, at this time . . You may continue to rest comfortably . . knowing that you can depend on your subconscious mind . . to do what needs to be done . . to enable you to live a happier, healthier and more peaceful life . .

You can experience . . with each of your senses . . a calmness, moving all through your body . . flowing into every fiber of your being . . And you may become more aware . . of your own inner resources . . And you are experiencing a lot of joy . . in discovering all that you can do . . to make the fullest use of your talents . . and skills . . to help yourself . . as well as to help other people . .

It only takes a moment of time . . to notice something beautiful . . As you keep noticing, more and more . . the beauty and the good things . . in life, all around you . . You will soon be seeing beauty everywhere . . You will keep realizing . . more each day . . that the world is a bright and beautiful place . . And most of the people in it . . are truly, overflowing with love . .

Get a picture in your mind of a child . . hurriedly going into a warm kitchen and asking, "Mom, is it soup yet?" . . That is a cute advertisement I have seen several times . . It is typical of a child . . Children, often, "Can hardly wait" . . for something good to happen . . Many adults are that way, too . . However, you are realizing that . . it takes time for good things to develop . . We walk out into a field . . and we see grass . . We see cattle eating that grass . . And the dairy farmer understands that the grass will soon become milk . . It just takes a little time . . Patience is important . . True patience is the art of doing something else . . while good things in life develop . .

And now . . for the next few minutes . . allow yourself to continue relaxing . . Your subconscious mind is absorbing . . everything we have talked about . . and is quite busy . . resolving those issues perfectly . . There are problems to resolve . . in your conscious world . . that are being resolved . . by your wonderful . . subconscious mind . . as you are lying here . . relaxing . . And that is all I want you to do . . It is all you need to do . . Relax . . just . . relax . . (Pause)

When I give suggestions to awaken you, from the hypnotic state . . you will open your eyes feeling happy, healthy, confident and completely relaxed . . Like a new person . . You will feel much better . . both mentally and physically . . You are in control of your life . . and each day, you become more aware of greater joy and happiness . . in all areas of your existence . .

I will begin my count now . . from ONE to FIVE . . And when you hear me say the number FIVE . . you will open your eyes, feeling good all over . . Feeling wonderful . . because you truly are . . a wonderful person . .

ONE

TWO

THREE

FOUR

FIVE

STROKE & PARALYSIS - OVERCOME
RELEARNING TO WALK
(Follow Relaxation)

You have been able to perform many functions throughout your life . . just by, consciously, making the decision . . to carry out certain actions . . When you make a decision to eat . . and put food into your mouth . . you chew it . . and swallow it . . automatically . . And in the past, you have been able to walk, talk, move your hands and fingers . . any time you wanted to . . All of these things became so natural for you . . that you could do them easily . . just by making the decision to do so . . In fact, it became so easy, that you could do it . . without even being consciously aware . . that you had decided to do it . . Then . . a short time ago . . you discovered that you were, suddenly, unable . . to do things you did for years . . so automatically . .

Since that time . . you've been experiencing some difficulty . . because of an experience you went through . . And, consciously . . you don't understand what caused it to happen . .

There is a lot of information . . stored in your mind . . Information you are not consciously aware of . . What I want to do now is . . ask your subconscious mind to begin sorting through that information . . to search through it all . . and discover just what happened . . that caused you to experience that problem . . When we find the cause . . it's easier to find the cure . .

When your subconscious mind discovers . . what caused that problem . . then I want it to review that information . . and work out the solution . . So that your body will be restored, completely and perfectly . . (Pause) When your subconscious mind understands . . that there is no need for you to continue experiencing that problem . . one of your fingers . . will lift up towards the ceiling . . and remain up, until I tell it to go back down . .

NOTE : STROKE OR PARALYSIS PATIENT MAY NOT HAVE ABILITY TO RAISE FINGER. DISCOVER ALTERNATIVE METHOD FOR SIGNAL.

IF FINGER RAISES, CONTINUE WITH : Your subconscious mind has indicated, there is no reason you need to continue experiencing that problem . . Now, when your subconscious mind knows the changes have begun . . and your body is being healed, completely and perfectly . . one of your fingers will lift up and remain up . . until I tell it to go back down . .

IF FINGER DOES NOT RAISE, THE FIRST TIME , CONTINUE WITH: Your inner mind, easily knows . . how to restore your skin . . if it is cut or bruised . . Your inner mind also knows . . how to cause a bone to grow back together . . if it is broken . . And it is normal and natural for your inner mind . . to cause the healing processes of your body . . to function properly . . and heal any part of your body . . including your brain . . Your mind is understanding that . . and is working out the solution . . to your problem . . All parts of your mind are cooperation . . and are healing your body . . rapidly and perfectly . . in a way that is pleasing to you . .

Think of your subconscious capabilities . . All of that power and energy in your mind . . Your brain has all of the potential it needs . . to fully restore every part of your body . . Your mind also has great powers of creativity . . And is, now, creating ways of restoring . . all of your body functions . . in an easy, natural manner . .

Your subconscious mind . . and your body . . are in strong communication . . and are working in harmony . . to rejuvenate and restore your body . . All of the cells . . the atoms and the molecules of your body . . are functioning, harmoniously . . to regenerate your body to perfection . . All of the chemical activities of your body . . are cooperating to renew your body . . to perfect health . .

In your own way . . you are creating an image in your mind . . of your body restored to perfect health . . And you are feeling that rejuvenation taking place . . Hold that vision . . strongly, in your mind . . Keep that image, of your body, in perfect health . . Hold that image in your mind . .

You are recalling, when you were a child . . just learning to walk . . You had to get up on your feet and make a concentrated effort . . to put one foot ahead of the other . . and take steps to get from one place to another . . And as you continued practicing your walking . . it became so automatic to you . . that you, soon, could do it . . without, consciously, thinking about it . . Your inner mind is remembering that now . . Your body and your brain . . has all of the knowledge needed . . to restore your ability to walk . . And to use all of the muscles, ligaments, tendons and nerves in your body, easily . . You even know how to walk backwards . . Your mind is revitalizing . . what you already know . . Bringing it to the forefront of your brain . .

Looking at it now . . from a new point of view . . Remembering that when you were a baby . . you had to learn . . how to walk . . because you had never done it before . . Now, your inner mind is helping you to learn . . to do it again . . Realizing that what you can learn to do once . . you can learn to do more easily now . . Now that you have had that past experience . .

Yes, you have already learned how to walk . . Therefore, you can now re-learn . . what you already know . . Your subconscious mind is searching out the information . . Put there from your previous learning experience . . and putting it into good use again . .

To enable your mind to do that searching, properly . . I need you to go into a much deeper state of hypnosis now . . DEEPER and DEEPER . . DEEPER now . . Go way down . . WAY down . . into the very basement of hypnosis . . As far down as you need to go . . to achieve what you need to achieve . . Continue to relax . . RELAX . . and go DEEP DOWN . . and relax . . (Pause)

Let all of your senses be clear . . as you re-experience the muscles, strengthening . . And the awareness of all that is . . for your subconscious mind to review . . and explore . .

As your subconscious mind is reviewing . . that previous learning time . . all of your muscles, tendons, nerves and ligaments . . are regaining their previous strength and coordination . . And your brain is rejuvenating to redirect the proper signals to be sent . .

What you are doing . . requires complete cooperation . . of your mind and body . . I want you to reinforce that cooperation, each night . . just before you go to sleep . . by visualizing, in your mind . . that you are walking . . and running . . easily and perfectly . . with great strength and agility . .

By doing this . . every night, before you go to sleep . . your subconscious mind will cause it to happen . . Having faith . . is what heals . . Faith in God . . and faith in yourself . . You will soon be healed . . completely and perfectly . . by your faith . .

I will begin my count now . . from ONE to FIVE . . And when you hear me say the number FIVE . . you will open your eyes, feeling good all over . . Feeling wonderful . . because you truly are . . a wonderful person . .

ONE, TWO, THREE, FOUR and . . FIVE . . You may open your eyes.

STUDY SCHOOL WORK - ENJOY
OR HOUSEWORK

(Follow Relaxation)

You have been resting . . Relaxing . . And that is good . . for you have earned it . . And now, you are ready to enjoy some very pleasant changes . . in the way you study /do housework . .

Many people have found that if something is boring . . tiring, monotonous or tedious . . just a slight change . . can make that same thing . . surprisingly pleasant, enjoyable and, even, inspiring . . Schoolwork (Housework) . . when completed . . can give a person a sense of accomplishing something . . and doing it well . .

When you are just beginning your schoolwork (housework) . . the feeling that it is going to be done . . is being done . . and has been done . . and has been completed . . will cause you to have a feeling of expectation . . that will enable you to concentrate better . . (Learn more rapidly and enjoy studying) And develop ways of doing your housework that makes it more enjoyable . .

Think it over . . Don't agree yet . . Think it over before you agree . .
(Pause)

You can actually enjoy doing (your class assignments / different types of work in your own home) And you can feel very proud in knowing (that you have completed your homework / that your home is really clean) . .

There are times when you really enjoy being you . . Being the person inside your body . . Feeling relaxed . . Feeling comfortable . . And in your own mind, you can explore thoughts and ideas . . that really give you pleasure . . They are all . . your thoughts . . Your ideas . . (Pause)

Now, getting back to the change . . A slight change . . can give you a sense of accomplishing something . . Of knowing that you have done a good job . . That you have completed something with a joyful sense of accomplishment . . Enabling you to go to bed . . and sleep peacefully and calmly . . knowing your (schoolwork / housework) is done for the day . .

The overall image of your (schoolwork / housework) completed . . is a good thing to accomplish . . And it keeps becoming easier . . and more enjoyable . . for you to achieve . . The nice feelings come as you are doing it . . Causing it to be all worthwhile . . Is that all right ? . . (Pause)

I expect your mind is going to translate everything I am saying . . into your own words . . Your own phrases . . And your own actions . . So, the changes are accomplished in your own ways . . Not in mine . .

Okay, now, I'm going to explain something else . . When I went to college . . I had a small apartment to live in . . I didn't like keeping it clean . . No, and I didn't like doing homework either . . I determined that . . if I was going to keep my apartment clean . . and pass the college courses . . I had to work out a system . . of getting my class work and my housework completed together . . I spent a little time, thinking this through . . And this was what I came up with . .

From the time I was a young child . . I had always enjoyed playing the trumpet . . and the guitar . . And I had always enjoyed playing basketball, football . . and other sports . . So, I developed a plan that caused me to learn . . to really enjoy cleaning my apartment . . and doing my school work, as well . .

According to my plan . . I would never study . . or do housework . . more than thirty minutes at a time . . At the end of thirty minutes . . if I wasn't finished . . I would stop and play my trumpet . . or my guitar . . for thirty minutes . . Then I would go back to my studies . . or my housecleaning . . for another thirty minutes . . And I continued this routine until my studies or housecleaning were completed . . And it kept becoming more enjoyable . .

I kept changing, every thirty minutes, from textbook or house cleaning . . to doing something I enjoyed . . and then back to school work or house work . . Shifting from one to the other . . every thirty minutes . .

Every time you shift from one pattern of activity . . you rest from the previous activity . . So, you can keep doing what you're doing, at top speed . . because when you change from doing one thing . . you are resting from the other . . You alternate from doing something tedious . . to another thing you enjoy . . Understanding that you are actually resting . . while getting your homework or house work completed . . And you learn to enjoy it . . because it all requires different patterns of functioning . . Do you understand ? . .

Now, you can put that into your own understanding . . And what you do will be your own accomplishment . . And you can be proud of that . . You can think about these things at your own convenience . . And decide to accept them and put them to your own advantage . .

It will bring you much pleasure and happiness . . with a real sense of self-worth and accomplishment . .

You are realizing that every task . . is important . . The surgeon who performs . . a successful open heart operation . . that saves a person's life . . considers his accomplishment as being very important . . But the nurse who handed him his surgical tools . . is just as important . . And the person who applies the anesthesia . . is just as important . . And the person who monitors the heart beat . . is also just as important . . The surgery would not be successful . . unless each person involved . . did his or her job . . Regardless of how small the job may seem to be . .

You will find pleasure in giving respect to doing (your school assignments) (each part of your house work) For it is all . . very important . .

Notice that you are already beginning to feel enthusiastic about it . . Already . . you are sensing the feeling of satisfaction that you will have . . in doing things you need to do . . Knowing that it will be . . your own accomplishment . .

You are already organizing the words you have heard here . . into your own actions . . And you will be pleased to find . . your actions taking place . . for your greater accomplishments . . after you awaken from the hypnotic state . . You will be very pleased and proud . . of your achievements . . And, rightfully so . .

In just a moment now . . I will begin my count, from ONE to FIVE . . When you hear me say the number FIVE . . you will open your eyes, feeling awake, alert and ready to take on the world . .

ONE
TWO
THREE
FOUR
FIVE   Open your eyes now . .

You are in a light relaxation now . . and you are doing very well . . Continue to relax . .

I want you to use your imagination . . It will help you to reach your goal . . I want you to imagine of yourself now . . riding in a comfortable car . . You are on your way to a meeting with a group of people . . who are thinking about forming a club . . Just for people who want to overcome . . the problem of stuttering . .

You arrive at the meeting . . and everyone seems to be sitting . . by themselves . . wondering what to do . . No one seems to be talking to each other . . Everyone feels a little hesitant to talk . . Perhaps they're afraid of being heard . . stuttering . . So, they just sit . . Finally, you speak up and ask . . "Who is in charge here ?" . . A young lady admits to having put the ad in the paper . . but says she stutters too badly to lead the meeting . . Someone else suggests that . . since you brought it up . . maybe you would be a good person to be in charge . . You try objecting . . fearing that you, too, would stutter too much . . But everyone agrees that you . . should be in charge . . So, you arise . . moving to the lectern at the back of the room . .

You begin by telling everyone, why you decided to attend the meeting . . after reading the ad in the local newspaper . . And you continue . . telling everyone how they . . might be helpful to each other . . And supportive, in overcoming the problem . . of stuttering . . You talk about five minutes . . when a young man raises his hand . . He says he has been listening to you . . but you have not stuttered one time . . And you suddenly become aware that . . he is right . . You were feeling so, at ease . . up in front of the others at the meeting . . that you were talking fluently . . You were talking confidently . . and you felt totally relaxed and at ease . . Your previous fears and tensions were gone . . when you got up in front of this group . . Your stuttering had been replaced . . by a smooth, easy flowing manner of speaking . . Even though everyone at the meeting . . had been strangers to each other . . you felt confident . . You felt secure . . And much more relaxed and at ease . . You felt quite proud of what you had accomplished . . You were pleased to find yourself speaking . . easily and naturally . .

In just a moment . . I'm going to ask you to repeat a sentence after me . . And you'll be amazed at how clearly you talk . . You'll be pleased to hear yourself speaking . . easily and freely . .

Now, repeat these words after me : "At a meeting - of a group of stutterers - I was asked - to lead the meeting - to determine - whether or not - we should form a club - to help each other overcome the stuttering problem - After talking to the group - about five minutes, without stuttering - my confidence kept increasing - We decided to form the club - and I was elected President - It helped me so much - that no one in the club - ever heard me stutter - I overcame the problem - my first night at the meeting . .

You can continue to relax . . as you move into a deeper . . more comfortable state now . . While your mind is reviewing . . what first caused you to begin stuttering . . It was a long time ago . . but your subconscious mind is remembering . . and is examining . . and exploring . . what caused that problem . . And is working out the solution . . Your subconscious mind is also realizing . . there is no reason . . the problem should continue . . When it first happened . . perhaps there was a reason for it . . Perhaps it protected you from something . . But now, that reason is gone . . And so, your subconscious mind is causing you to experience . . very pleasant changes . . that are getting rid of the problem . . for now and forever . .

When your subconscious mind understands . . what has been causing that problem . . and knows that you don't need it anymore . . and changes have started, so you are getting rid of that problem completely . . one of the fingers on your right hand will lift up . . towards the ceiling . . and will remain up . . until I tell it to go back down . . (Pause for response)

NOTE : IF FINGER HAS NOT LIFTED, GO TO "THERAPY -FINGER RESPONSE" BEFORE AWAKENING CLIENT.

As you continue relaxing now . . your mind is peaceful . . and is open to awareness and understanding . . You are becoming more aware . . of a spirit of power within you . . that enables you to overcome obstacles . . and improve all areas of your life . . You came here . . from the same creator . . that everyone else came from . . And you are here for a purpose . . You are here because you are very special . .

You do not need to measure up . . to anyone else's expectations of you . . you are not here for the purpose of being . . what someone else expects you to be . . You are YOU . . And you are unique . . Your main purpose is to be . . what you want to be . . Each day . . your self-confidence grows stronger . . Your self-acceptance is increasing . . And your self-reliance . . becomes more and more real in your life . .

Just continue to relax . . In just a moment . . I'm going to count from ONE to FIVE . . With each number I say . . your mind will become more alert . . And when you hear me say the number FIVE . . you will awaken and open your eyes . . feeling refreshed, calm and very comfortable . .

I will begin my count now . .

ONE

TWO

THREE

FOUR

FIVE   Open your eyes now . .

(follow Relaxation)

Research conducted by psychologists . . has revealed that all of us . . use only a small fraction of our total . . mental and physical ability . . It has been found that the average person . . uses less than five percent . . of his mental capacity . . And even the greatest geniuses . . rarely use more than fifteen percent . . of their mental abilities . .

These facts indicate . . that we are all capable of achieving outstanding accomplishments . . merely by learning how to use . . our physical and mental abilities . . more efficiently . .

Hypnosis is one of the best known methods . . for developing your mental abilities . . and enabling you to use . . your natural, inborn talents . . And help you to become more successful . . than you ever believed possible . .

Hundreds of books have been written . . and thousands of articles have been published . . telling about the tremendous power of your mind . . Those books and articles . . tell how to use your mind . . to "win friends", "improve your health", "attain wealth" or to "be successful" . . in all other areas of your life . .

People who have studied the techniques . . taught in those books . . and who have put the instructions into action . . have discovered that the mind . . is an amazingly powerful asset . .

After many years of research and . . hypnotizing many people . . I have found that the best way to get your mind to work for you . . and enable you to use your natural inborn abilities . . is through hypnosis . . Just as you are doing now . . When you are in a hypnotic state . . as you are in now . . all of the suggestions, thoughts, ideas and instructions . . go directly into the storehouse of your mind . . And they begin working immediately . . to help you achieve a healthier, happier, more successful . . and more rewarding life . . than ever before . . So, what we are doing now . . will cause your natural, inborn talents, skills and . . mental abilities . . to keep emerging more, each day . .

Your subconscious mind is comparable to a computer . . in that it records everything you see, hear and experience . . as you go about the activities of your daily life . . And it has been doing that . . ever since you first came into existence . .

You have accumulated tremendous amounts of information and knowledge . . Far beyond what your conscious mind has been aware of . . And you have the ability to extract . . and use that knowledge . . for your own personal well-being . . For your own benefit . . And for your own advancement . .

You are drifting . . into a more peaceful hypnotic state of relaxation . . as I talk to you . . Your confidence is increasing . . and you are becoming more aware . . that you possess outstanding capabilities . . You are learning to be more calm and relaxed . . during your daily life . . And you are realizing . . that it is your own mind . . that is helping you develop the talents and abilities . . that you possess . .

Your subconscious mind . . and all levels of your inner mind . . are your most powerful sources of energy . . And they are at your disposal . . History reveals that the power of the mind . . has shaped the destiny of mankind . .

All scientific progress in our world today . . such as electricity, telephones, cars, appliances . . and other luxuries we use and enjoy . . have come to us . . as the result of people . . making use of their ability to think . .

Everything we have was formed as a thought . . in some person's mind . . before it was produced for us to use . . And you are also capable . . of outstanding thoughts and accomplishments . . by using the power of your own mind . .

Your ability to think . . can help you achieve any goal you set for yourself . . because your subconscious mind will cause you . . to put your thoughts into actions . . You will use the power of your mind . . to produce original thinking . . which will result in producing success . . in all areas of your life . .

You are continuing to drift . . into a deeper . . DEEPER . . hypnotic state now . . Go deeper now . . These suggestions and instructions . . are going directly into the storehouse of your mind . . And will help you on both the conscious . . and the subconscious levels . . of mind activity . .

These principles of relaxation are clear . . And you will use these principles of relaxation . . which you are experiencing now . . during your daily life . . You will be relaxed and calm . . in every situation or circumstance . . in which you find yourself . . Whether you are alone or with others . .

Regardless of what you are doing or who you are with . . you will remain relaxed and calm . . and will be able to concentrate your mind . . Enabling you to be more efficient, in everything you do . .

Your ability to use your sense of observation . . is continuing to improve . . And you will be able to evaluate things more thoroughly . . And will be able to make wise decisions . . more easily . .

You are developing the ability . . to concentrate with your subconscious mind . . You will use your subconscious mind . . to direct your life properly . . And you'll have complete control . . over your emotions . . Your ability to concentrate . . is continuing to improve more, each day . . That enables you to think more clearly . . And gives you more control of your own destiny . . You can see things in their true perspective . . without magnifying them . . And without letting them get out of proportion . .

Your mind is more dependable than your emotions . . And you are learning to use your mind for wise guidance . . You can reason your way around emotions . . that are unpleasant or harmful . . You avoid gossip . . and you will be successful . . in overcoming emotional burdens . . in a peaceful, loving way . .

In every situation or circumstance . . that comes up in your life . . you can be calm and relaxed . . That enables you to get a good comprehension of all the facts . . You can evaluate things, thoroughly and completely . . and will be able to make wise decisions, easily . . Then you will have the courage and confidence you need . . to act efficiently and effectively . . Guided by your ability to think, reason and understand . .

You continue moving into a deeper . . and DEEPER hypnotic state . . as these suggestions and instructions continue . . becoming more effective in your mind . . You continue progressing more each day . . and you will be the successful person you are capable of being . . Your subconscious mind understands . . that you have been absorbing countless impressions . . learning many facts . . storing ideas, symbols and all kinds of information . . in the storehouse of your mind . . ever since you first came into existence . . So, your mind possesses great amounts and varieties of wisdom . . far beyond what your conscious mind . . has been aware of knowing . .

All of that knowledge and wisdom . . is in the storehouse of your mind . . and is a part of your own development . . It is the result of the many experiences you have gone through . . And you can access and use that knowledge . . to enable you to continue advancing . . in all areas of your life . .

Realizing that you possess enormous amounts of knowledge . . causes your self-confidence and self-acceptance . . to keep increasing . .You understand that you have . . remarkable capabilities . . So you will set up goals for yourself . . And you will challenge yourself in everything you do . . knowing that you have the ability to achieve . . any goal . . or any destiny . . you set for yourself . .

All of your qualities and characteristics . . continue to develop more strongly for you each day . . Because your subconscious mind knows they are true . . And because you have the courage . . and determination . . to be successful . . in all areas of your life . .

Just continue to relax . . In just a moment . . I'm going to count from ONE to FIVE . . With each number I say . . your mind will become more alert . . more clear . . And when you hear me say the number FIVE . . you will awaken and open your eyes . . feeling refreshed, calm and very comfortable . .

I will begin my count now . .

ONE

TWO

THREE

FOUR

FIVE   Open your eyes now . .

It is your God-given birthright . . to be successful . . In other words . . you are on this Earth to experience a happy, joyous, prosperous life . . You have as much right to happiness and prosperity . . as any other person . . on this Earth . . The good things created by God belong to you . . just as much as to any other person . . And they are available to you . . merely by developing your talents, skills and abilities . . And by putting your inborn knowledge and wisdom into action . .

As you continue relaxing . . and listening to what I am saying . . you are realizing that you already have the capability . . of attaining everything you need . . Wealth, friends, a lovely home, a healthy body . . and anything else you desire for yourself . .

It is natural for you to desire prosperity, success and recognition . . It is natural for you to want enough money . . to do things you desire to do . . whenever you want to do those things . . So, you are a normal person . . in wanting to be successful . .

As you accept the suggestions and instructions I am giving you . . and follow the simple techniques I describe to you . . you will find that you can use your own mind . . to bring to yourself . . an abundance of wealth . . and a highly successful life . .

You deserve to have . . the best food, good clothes, a beautiful home . . and all the money you need . . to buy things that will make you happy and comfortable . .

So, listen to what I am saying now . . and you will learn techniques . . that will increase your ability to be successful . . If you don't seem to be hearing everything I say to you . . it's okay . . Your subconscious mind is hearing and absorbing everything . . and will cause you to put it all . . into your own actions . . Just relax . . Relax as I continue . .

Many people do not agree . . with everything written in the Bible . . And that is okay . . But psychological research has proven . . that there are many things written in the Bible . . that are scientifically correct . .

For example : The Bible says . . "As a person thinks in his mind . . so is he" . . That statement has proven to be true . . It's a fact that the thoughts in our minds . . cause us to be . . what we are . .

Another statement found . . in Romans 12 :2 says . . "You can be transformed by the renewing of your mind" . . And that, too, has proven to be true . .

By learning to experience these principles of relaxation . . as you are enjoying now . . you are . . at the same time . . learning to use the tremendous power . . of your own mind . . to solve any problem or difficulty that comes up in your life . . You can use your own mind to work out solutions . . that will enable you to experience a more productive . . happier, more fulfilling life . . than ever before . .

You are choosing harmony, success, prosperity, abundance and security for yourself . . Your own creative abilities . . will keep emerging more and more . . each day . . Revealing better ways to enable you . . to give greater service to others . . and receive greater rewards for yourself . .

The words I am telling you are going directly into the storehouse of your mind . . And they keep becoming more effective each day . . as you proceed to use these ideas and thoughts . . in a positive, active way . .

I want you to relax . . a little deeper now . . You are resting . . comfortably . . and going deeper . . You are deeply relaxed . . And you are continuing to progress, spiritually . . and will prosper in all areas of your life . . You are constantly maturing . . mentally, physically, emotionally and spiritually . . So, it is easy for you to relax . . Deeply . . relax . .

Combining these principles of positive thinking . . and hypnotic relaxation . . will automatically increase your energy level and vitality . . Every cell in your body is continuing to function more perfectly . . And your body will express increased vitality, energy and power . .

The work you do is a divine activity . . Therefore, your work will keep becoming more prosperous and successful . . Remember that you become successful . . by doing commonplace things in life . . with a spirit of enthusiasm . . and with a genuine desire to help others . . Regardless of what your work might be . .

As you put your best efforts into actions . . coupled with persistence . . you will be rewarded with an abundant life . . A life filled with happiness, joy . . and rich living . .

You will use the creative ability of your mind . . And will be aware of good ideas emerging . . that will enable you to increase your standard of living . .

You will be constantly aware that your thoughts are creative . . And every thought tends to become a reality . . It causes your subconscious mind to respond . . according to the nature of your thoughts . . So you will always think good, positive, uplifting thoughts . . that lead to success . .

Your thoughts are comparable to driving a car . . You can steer them . . and guide them . . in the direction you want to go . . Your ability to think wisely . . will pay off in great dividends . . as you guide your thoughts in a constructive way . .

Remember, that all the good things we enjoy in life . . the luxuries: such as, television . . radio, automobiles, airplanes, furniture and appliances . . all began as a thought . . in someone's mind . . before they became a reality for us to use . . And as you focus your thoughts on the goals . . you desire to achieve . . your thoughts will grow . . and become a reality . . that will bring you health, happiness, prosperity and peace of mind . .

Right now . . I am going to give you the keys . . that will unlock the doors to your future prosperity and success . .

The first key . . is to get a clear image in your mind . . of what you want to achieve . . (Pause)

The second key . . is to believe . . that you can and will succeed . . in accomplishing your goal . .

And the third key . . is to begin working now . . And continue working toward your goal . . regardless of any obstacle . . And it will be accomplished . .

There are hundreds of books available today . . explaining how to be successful . . Nearly all of the books clearly emphasize . . that the most important key . . in achieving success . . is to set a goal to achieve . . You begin by getting a clear idea in your mind . . of what you want to achieve . .

Refuse to be like the man who shoots an arrow into the sky . . not knowing where it will land . . Have a bulls eye to shoot at . .

494

Decide what your target is . . And then . . start aiming . . and moving toward your target . .

A person may have a goal . . but no ambition to follow through with . . That person is wasting his time . . He may as well not have a goal . . A person who has no goal . . may start out in the right direction . . But when he comes to an intersection . . he doesn't know which way to turn . . Because he doesn't know where he is going . . So, always have a goal set in your mind . . That will enable you to make decisions wisely . . any time you have a decision to make . . Because you will know where you are headed . .

You wouldn't get into your car and start on a trip . . to a distant city . . if you knew you would never reach your destination . . You take a trip . . believing . . that you will arrive safely . . at your destination . . And it's the same thing when you set a goal to achieve . . You set a goal because you believe you can attain that goal . . Having a goal in your mind . . causes you to be persistent and patient . . enabling you to keep advancing toward your goal . .

Success comes, as a result of making things happen . . Success is the result of achievements . . every day achievements . . that are accomplished, one step at a time . .

You are successful . . when you set a goal . . and then, persistently perform the necessary actions to achieve your goal . . Each action you perform . . and each effort you put forth toward achieving your goal . . is rewarded . .

As you continue moving forward . . toward prosperity and success . . you always keep in mind, the goal you are aiming at . . You always know your purpose . . And organize your efforts . . so you perform efficiently and effectively . . in everything you do . .

You will always think positive . . and that will cause you to use your mind wisely . . realizing that everything you do . . is directed and controlled by your thoughts . . through the power of your own subconscious mind . . The presence of a thought . . or an idea in your mind . . produces an associated feeling . . And causes you to transform that feeling . . into an equal action . . that is in harmony with the nature of your thought . .

So, by setting a goal, you want to achieve . . your mind becomes alert . . for facts, information and knowledge . . that will enable you to achieve your goal . .

You are now ready . . to put these precepts into action . . You are going to transform your goals into realities . . You will begin by writing out plans . . of what you can do . . to achieve your goal . . Write out a clear, concise statement . . of the goal you want to achieve . . Follow that by listing . . a number of items you can do . . to help achieve that goal . . Construct a time-frame schedule . . Then decide what information or knowledge you need . . and consider how you will get it . . And, of course, consider the type of associations you need . . to enable you to attain your goal . . Each night, read what you have written . . And meditate on that . . before you go to sleep . . Soon you will see your goal . . become reality . . Duplicate these efforts . . for each goal you set for yourself . . and you will be successful . . in all aspects of your life . .

All of these thoughts and ideas . . are in the storehouse of your mind . . They are a part of you now . . and are being used by you . . automatically . . to make your life more prosperous, more successful . . more useful . . And they will make you much happier . .

Each day, your desire and determination to succeed . . keeps becoming stronger . . And you have the confidence you need . . to accomplish each and every goal . . you establish for yourself . .

EMERGE

SUCCESS - IN LIFE

Continue to relax . . You are doing very well now . . I want you to be very comfortable . . Nothing disturbs you and nothing bothers you . . Just continue to relax . . and allow yourself to ink into a deeper . . and DEEPER . . relaxed state . . Allow yourself to let go . . as you sink deeper . . DEEPER . . Very deep now . . A little deeper with each breath you take . . Your body completely relaxes . . all over . . and you feel yourself drifting . . drifting on a cloud . . And you know you are safe . . Safe and secure . . Let yourself drift outward now . . You are in good hands . . Your mind is focused on the sounds of my voice . . You will hear no other sounds but what comes from my voice . . You will heed my words . . and cause my words to form into your own actions . .

Your mind is interested only in the words from my voice . . And you listen . . expectantly . . for the suggestions I am about to give you . . For you see, your sense of imagination is heightened . . So you will easily visualize whatever I suggest to you . . as you become more and more relaxed . . with every breath you take . .

First, I want you to see yourself as a success . . Imagine yourself to be successful . . only, more than you have been in the past . . You can be far more successful . . because now there is strong reason to believe it . . You truly want to be successful . . That's one of the reasons you are here . .

And so, you will continue to envision yourself . . to be a success . . in every way . . In order for you to be a success . . you must first visualize yourself to be successful . . And since you are what you believe yourself to be . . you must believe yourself to be a success in every way . . Picture yourself successful . . And since you become what you think about all day . . you think success . . you feel success . . And you concentrate your every thought . . on being successful . .

Now, you know . . when a concert pianist plays the piano . . he concentrates his mind only on playing the piano . . He is not wondering if he will hit a wrong note . . or what is going on in the audience . . He is concentrating his entire mind on playing the piano . . He is not concentrating part of his mind on playing . . and part of his mind on the fear of not doing it right . . His entire being is concentrated on playing the piano . .

Not long ago . . there was a 14 year old girl who became . . the youngest to ever succeed . . in swimming across the English Channel . . How did she do it ? . . She concentrated her mind so much on swimming . . before she started . . that she had already swam the channel . . in her mind . . before she ever got in the water . . Swimming the English Channel was already an accomplished fact . . in her mind . . before she ever began . .

Henry Ford . . had to conceive the automobile in his mind . . before he ever built it . . Thomas Edison . . had to see the electric light in his mind . . before he ever designed it . . And, for you . . it's the same . . Being a success . . in your chosen field . . or your smallest goal . . is an accomplished fact, in your mind . . before you ever begin . . Just as in the case of that young swimmer . . if part of her mind had been concentrating on fear . . of what might happen if she didn't make it . . then she would have been sapping her own strength . . She would have been reducing her own power . . and her own ability . . The truth is, that each of us . . saps our own strength . . to a certain extent . . depending on the amount of fear . . we allow to creep into our minds . . And sometimes . . we even become afraid of letting go of fear . . We fool ourselves into thinking that . . perhaps fear . . is a good thing . . Maybe it will protect us . . or motivate us . . We say, "Maybe, if I am afraid I am going to be poor . . then I will have to strive to be rich" . . But, nothing could be further from the truth . . Now, I am going to ask you a question . . And I want you to, silently . . think of the answer . .

When . . can you accomplish . . what you want to do? . . When can you accomplish, what you want to accomplish ? . . (Pause) Well, the answer is . . When you get rid of the fear . . that you may not accomplish it . . But 'fear' is not the only obstacle . . There are Three . . negative emotions . . Any one of which can keep us . . from accomplishing our goals . . These Three negative emotions . . must be eliminated . . They must be eliminated from your mind . . NOW . . Eliminated, right now . . before we can even get started on self-improvement . . These three negative emotions don't do anything except . . hold you back . . Let's talk about what they are . .

The Three Negative Emotions . . we need to deal with are . . Fear, Anxiety and . . Guilt . . or FAG --- F. A. G. . . Fear, Anxiety, Guilt . . In fact, you are so desirous to be rid of them . . that we are going to remove them from your mind . . But, before we remove them . . I will show you how to recognize them . . so they will never be allowed . . to creep back into your thoughts again . .

Now, the first negative emotion . . is, FEAR . . "I'm afraid of" . . whatever . . You see, fear . . usually creeps back in the form of motivation . . You say to yourself, "Oh, It's good for me to be afraid . . It motivates me" . . That brings us back to the earlier example . . "Maybe if I'm afraid I am going to be poor . . then I will have to strive to be rich" . . Well, that's ridiculous . . For you know . . fear only motivates people to panic . . Oliver Wendell Holmes once said . . "One should not allow a man to yell, fire, in a crowded theater" . . Obviously not . . Because it makes people afraid . . And what do they do when they become afraid ? . . They panic . . They lose their reason . . They rush for the exit . . Fear . . is a suggestion of the unknown . . It is a negative . . suggestion . .

As you can see . . fear doesn't motivate people . . it paralyzes them . . Emotion takes over . . And when that happens . . reason . . and logic . . fly out the window . . So, right now . . you must allow yourself to accept the suggestion that . . all fear must go . . I don't care what you are afraid of . . all fear must go . . It does no good at all . . to hold onto fear . . Any kind of fear . . Let it all go . .

Now . . Anxiety . . as you know . . is just another word for . . worry . . And you'll find that . . really successful people . . have no need to be anxious . . Why ? . . Because they've learned to channel their energy into positive attitudes . . positive planning . . rather than let it go to waste in the form of anxiety . . or worry . . Anxiety just clutters the mind . . It adds confusion to the mind . .

Think of the person on a television quiz show . . who knows the answer . . but because he is so anxious . . the answers are blocked from entering his conscious mind . . and he misses the question . . Then, immediately after leaving the stage . . he recalls the answer . . You see, anxiety was blocking his recall . . and it made him inefficient . . You may have had the same thing happen to you . . Perhaps in a group meeting . . when you wanted to introduce someone but couldn't recall his name . . You became anxious and your mind became confused . . Just enough for you to forget . . when you needed to recall it the most . . Many a business man has spoken in front of a group and . . after sitting down . . finishing the speech . . he, then, remembers a lot of good points he intended to say . . which would have made his speech more effective . .

Now, why does this happen ? . . Because we allow this negative emotion called, anxiety, to slip in and confuse our thinking . . The amount of energy we waste . . through anxiety . . could make us a lot more effective and successful . . The way to combat this problem is simply this . . Anxiety has got to go . . Fear and Anxiety are emotions that do nothing but injure you . . And you can't afford them any longer . . So, we are going to remove them . .

But, you know . . the most insidious negative emotion of all . . is Guilt . . Now, guilt comes in later . . Guilt is, kind of a . . after-the-fact emotion . . You say to yourself . . "I feel guilty because I made a wrong decision" . . Then you conclude, "Therefore, I should punish myself" . . Because . . guilt calls for punishment . . We know this is true from our court system . . When a man is found guilty . . punishment follows . . Sometimes, this guilt-emotion is very subtle . . It's almost forgotten from the conscious mind . . But not from the subconscious mind . . Guilt brings out shameful feelings, like . . I feel guilty because of something that happened, a long time ago in my early childhood . . I didn't do the best for my Mother . . I didn't do the best for my Father . . or my Brother . . or Sister . . I could have done this . . but I didn't . . I should have done that . . but I didn't . .

Now, what are we going to do about all this guilt ? . . Guilt tells us, we should be punished . . This feeling of guilt . . makes us feel certain . . that we don't deserve all of the good things in life . . Guilt makes us certain . . that we don't deserve to be a success . . And, if I don't deserve to be a success, then somehow . . I have to prevent it from happening . . Do you see how insidious that emotion is ? . . It comes on later . . It's kind of a 'after-the-fact' emotion . . It gives you the, 'I don't deserve' complex . . It gives you the, 'I must punish myself' complex . . Yes, and how can I punish myself ? . . By never achieving the goals for which I am striving . . So, right now . . you allow yourself to realize . . that you can well do without Fear . . You can do without Anxiety . . And you can surely do without Guilt . . For you now realize that you can't start your car on the road to success . . if you have three pieces of baggage, dragging behind you . . So, right now . . you're ready to remove that excess baggage . .

You are ready to remove . . those three negative emotions . . which have only been holding you back . . So, I am going to count . . from

ONE to TEN . . And as I count to TEN . . I am going to remove all Three of those negative emotions from your mind . . Never to return . .

Now, you know how to recognize them . . You can recognize them, right away . . And you are not going to let them return, once I remove them . . You are NEVER going to allow them to return . . once I remove them . . Now I am going to count to TEN . . and at the count of TEN . . the Three negative emotions are completely removed from your mind . . You don't need them at all . . You never did need them . . And even if you felt a need for them in the past . . The reason for needing them has outlived its usefulness . . That's all behind you now . . It's all in the past . .

At one time, you may have felt you had to be afraid of something in your past . . Well, if you ever did . . the reason has long outlived its usefulness . . And maybe . . you thought you had to feel guilty . . Those emotions may have been useful, at one time . . but their usefulness has expired . . Their usefulness has passed . . Their usefulness has collapsed . . and melted away . . It's true, you used to worry . . but you now realize . . you don't need to worry anymore . . You used to feel anxious . . Yes, and you used to feel guilty . . Those were the punishments . . you bestowed upon yourself . . But now, you realize . . you don't have a need . . to be punished any longer . .

So . . on the count of ONE . . these emotions are now going to be removed . . permanently . . from your conscious and subconscious minds . . TWO . . These emotions . . have been holding you back . . THREE . . They have been holding you back because you were afraid to recognize them . . FOUR . . Fortunately . . you, now, realize that you have allowed them to interfere in your life, long enough . . FIVE . . Once they are removed from your mind . . you're never going to allow them to creep back in again . . SIX . . You're going to be surprised and amazed at just how easily and quickly this is going to work for you . . SEVEN . . You realize that never before have so many blocks been removed, so quickly and so easily . . EIGHT . . And you're anxious to be getting rid of them . . Right Now . . NINE . . Just feel them, pouring out of your system . . You can feel them leaving you . . and you are letting them go . . We are getting rid of every single one of those negative emotions right now . . Breath deeply . . That's it . . Breath deeply . . All the way in . . and all the way out . . as you relax and Let go . . Let go . . Let go . . Let go . . and . . TEN . .

501

Relax completely now and breath normally . . Relax your entire body . . as those negative emotions leave you for good . . Now relax deeply and completely . . You're going to be amazed at how efficiently you will operate in the next coming weeks . . Now that you have allowed those three negative emotions to leave you completely . . You will carry on with confidence from here . . You are in control . .

Continue to relax for a few minutes longer . . I will give you a little time of silence now . . for your subconscious mind to absorb everything we have discussed today . . Just relax in silence . . (pause)

We can work further on these issues together . . or any others . . whenever you'd like to make an appointment with me . . I know how much you enjoy having me hypnotize you . .

And now, I am going to begin my count . . from One to Five . . and when you hear the number Five . . to an alert, waking state . . feeling clear of mind . . relaxed . . and feeling wonderful . . I will begin . .

One . . You will remember everything you have experienced here today . . with clarity and complete understanding . .

Two . . You will remain connected to your spiritual and inner supporting strength . .

Three . . Everything I have told you is true . . and is already happening . . Feeling wonderful . . For you truly are a wonderful person . .

Four . . Beginning to be more aware of your body as it wants to stir and fully awaken . .

Five . . Move your fingers and toes now . . Stir and stretch as you open your eyes . . feeling clear, rested and ready for your next great experience.

You are continuing to relax . . And as you listen to the sound of my voice . . while letting your mind simply relax . . I want you to allow your mind to be fertile . . In fact, let it be . . creative . . And feel your ability . . in this creative atmosphere . . become greater and greater . . with every day that passes . . You're going to find that your ability to visualize, creatively . . actually increases . . and becomes more profound . . with each day that passes . .

You have learned, quite well . . how to relax . . You have learned how to relax your mind . . and you have learned to visualize . . More importantly . . you have learned how to remove those negative emotions . . of Fear, Anxiety and Guilt . . And in addition . . you have learned how to prevent . . their re-acceptance, into your being . . because you have learned how to recognize negative suggestions . . when they come your way . . You have learned how to reject negative suggestions . . positively . . And you have learned how to reject them, out loud, too . . So, as you continue to relax your mind . . you allow your imagination free reign, for creativity . .

It is imperative . . that you develop an unbounded confidence . . in your own ability . . to accomplish . . whatever you set your mind to do . . Because, you see, confidence . . in your own ability to do something . . has a great deal to do with your actually accomplishing it . . You simply must have the confidence . . in your own ability . . to accomplish your goal . . Which brings up my question for you . . I don't want you to answer it out loud . . I just want you to think about it, silently . . and contemplate what I am asking . . The question is . . "How do you get the confidence ?" . . Think about that now . . How do you get the confidence ? . . If you think about it . . you'll realize that you're already on the road . . to achieving confidence, right now . . For you know that confidence . . depends entirely . . upon you own state of mind . . And, of course . . your own state of mind is . . the most important thing you possess . . It's the most influential thing about you . . Now, let me rephrase that . . Your most important asset . . for achieving success . . is your own state of mind . . Because, you realize . . that before you can convince anyone . . of anything . . you must, first . . convince yourself . . And before anybody else . . can have any confidence in you . . you must display confidence in yourself . . You understand that . . And you understand that any . . really . . effective salesman . . must be awfully satisfied . . with the product that he sells . . He must be completely satisfied with his own product . . before he can effectively convince anyone to buy the product . .

But, besides the product, there is one other thing you are selling everyday . . It doesn't make any difference whether you are a salesperson . . or a doctor . . or a mechanic . . Every one of us is selling it every day . . to every one we meet . . That's right . . We are selling ourselves . . So, you see . . you must, first be satisfied with yourself . . before you can effectively sell yourself to anybody else . . You must, first, appreciate yourself . .

You're the only one there is . . like yourself . . So, appreciate yourself . . for what you are . . You must appreciate yourself for your honesty . . You must appreciate yourself . . for your integrity . . You must like yourself . . Like yourself for all the wonderful characteristics . . that you know you possess . . And there should be no question in your mind . . about your own honesty . . or your integrity . . or any of your own capabilities . . No question at all about your own . . trustworthiness . . Or even about your ability in any interpersonal relationship between you and another person . .

Of course, you like yourself . . You like what you do . . and how you are . . And you accept the challenge . . of your own daily duties . . For you realize, there aren't any lowly jobs . . Just inefficient employees . . You realize that if a person has the wit to recognize it . . there is a challenge in any job he holds . . That's why you like the job you hold . . because it has a real personal challenge . . It's a challenge to do a better job than anyone has ever done . . Of course, you have a good job . . But did you ever think you held a lowly job in the past ? . . Well, let me remind you that every job is essential . . And, should it ever befall your lot . . to be assigned a job that seems . . perhaps, beneath your dignity . . you might recall this one, simple, truth . . Every job . . is essential . .

A long time ago, in Greece . . there were some politicians . . who thought about playing a joke . . on one of their members . . So, they got him appointed as . . Chief Garbage Collector . . Well, instead of being embarrassed . . as they had planned . . this man decided to show . . what a man could do . . with such an assignment . .

He set his mind on becoming the best garbage collector there was . . And, of course . . we recognize today, that our garbage collectors . . are an essential part of the community . . But, in those days . . unsanitary conditions . . encouraged mice and rats and pestilence, for decades . .

Soon, however, those conditions were eliminated . . Habits of cleanliness were promoted . . and civic pride was developed . . In a few years . . people came to look upon the office of . . public scavenger . . as being one of dignified responsibility . . And, thereafter . . only men of high esteem . . and integrity . . could aspire to hold such a position . .

In our minds . . a job seems to be important . . or unimportant . . depending upon the attitude of the men who would till them . . So, you allow yourself to develop confidence in your own abilities . . to accomplish whatever challenge is put before you . . And you are going to allow yourself to visualize . . yourself . . right now . . accomplishing whatever you set your mind to accomplish . .

Visualize that, in your mind's eye, right now . . (Pause) You are going to be surprised and amazed . . as you see your confidence . . and your abilities . . grow rapidly . . You have already seen it improve . . And it's going to improve, even more . . because of your new state of mind . .

You are going to allow yourself to accept a suggestion . . That you are going to visualize yourself . . daily . . as being successful . . I want you to visualize yourself . . in your most successful moment . . right now . . Go ahead . . Get that image firmly in your mind . . (Pause) Let this become an accomplished fact in your mind . . right now . . You are going to be amazed at just how successful you are going to be . . And how rapidly you become completely successful, in every way . . You have been working hard toward that goal . . so . . let yourself feel comfortable . . Feel that surge of confidence come over you . . Allow yourself the luxury of feeling self-assured . . knowing you are completely self-reliant . . Visualize your self-discipline increasing . . And visualize yourself as being the most successful person that you know . . And do it, right now . . vividly, in your mind's eye . . (Pause)

Now, relax, completely . . Sink down deeper . . and deeper and DEEPER . . Relaxing more and more . . with every breath you take . . Relax . . and let every suggestion . . that you hear from my voice . . be reinforced . . over and over again . . Every suggestion is being reinforced . . and is going directly into . . the storehouse of your subconscious mind . . Continue to relax for a few more minutes . . while your subconscious mind absorbs . . everything we have talked about . .
(Pause)   EMERG

505

(Follow Relaxation)

You are resting and feeling very good about yourself . . and about being here . . Being under hypnosis is very peaceful and relaxing . . Just continue relaxing now . . Allow your conscious awareness to keep narrowing down . . as the subconscious part of your mind . . is receiving . . and absorbing . . everything I am saying to you . .

You spend a large part of your life . . at work . . and for good reason . . From now on . . you will look forward to being at work . . and to doing your work . . There are obstacles there . . to overcome . . But your work will keep becoming more enjoyable and more exciting . . And you will handle every situation . . that comes up in your work . . in a relaxed, calm and logical way . .

During your working hours . . you will be able to make decisions calmly and wisely . . You will always be able to think clearly . . and be relaxed and at ease . . in every situation . . Your self-confidence and self-reliance keep increasing . . enabling you to make decisions at work . . wisely and confidently . . You will have confidence in every decision you make . .

Your concentration keeps improving, more each day . . enabling you to do your work more perfectly . . You will anticipate great success in your work . . and you'll find that your energy and enthusiasm for your work . . continues becoming stronger . .

You will radiate a very pleasant personality . . and find that your talents, skills and abilities keep increasing . . That helps you to continue doing a better job . . Your interest in your work and your knowledge about your work . . keep increasing . . The subconscious level of your mind . . will cause your creative abilities to keep emerging . . enabling you to come up with better ideas . . that you will put into your own actions in your work . . You will always perform to the best of your ability . . And will keep becoming more and more successful . . in doing the work of your choice . .

Your success keeps increasing . . You enjoy achieving greater and greater success . . One of the things that keeps increasing your success . . is managing your time efficiently . . You plan your time wisely . . You plan your projects wisely . . You use wisdom and logic in putting your plans and projects into action . . And get tremendous pleasure in seeing them completed successfully . .

You are always sincere and honest in doing your work . . knowing that it will bring you great rewards . . and enabling you to achieve outstanding accomplishments . .

You have tremendous capabilities . . You have the talents, skills and abilities you need . . to be an exceptional success . . Your creative mind will help you make wise decisions . . that enable you to make the very best use of your talents, skills and abilities . .

You remain relaxed and calm . . as you go about your daily activities . . You are in control of all areas of your life . . Every day you will notice yourself becoming more successful . .

You are an excellent worker . . and you have great pride in your work . . You get great pleasure in continuing to improve in everything you do . . Your confidence keeps increasing . . and your happiness continues increasing . . as you become more and more successful . . in your work life and in all of your other activities . .

Continue now, to relax . . as I begin my count . .

EMERGE

NOTE : MOST SUICIDAL IMPULSES ARE TEMPORARY. MANY ARE BRIEF.
ESPECIALLY IF THERE IS SOMEONE AVAILABLE WITH WHOM THE PERSON
CAN DISCUSS THE PROBLEM (S). IF THE SUICIDAL PATTERN CAN BE
INTERRUPTED . . OR IF THE CLIENT CAN BE GIVEN A "FACE SAVING"
WAY OUT, THE SUICIDAL DANGER WILL PROBABLY LAPSE. THE
THERAPIST NEEDS TO REMEMBER THAT THE SUGGESTIONS HEREIN ARE
NOT AN ATTEMPT TO SOLVE THE PROBLEM. INSTEAD, THEY ARE
DESIGNED AS A DETERRING DEVICE ONLY IN ORDER TO HELP THE
CLIENT ACHIEVE PERMANENT AND LASTING RESULTS, YOU WILL
NEED TO "PRIORITIZE" UNCOVERING THE CAUSE OF THE PROBLEM, THEN
GET CLIENT RELEASED FROM THE CAUSE .
(Follow Relaxation)

You are resting comfortably now . . Continue to relax . . as your
subconscious mind receives and absorbs . . everything I am saying to
you . . You are having a problem with your life . . and so, we are
going to talk about this problem . . In the future . . if you ever have
any thoughts, or ideas . . feelings or impulses . . about suicide . .
those thoughts or feelings . . will be an automatic signal . . that will
cause you to call me, at once . . And you will keep doing everything
you can to get in touch with me . . until you are successful . . Do
you understand ? . .

MAKE SURE CLIENT RESPONDS AND UNDERSTANDS COMPLETELY. IF
CLIENT DOES NOT UNDERSTAND AND AGREE, EXPLAIN IT FURTHER.

As you are attempting to call me . . you will keep feeling more
comfortable and at ease . . And when you reach me, and hear my
voice . . you will become calm and relaxed, quite easily . . You will
go into a hypnotic state, quickly . . any time I tell you to . . even if
you do not want to at the time . . Do you agree to that ? . .

WAIT FOR RESPONSE. IF CLIENT SAYS, "NO", TELL CLIENT THE
FOLLOWING STATEMENT : You will still have the freedom to do whatever
you want to do . . after you come out of the hypnotic state . . So, I'm
sure you will find it agreeable . . to go into an hypnotic state, whenever I
tell you to . . You agree with that, don't you ? . .

WAIT FOR RESPONSE. ONCE YOU GET THE CLIENT TO AGREE , HE / SHE
WILL ALWAYS KEEP THEIR PROMISE.

You are understanding, clearly . . that if you ever have any impulses or
feelings . . about committing suicide . . you will immediately go to a
telephone and call me . . As soon as you begin pressing the numbers . .

you will feel better and more relaxed . . And you will be, positively, unable to commit suicide . . until after you have actually contacted me . . and informed me . . that you want me to hypnotize you . . because you have been thinking about suicide . .

If, for whatever reason, I am not available . . you will continue to relax . . and you will, automatically, go into a deep hypnotic state . . You will remain in the hypnotic state . . and continue feeling calm and peaceful . . as long as you need to . . until I am available . . However, when your mind is aware . . that your desire to commit suicide, has faded away . . In about five or ten minutes . . you will awaken from the hypnotic state . . feeling peaceful and serene . . You will continue to try to contact me . . even if it is the next day and the situation has passed . . I still want you to inform me of the experience . . and everything that occurred . .

During the time you are in the hypnotic state . . you will experience a strong sense of awareness . . of the fact that you were created . . by the same creator . . that created every other person on this planet, Earth . . You will realize that you are just as good, and just as deserving of a happy, enjoyable, prosperous life, as any other person . . You will accept the thoughts and ideas . . coming out of your inner mind, into your conscious awareness . . And you will experience a sense of love, joy, forgiveness and oneness with your creator . . You will experience a feeling of tranquility and well-being . . You will find yourself thinking, saying and doing, the right thing at right time and in the right way . . Whatever you need to know, you will realize, your inner mind already knows . .

EMERGE

SUICIDE - OVERCOME
BEFORE REASON IS REALIZED

(Follow Relaxation)

As you continue to relax . . I want you to begin sinking deeper . . and DEEPER . . More and more relaxed . . as you go down deeper . . DEEPER and DEEPER now . . Relax as you go down DEEPER . . Relax . . I am going to give you some suggestions now . . And these suggestions are going to take complete and thorough effect upon you . . immediately . .

For the first time in your life . . you have some idea, some inkling . . of why you thought about committing suicide . . It doesn't matter why you thought about it in the past . . it was wrong . . And we know it was wrong because, otherwise . . you would have realized that, suicide, was not the answer to the problem . . And you wouldn't have thought of it . . Therefore, you have considered that suicide is . . a sort of an answer to the problem . . The only reason people do things . . is because they feel that it is an answer to a problem . . And though they don't think so . . in their conscious mind . . they do believe it . . in their subconscious mind . .

The truth of the matter is . . your reason for contemplating suicide . . is because you believe, in your own mind . . that you are already dead . . I realize that sounds fantastic . . but that is exactly what you had in your mind . . And to an extent . . you still do . . Because you were trying to bring your body into conformation . . with the belief that was in your mind . . Now, this has to be distinguished from a 'Death-Wish' . . A person who 'wishes he were dead' . . does so because the pain is too great . . Or this situation is just too bad or, that's too 'something else' . . No . . A death wish is something entirely different . .

You have probably heard people say, "Oh, my God, I can't stand any more of this . . I wish I were dead" . . Dead, in order to get away from the simple problems of every day life . . The slings and arrows of adversity . . But you remember, in Shakespeare's, "Hamlet" . . When Hamlet considered suicide . . on the basis of, "To be or not to be ? That is the question" . . He also considered . . "Perchance to Dream . . Aye, That is the rub" . . What kind of dream would there be in this, 'Sleep of Death' ? . . You see, one never realizes . . One never knows . . It just might be . . that in the Sleep of Death . . the situations would be even worse, than they are in life . . And in this, Sleep of Death . . you really would endure 'All sorts of Hell' . . And that's what comes to everyone's mind . . who considers suicide on the basis of . . a 'Death Wish' . . And that is why . . once that is considered . . the idea of attempting suicide . . is quickly forgotten . .

I'm talking now, about a genuine suicide attempt . . Not about the attempts, in order to get attention . . Not about the attempts . . in order to have someone run to you and be sympathetic . . I'm talking about genuine attempts . . to end one's life . . So, genuine attempts . . to end one's life . . are not conducted . . on the basis of . . a Death wish . . And, they are not on the basis of getting attention . . They are based on perfect logic . . If a person believes, in his own mind, that he is already dead . . then it makes perfect sense to attempt to get the body to conform . . to the belief which the mind already has . . After all, if you believe yourself to be a plumber . . you're going to buy overalls . . so you'll look the part . . If you believe yourself to be a doctor . . you'll buy a business suit . . or maybe a white coat . . You clothe your body with the type of clothing . . that corresponds to the belief your mind has, of what you, yourself, are . . And this is just as true, whether it's a belief that you are dead . . or whether it's a belief that you're a physician . . So, now you know . . this is not a Death Wish . . because you want to live . . If that is agreeable to you, you might say, "Well, Why can't I just change my mind . . and conform my thinking in line with what my body is ? . . My body is alive . . so I'll just make my mind alive . . That's an easier way . .

The answer is . . Of course, it's an easier way . . And that's exactly what we're going to do . . But it's not so completely easy . . because we don't know exactly how you got the idea in your mind . . to begin with . . that you were dead . . When, consciously, you know very well . . that you are alive . . If I ask you, right now . . "Are you alive ?" . . You will say, "Well, Yes . . I'm alive" . . But your subconscious mind would say, "NO" . . Because your subconscious would reason, "There was a time in my life when I knew I was dying . . and I accepted that belief . . I could not help myself and no one else could help me . . And, at that particular age level . . and at that particular time . . I really felt that I was dying . . And so, I accepted the thought that I was dead . .

511

There is only one way to get a thought out of the subconscious mind, and that is . . Get it out, the same way it went in . . When it went in . . you were hypnotized . . if you want to use that word . . Hypnotized into the belief . . that you'd accepted yourself . . to be dead . . And your symptoms . . the symptoms for which you came in here . . began, at that time . . And you've been trying . . one way or another . . to make your body conform to that belief, ever since . . And we're now going to remove that idea . . from the deepest part of your subconscious mind . . Just as soon as we can get you back here . . and age regress you . . back to that particular time in your life . . when all of this started . . But, that is not all we're going to do . . The first and foremost thing to be done . . is to give you a strong suggestion, right now . . And that is to absolutely prevent . . any further suicide attempts or thoughts . . Absolutely and unconditionally . . prohibit you from attempting suicide, in any way . . Until we can get this straightened out . . And here is how it works . .

From this moment on . . if even the slightest urge comes over you, to think of doing away with yourself, at all . . Immediately, in your mind's eye . . you will recall that the only reason you want to do this . . is to conform your body with your mind's idea of yourself . . And your mind has accepted the concept that you are dead . . You have a therapist who is curing this problem . . And you are leaving it in his hands . . You are not going to be your own therapist and do yourself in . .

Instead, you are going to say . . "Wait . . That is something for the therapist to do . . He will take care of that . . That is why I am paying him . . That is why I am going to him . .

So, from this moment on . . you are, absolutely, unconditionally prohibited . . from any suicidal attempt whatsoever . . Direct or indirect . . disguised or undisguised . . But that doesn't mean you are through . . Oh, NO . . You have just begun . . Because we have yet to get to the very time . . the very incident . .

There was an incident in your past . . in which your mind had accepted the notion that you are dead . . And now, you believe yourself to be dead . . And you have believed yourself to be dead . . from that first moment . . Because you realized, at that moment . . at that time in your life . . at that age and with the mind of that person, at that age . . that you were in such a position that you were

512

totally helpless . . You couldn't help yourself and no one else could help you . . You thought you were dying and you thought . . you did die . . And that suggestion . . under your self-hypnosis . . sealed itself into the deepest part of your subconscious mind . . And so, we are going to remove it . . as soon as we can find it . .

And so, I now give to you, this suggestion . . That you are going to have a dream . . You are going to have a very vivid dream . . A dream so vivid, that it wakes you up in the middle of the night . . And that dream is going to be about . . that death incident . . The incident where you really thought you had died . . Not only is it going to come to you in a dream . . but you're going to write it down . . as soon as you wake up . . You're going to get up and write it all down . . And you can't go back to sleep until you write it all down . . You write down every detail . . Writing on one side of the page only . . And writing clearly . . And you bring it to me, the next time you come in . . And the same incident will pop into your head . . later on . . in the waking state . . You may have only one incident . . or you might even have two . . There may be more than one . . But there is, at least, one . . And it will pop into your mind, from the deepest part of your subconscious . . when you least expect it . . In a dream or in the waking state . . Write it down, complete in every detail . . We are going to take you back . . to that time . . to that incident . . You are going to relive it . . And you are going to realize that you did, indeed, live through it . . surprisingly enough . .

And now, I want you to rest . . And I want you to sleep . . And I want you to relax . . Really relax . . completely, in every way . . Five minutes from now . . you will go to sleep . . A very deep, restful sleep . . You will not consciously remember anything but a very deep, peaceful sleep . . After one hour of pleasant sleep . . you will wake up, refreshed . . and feeling good about yourself . .

Right now, I am going to give you a period of silence . . And during this period of silence . . These suggestions I have given you . . will take complete and thorough effect . . upon your mind, body and spirit . . And that period of silence begins . . now . .

Client will SELF-EMERGE after approx. one hour.

513

SURGERY PREPARATION
UNDER HYPNOSIS
(Follow Light Relaxation)

You are resting easy now . . and you will continue feeling the sensations of comfort . . and relaxation . . while your subconscious mind is listening . . to each word I say to you . .

As you continue relaxing . . your conscious mind keeps becoming more peaceful . . Each time you inhale . . you bring the breath of life into your body . . And you feel your oneness with God . .

Every time your heart beats . . it pumps blood through your circulatory system . . in a perfect way . . Like a song of health and strength . . and life . .

Your entire body continues becoming more relaxed . . more peaceful and more at ease . . And you realize that everything is being worked out . . for your perfect health . . Your perfect well-being and happiness . .

Your doctor believes your physical condition can be corrected . . And that means your body will respond properly . . And you will soon experience complete and perfect recovery . . And your body will be totally rejuvenated . .

You have selected a doctor that you have great confidence in . . So your mind is at peace . . and your faith is strong . . Your confidence is increasing . . and you know everything will go smoothly . .

Each time you see water . . Each time you touch, think of . . or imagine water . . or hear the word, water . . that will be a signal for you to become more relaxed . . calm and peaceful . . Your subconscious mind will cause the signal you have been given . . to work at all times . . And keep you calm and completely relaxed . . regardless of where you are or what is going on around you . .

God's will is that you always have a healthy body . . Your mind is understanding that . . and is causing the processes of your body to function properly . . and restore your health in a perfect way . .

You are feeling more comfortable now . . and are experiencing restful, calming sensations of relaxation . . in every part of your body . .

When the time comes that they begin preparing you . . to enter the operating room . . your subconscious mind will recall . . how comfortable and peaceful you are now . . And will automatically cause you to continue . . to experience this same feeling of calmness and relaxation . .

Being prepared to enter the operating room will be a signal . . that will cause you to relax completely . . And you will remain comfortable and at ease . . throughout the operation . .

At all times, you will feel safe and secure . . Your mind is at ease . . You have faith and confidence in your doctor . . And you know everything will go smoothly . . You will be pleasantly surprised at how relaxed and calm you will be . . You will be able to breath easily . . because you will be peaceful . . and at ease . .

As soon as they begin preparing you . . to enter the operating room . . that will be an automatic signal . . to cause your muscles . . and your nerves . . to relax . . You will be completely relaxed during surgery . . and will remain relaxed . . after the surgery has been completed . .

Your breathing will be regular, strong and easy . . Your heart will continue pumping . . and will remain strong and regular . .

When the surgery has been completed . . all of the activities and functions of your body . . will work normally . . and will cause your body to heal rapidly . .

Your body will heal so quickly and so perfectly . . that you will be able to look back on this whole experience . . and be pleasantly surprised, at how easy it was . .

Your mind is peaceful and at ease . . And you will remain relaxed and calm . . even after you awaken . . from this hypnotic state of relaxation . .

Your mind will be thinking only good, uplifting thoughts . . at all times . . And your mind will receive only good thoughts . . and energy vibrations, from others . . before surgery . . during surgery . . and after surgery . .

You will continue to relax . . as instructed . . You are now ready to come up . . to a wide awake, fully alert state . . Feeling comfortable, confident and happy . . On the count of THREE . . you will be fully awake . . feeling good about everything . .

ONE . . Coming up now . . Coming closer to the surface . .

TWO . . Feeling much better . . Breathe the breath of life into your body . .

THREE . . Fully awake and alert . . You may open your eyes now . . You are doing very well . .

There was once a young rattlesnake named, Seymour . . Now, Seymour was a very clever snake . . who loved to drink lemonade while wearing his 'cool' sunglasses . . whenever he went up to ground level . . for basking in the sunshine . .

"You'd better take off those cool shades, young snake", his mother would scold . . "If that farmer comes around, you may not see him in time . . and you'll be in big trouble!"

But Seymour knew what he wanted in life . . He was old enough, he thought . . He didn't need advise all the time . . He would get along in the world just fine . . He was quite comfortable with things, just as they were . . And, It wasn't long before Seymour was snoozing peacefully . .

Quietly, the farmer tippy-toed up . . as close to the sleeping rattler as he dared . . He raised his shovel high into the air . . and yelled, "I got'cha, little rattler !"

Seymour jumped and rolled . . screaming back down into his hole . . just as the shovel buried itself into the dirt . . where he'd been sunning . . As he slithered down deep into the chamber . . he shouted excitedly, "Mom! . . That old farmer almost caught me napping . . That was really close" . .

"It was close, all right," Mom agreed, then asked . . "Where's your tail?"

Seymour looked in disbelief . . My TAIL ! He chopped off my tail ! . . He can't do that to me"! he cried . . "Can he" ? . .

His mother advised, "I know just what you're going through, son . . Almost the very same thing happened to me . . when I was your age . . She was very sympathetic and suggested . . "Lay on the bed and I'll get the plastic surgeon . . Maybe he can do something for you." . .

After examining little Seymour . . the plastic surgeon wagged his tongue and said . . "I'm afraid the best I can do is to cover it over . . with old molten skin . . Would you like that, Seymour?" . .

"No way", cried the little snake . . "I don't want to be sewn up like a crazy quilt blanket" . .

The plastic surgeon wagged his tongue a few more times and left the family to ponder what to do . . knowing they would do all they could for him . .

Big Jake the Snake pushed his way into the bedroom . . where his young friend lay in anguish . . "I just heard about your problem, Seymour . . and I have a suggestion for you . . Without your rattles . . you can curl yourself up and roll like a Hoop Snake . . You'll travel a lot faster" . .

"But I don't want to be a Hoop Snake, Jake", Seymour cried. "I just want to be a rattler". .

Seymour's sister, Slitheri . . had been quietly taking it all in . . Finally, she spoke up . . "I've been talking with my teacher, Seymour . . She would like you to enroll in the Special Add Class . . I don't know why but . . she thinks you're bright enough to become an ADDER."

Again, Seymour shook his body in revulsion's . . "No, no, NO! I don't have rattle buttons to count on now . . So I am positively Not going to be an Adder . . Somehow, I'm going to be a Rattler . . I'm go to the rubbish dump to think this out . . Come on, Big Jake . . You can give me a fang" . .

Together they slithered through the grass to where the farmer dumped his rubbish . . They dove down deep into the mess . . not knowing what they were looking for . . Stopping to catch their breath . . Seymour suddenly noticed little Squeegy . . the field mouse . . peeking at them from under a corn stalk . .

"Go away, Squeegy", Seymour snipped at her . . "I'm in big trouble . . and there is nothing a little mouse like you . . can do to help" . .

Squeegy smiled and replied, "Maybe there isn't . . Or maybe there is . . Just because I'm different than you are . . doesn't mean I can't understand . . what your needs are, Seymour . .

"What do you know"? Seymour replied . . "You're just a mouse . . A gray, furry little mouse . . And besides that . . You're a girl"! . .

Squeegy just smiled and asked, "How would you feel if I showed you . . just the thing you need most in life ?"

Seymour thought for a moment. Then he answered . . "If you can give me the one thing I need most in life . . I promise I will NEVER invite you home for dinner" . .

With that she scampered over, tugging him by the nose . . "Come on", she said. "Just follow me" . .

Single file, Squeegy led them through the maze of broken items; dishes, toys . . and piles of junk from bygone days . . She stopped at an old baby carriage . . and looked up at it with gleaming eyes . .

"Up there, Seymour . . Up in this old carriage is where you'll find the answer to your dreams" . .

"A Baby Carriage ? . . Okay", Seymour was confused but finally agreed, "This had better be good" . . Stealthily, the little snake wound his way to the top of the carriage . . disappearing over the edge and down inside . . Several moments of silence passed . . Then, a great rattling noise came from up above . . Seymour's smiling face appeared . . at the rim of the pram, as he yelled . . "Squeegy! We were meant for each other . . I love you, Squeegy!"

Then to his friend, he yelled, "Big Jake . . find me some masking tape . . Quick! . . Oh, this is gon'na be So-o Cool."

Okay", Jake replied . . "I'll get some tape for you but . . What did you find up there ?"

Seymour leaped from the top of the pram . . in parachute-like fashion . . Slowly, drifting down to his dearest friends . . tightly clinging onto his newest prize . . a baby's RATTLE . .

After taping it onto his tail . . Seymour came to realize . . that he would have been much better off . . to have listened to his parents when they offered advise . . They had similar experiences when they were young . . So, he vowed to thank them . . and his sister and Big Jake, his friend . . for offering their help . . He began to understand that everything in life changes . . And it was up to him to adjust to the changes . . Most importantly, he began to see how he had misjudged . . his new friend, little Squeegy . . Sure, she was different than he was . . She didn't have tough Rhino skin . . all green with orange stripes . . She looked kind of gray . . with pink ears . . But the important thing was . . she was kind of . . smart . . In fact, they thought a lot alike . . about a lot of things . . They really did have a lot in common . . That was when he made up his mind . . to think for himself . . and not make judgments about others . . from useless gossip . .

Seymour suddenly had a thought . . Hmm . . A rattle snake and a field mouse as good friends ? I wonder what the farmer would think of that . .

EMERGE

(Follow Relaxation)

You are resting easy now . . and you will continue feeling the sensations of comfort . . and relaxation . . while your subconscious mind is listening . . to each word I say to you . . As you continue relaxing . . your conscious mind keeps becoming more peaceful . . Each time you inhale . . you bring the breath of life . . into your body . .

Your body is one of your most prized possessions . . You realize the importance of your body . . And you are aware that only you can take care of it . . You respect your body and you desire for it to always be healthy . . In addition to wanting your body to be healthy . . you want your appearance to be good . . You will look much better wearing those new dentures . . and you will be more calm and relaxed, when you are eating . . It will be easy for you to chew your food, enabling your food to digest properly . . You will also feel more at ease, when you smile . .

Notice how good you feel, right now . . You are breathing much more easily and freely . . Every muscle, from the top of your head to the bottom of your feet . . is relaxing peacefully and comfortably . .

I lived in a forest area at one time . . And as I would drive through the beautiful hillsides . . I would often marvel at how beautiful they looked . . Then one day, there was a terrible fire . . that destroyed nearly all of the area . . The hills turned black and the trees were gone . . Hardly what one would call, 'beautiful' . . And I thought how terrible it was, to have all that beauty ruined . .

However, as time passed . . I began to witness a miracle . . I began to notice little patches of green, here and there . . Little trees began growing . . The lost beauty was returning . . The last time I drove over that road . . I thought of life . . It doesn't matter what happens . . Injuries may occur . . Teeth may decay . . They may even need to be replaced . . Yet, life continues to go on, in everything we do . . We may develop a few scars . . but we continue to recuperate . . Maybe not exactly the same as before . . yet, sometimes, in a new and better way . . What a miracle this is . .

Whenever I recall that forest fire, a few years ago . . I also recall the transforming power that brought newness and beauty . . to that area once more . .

You are feeling calm and peaceful now . . And realizing a new and wonderful feeling of confidence and pride in yourself . . This relaxation . . that you are experiencing . . is enabling you to realize that . . even though the teeth you were born with, have been removed . . they have now been replaced with new teeth . . And your mouth and gums can adjust to those new teeth . . just as easily and comfortably . . as it adjusted to the teeth that were removed . . In fact, you can enjoy your new teeth, even more . . Knowing that they will never wear out and will never get any cavities . .

I want you to do something for me now . . I want you to hold your (L / R) arm, straight out in front of you . . and make it rigid and stiff . . Make it just as stiff as you can make it . . Now, notice the feeling of energy and strength in that arm . . Okay, now, let the arm relax and feel very comfortable . . Just put your hand down on your lap again . .

Now, just by deciding . . to make your arm, rigid and stiff . . you were able to do that . . You controlled it easily . . just by listening to what I told you, and responding . . Because you were willing to respond . . And just as easily . . you can control any other part of your body . . including the muscles in your mouth and throat . .

Your subconscious mind is realizing that you are in control . . And any time you decide to put your teeth in your mouth . . they will always feel comfortable . . In fact, your teeth will soon feel so comfortable . . that you won't even think about them being in your mouth . . They will feel normal and natural . .

You will always feel good about your appearance . . with the teeth in your mouth . . The dentures will function easily . . And you will be able to eat any kind of food you desire to eat . .

In just a few moments, we will be concluding this session . . And you will awaken from the hypnotic state, feeling rested and refreshed . . You will feel as though you have just awakened from a long, restful, enjoyable nap . . Your whole body will feel vibrant and alive . . And you will be full of energy and vitality . .

Continue to relax . . as I begin to count , from ONE to FIVE . . When you hear me say the number FIVE . . you will open your eyes, feeling good about everything in your life . .

I will begin my count now . .

ONE . . TWO . . THREE . . FOUR . . FIVE . .

You will continue drifting into a deeper . . and more peaceful state of relaxation . . Your subconscious mind is aware and absorbing the suggestions . . and the guidance I am giving you . .

These suggestions along with the instructions I am giving you . . will enable you to get rid of that problem . . of teeth grinding, completely . . We are going to help the muscles in your jaws to relax . . during the night, while you are sleeping . . And, during the day . . as you go about your daily activities . . You will avoid stressful situations, during the day . . and allow your jaws to be slack and loose . . As relaxed as possible . . At night, you will want to keep your mouth relaxed . . but slightly open . . wide enough to place your tongue between your back teeth . . That will keep your jaws loose and flexible . . And do what you can to avoid . . stressful dreams . .

When you are ready to sleep . . take a deep breath . . through your nose, and hold it . . Then, release it slowly . . Do this three times, and you will relax . . This will be a signal for your jaws to remain relaxed . . through the night . . You are learning to be relaxed and calm . . at all times . . When you are sleeping at night . . as well as when you go about your activities, during the day . .

Your subconscious mind has capabilities, far beyond what you have been consciously aware of . . And your mind is remembering everything it needs to . . for keeping your jaws . . and your entire body . . relaxed and calm . . during the night, when you are asleep . . Or during the day . .

From now on . . you will be completely relaxed and calm . . during the night, when you are sleeping . . After you breath deeply, three times . . just before you go to sleep . . Your mind will hold the thought . . "Lips together -Teeth apart" . . That will have the effect of enabling your lips to stay together . . and your teeth to remain apart, during the night . . while you are sleeping . . The only time your lips will need to part, during the night, while you are sleeping . . is in a normal way to enable you to breath easily and freely . . and to keep them moist . .

You are deeply relaxed now . . DEEPLY RELAXED . . And you will notice a feeling . . of a calming peacefulness . . coming over your whole body . . That calmness . . and peacefulness . . will continue, during your daily life . . and during the night, when you are sleeping . .

Each night, just before you go to sleep . . I want you to close your eyes . . gently inhale, through your nose . . and think the words . . "Lips together - Teeth apart" . . As you continue doing that . . each night . . you keep reinforcing the idea in your mind . . And your subconscious mind will cooperate . . and cause it to become normal and natural . . as you sleep peacefully and calmly . .

You will also find your self-confidence and self-acceptance growing stronger . . And you will continue improving . . in all areas of your life . . physically, mentally, emotionally and spiritually . .

All of the suggestions and instructions I have given you . . are in the storehouse of your subconscious mind . . They are already working . . and will keep becoming more effective each day . . They will continue influencing your feelings and actions in a positive, helpful way . . You will notice the improvements . . and be very pleased with your continuous progress . .

In a moment, we will be concluding this session . . I will begin my count . . from ONE to FIVE . . and when you hear me say the number, FIVE . . you will open your eyes . . awake and alert . .

Now, I will begin my count . .

ONE, TWO, THREE, FOUR, and FIVE.

(Follow Relaxation)

You will continue drifting into a deeper . . and more peaceful state of relaxation . . Drifting deeper now . . DEEPER . . DEEPER . . and DEEPER . . All other sounds are in the far distance . . except for the sound of my voice . . There may be times when you don't hear my voice . . and that is okay . . Your subconscious mind is aware of everything I am saying . . As you go DEEPER . . and DEEPER into a restful state of complete relaxation . . It is so peaceful . . as you sink down deeper and DEEPER . . into a blissful state of relaxation . . Going just a little deeper . . with every breath you take . . It is so good . . to be calm . . and sedate . . So peaceful here . . Just relax . . (Pause)

It feels so wonderful, doesn't it . . to be so loose . . letting it all out . . Resting this way . . Relaxation is simply wonderful . . Now, tension . . is just the opposite of relaxation . . No one can ever relax and feel comfortable . . when they are tense . . One must relieve and release tension . . in order to relax fully and completely . . Talking about it, won't do it . . You have to really . . let go . . You have to feel the emotion, flowing right out of you . . You have to relieve yourself of energy . . by releasing it out from you . . Otherwise, it overflows inside . . causing many kinds of symptoms . . So, you acquire an excess accumulation of symptoms and of energy . . These excess symptoms lead to excess tension . . in the very body organs that need to be relieved of tension . .

Of course, there are many ways you can release tension . . You can express hostility in a socially acceptable manner . . Like punching a bag or beating on a drum . . or painting a picture . . You can throw things or beat on things . . Or you could vigorously clean your house . . If you think about it, there are hundreds of things you can do . . to release tension . .

Perhaps one of the best ways is through sexual intercourse . . As the old saying goes . . Sex does release tension . . And the more of it you have . . the more tension is released . . It is very difficult to find a tense person who has an active sex life . . It is not possible to reach four or five climaxes a day and still remain tense . . Likewise, one cannot remain tense if they are running a mile or two . . playing a set of tennis or having a vigorous swim . . Good, strong, physical exercise relieves tension . . and enables the mind, the body and the spirit to relax . . Relaxation is good for you . . but in order to attain a state of relaxation . . you must, first, release tension . . And rather than relieving tension by only one method . . it is better to combine a number of methods . .

Therefore, you should, FIRST . . express whatever hostility and anger you hold . . in a socially acceptable way . . TWO . . Engage yourself in a healthy but strenuous exercise . . in which you can become joyfully tired . . THREE . . Keep yourself physically fit by exercising regularly and working out . . FOUR . . Make certain that you have a full and active sexual life . . Seeing to it that you reach an adequate number of climaxes for yourself, and your partner . . daily . . This channels your emotional energy away from internal symptoms . . and allows you to express yourself, externally . . in a socially acceptable manner . .

These suggestions will enable you to relax fully and completely in every way . . And there will be a halt to the production of internal symptoms . . brought about by the internalization of tension . .

I want you to relax for another moment . . then I am going to give you suggestions . . that will help you alleviate this problem you are having . . with tension . .

You are ready now, so I will begin . . I am going to count, from ONE to FIVE . . And as I count to FIVE . . I want you to apply tension to every single muscle in your body . . Just as tight and strenuous as it is possible for you . . to tense yourself . . Extremely tight . .

ONE . . Feel yourself tightening . . tightening up . . Your hands tighten up . . Your arms tighten up . . Your elbows . . Everything . . Your legs tighten up . . Your feet tighten up . . and stiffen . . Every single muscle tightens . . Even your neck pulls back as every single muscle tightens . . And you feel yourself being drawn up into a knot . . TWO . . Every single muscle tightens . . Every single muscle in your body tightens . . Tighter and tighter and tighter . . Pulling against each other, tightening . . Very, very tight . . THREE . . You've never been so uptight before . . Very, very tight and tense . . in every way . . Almost like you were going to jump right out of your skin . . FOUR . . Extremely tight and tense . . And now, FIVE . . Very, very tense . . very tense . . Tense as you have never been in your life . . And, in a few moments . . In a few moments . . I am going to clap my hands . . And when I do . . you're going to release . . all this tension completely, in every way . . But you're very tight and very tense, right now . . Very tight and tense . . And you'll hold onto it longer . . than you'd think is possible for you to do . . And, in just a moment, I'm going to clap my hands . . And when I do . . you'll release all of that tension completely . .

Now, get ready, and . . RELEASE ! (CLAP) Release completely, in every way And let all your muscles completely relax and let go . . For you're going to relax completely now . . Let all that tension flow . . out of your hands and your feet . . All of the muscles in your entire body are completely relaxing in every way . . And you sink down deeper . . and DEEPER and DEEPER . . DEEPER . . and DEEPER . . and DEEPER . . Into the deepest, most profound hypnotic state you have ever been in . . As deep as you are now . . Soon, you will begin to level off . . and you will enjoy this peaceful, comforting state of complete relaxation . . And all of these suggestions . . take complete and thorough effect on you . . On your mind, your body and your spirit . . Deeply relaxed . . Deeply relaxed . .

I am going to give you a few moments of silence now . . as your subconscious mind absorbs everything we have talked about today . . And giving your body a chance to enjoy . . and appreciate this comforting state of relaxation you are in now . . Just relax . . Relax . .   (pause)

Your mind is peacefully at ease . . And you will remain relaxed and calm . . even after you awaken . . from this hypnotic state of relaxation . .

Your mind will be thinking only good, uplifting thoughts . . at all times . . And your mind will receive only good thoughts . . and energy vibrations, from others . . You will continue to relax . . as instructed . . You are now ready to come up . . to a wide awake, fully alert state . . Feeling comfortable, confident and joyful . .

On the count of THREE . . you will be fully awake . . feeling good about everything . .

ONE . . Coming up now . . Coming closer to the surface . .

TWO . . Feeling much better . . Breathe in the breath of life . . into your body . .

THREE . . You may open your eyes now . . Fully awake and alert . . You are doing very well . .

525

147 Prescript.   THERAPY - FINGER RESPONSE

QUESTIONS FOR THERAPY BETWEEN SESSIONS
(TO BE USED WITH FINGER-RESPONSE)

NOTE : THE FOLLOWING QUESTIONS ARE SOME THAT CAN BE ASKED TO DISCOVER THE CAUSES OF THE PROBLEM. THEY ARE NOT IN ANY ORDER AND ARE GUIDELINES ONLY. THEY ARE TO BE USED ESPECIALLY WITH 'OBESITY', HOWEVER, THE ONES WITH * IN FRONT OF THEM CAN BE USED FOR FINDING CAUSES OF OTHER PROBLEMS BY MERELY EXCHANGING THE QUESTION (WORD) FROM, OVERWEIGHT, TO WHATEVER PROBLEM (WORD) YOU ARE DEALING WITH.

1. IS THERE SOME EMOTIONAL REASON CAUSING YOU TO BE OVERWEIGHT ?

2.   IS YOUR SUBCONSCIOUS MIND WILLING FOR YOU TO CONSCIOUSLY KNOW THE REASON YOU ARE OVERWEIGHT ?

3. * IS THERE SOME IMPRINT OR IMPRESSION IN YOUR MIND CAUSING YOU TO BE OVERWEIGHT ?   (IF ANSWER IS "YES", EXPLORE . FIND OUT IF THERE IS MORE THAN ONE.)

4. * IS THERE SOME THOUGHT OR IDEA IN YOUR MIND CAUSING YOU TO BE OVERWEIGHT ?   (IF ANSWER IS "YES", EXPLORE. FIND OUT IF THERE IS MORE THAN ONE.)

5.* IS THERE SOME BELIEF IN YOUR MIND CAUSING YOU TO BE OVERWEIGHT ? (IF ANSWER IS "YES", EXPLORE.   FIND OUT IF THERE IS MORE THAN ONE.)

6. ARE YOU IDENTIFYING WITH SOMEONE , PERHAPS A PARENT OR OTHER RELATIVE, WHO IS OVERWEIGHT ?

7. *ARE YOU USING EXCESS WEIGHT AS A WAY OF PUNISHING YOURSELF ?

8. *ARE YOU USING EXCESS WEIGHT AS A WAY OF HARMING YOURSELF ?

9. IS THERE SOME CONFLICT IN YOUR MIND, OVER SEX, THAT CAUSES YOU TO BE OVERWEIGHT ?

10.*ARE THERE FEARS, IN YOUR MIND, CAUSING YOU TO BE OVERWEIGHT ?

11. ARE YOU USING YOUR EXCESS WEIGHT FOR SOME PURPOSE ?

    A .   TO AVOID A RELATIONSHIP WITH THE OPPOSITE SEX ?

    B .   FOR REVENGE ? TO GET EVEN WITH SOMEONE ?

    C .   TO COVER UP FEELINGS OF BEING INFERIOR TO OTHERS ?

12. ARE YOU OVERWEIGHT BECAUSE YOU WANT TO HURT YOURSELF ?

13. ARE YOU OVERWEIGHT BECAUSE YOU WANT TO HURT SOMEONE ELSE ?

14. ARE THERE ANY OTHER MOTIVES OR REASONS YOU ARE OVERWEIGHT ?

NOTE : WHEN SOME OF THE QUESTIONS HAVE BEEN ANSWERED, IT MAY BE NECESSARY TO LEARN MORE. CONTINUE ASKING QUESTIONS UNTIL YOU GET CLIENTS SUBCONSCIOUS TO AGREE THAT CLIENT IS RELEASED AND FREE FROM CONTROL THAT IMPRINTS / IMPRESSIONS HAVE HAD OVER THEM.

FOR EXAMPLE, IN QUESTION # 7 , IF THE ANSWER IS YES, YOU MAY NEED TO CONTINUE ASKING QUESTIONS TO DISCOVER WHY CLIENT FEELS A NEED TO BE PUNISHED. IT MAY BE DUE TO GUILT FEELINGS. IF SO, THAT NEEDS TO BE ADDRESSED SO CLIENT CAN BE RELEASED FROM THE CONTROL IT IS HAVING. THERE MAY BE AN OCCASIONAL CASE, EVEN AFTER ALL THE CAUSES SEEM TO HAVE BEEN UNCOVERED, IN WHICH A CLIENT HAS A RELAPSE. IF THIS HAPPENS, VERIFY THE CLIENT'S METABOLISM (DIGESTIVE & ELIMINATION SYSTEMS) TO ENSURE THEY ARE FUNCTIONING PROPERLY TO CLEANSE ALL EXCESS WASTE PRODUCTS OUT OF THE BODY, SO IT DOES NOT TURN TO FAT. THIS CAN ALSO BE ACCOMPLISHED BY USE OF THE FINGER - RESPONSE TECHNIQUE.

NOTE : INSIGHT REGARDING THE CAUSES OF OVERWEIGHT, OVEREATING, OR ANY OTHER PROBLEM, IS IMPORTANT IN OBTAINING PERMANENT RESULTS.)

15. DO YOU OVEREAT WHEN YOU FEEL LONELY ? REJECTED ? UNLOVED ?

16. DO YOU OVEREAT WHEN YOU FEEL TENSE ? ANXIOUS ? WORRIED ?

17. DO YOU OVEREAT TO FEEL MORE SECURE ?

18. DO YOU USE YOUR EXCESS WEIGHT (FAT) TO HIDE YOURSELF FROM SOMETHING ?

19. IS ONE OF THE REASONS FOR YOUR OVEREATING BECAUSE YOU FELT BETTER WHEN YOU WERE BEING FED, WHEN YOU WERE A BABY ?

20. IS FOOD EVER EATEN, BY YOU, AS A REWARD OR AS A BRIBE ?

21. DO YOU THINK ABOUT FOOD, WHEN YOU ARE EMOTIONALLY UPSET ?

22. DO YOU LIKE THE WAY YOUR BODY LOOKS NOW ?

23.   DO YOU TEND TO DISLIKE THE WAY YOU LOOK ?

24.   DO YOU DISLIKE YOURSELF, IN OTHER WAYS ?

25.   ARE YOU OVERWEIGHT TO MAKE YOURSELF UNATTRACTIVE TO MEMBERS OF THE OPPOSITE SEX ?

26.   DO YOU SUBSTITUTE FOOD, TO AVOID HAVING SEXUAL INTERCOURSE ?

27.   IS THERE SOME CONFLICT IN YOUR MIND, OVER SEX, THAT CAUSES YOU TO EAT MORE FOOD THAN YOUR BODY NEEDS ?

28.   ARE THERE ANY OTHER MOTIVES, OR REASONS, YOU OVEREAT ?

29.

30.

31.

32.

Add your own questions above.

(Follow Relaxation and/or other Prescription)

Now that you are resting peacefully . . and you are in a deep, hypnotic state . . I am going to explain something that your subconscious mind will understand . . And what I explain, will make it much easier . . for your subconscious mind . . to work out a pleasant solution to that problem . .

Therapy, through hypnosis . . can be compared to when you first began learning to read . . You started, by learning to recognize the letters of the alphabet . . Then you learned . . that the letters of the alphabet . . are arranged in different combinations . . to form different words . . You continued learning more and more . . about the different combinations of letters . . And it kept becoming easier for you to recognize words . . Then, you began learning to recognize combinations of words . . put together to make sentences . . And then you learned to read paragraphs . . Soon, the time came when you could read stories and books . . And you could understand the meanings of what you read . .

That is comparable to the way, therapy through hypnosis, works . . Except, in a hypnotic state . . as you are in now . . your subconscious mind is able to learn and understand things . . much more quickly . .

Your subconscious mind can review things . . you already know . . even though you are not consciously aware . . that you know them . . By reviewing the information in your mind . . that points to what has caused the problem . . your subconscious mind can assess that information . . and understand it from a different point of view . . than you had, when the information first went into your mind . . And it can work out a pleasant solution . . and develop pleasant ways of completely resolving the problem . .

It is similar to knowing how to read . . Once you know how to read . . and you come to a word that is unfamiliar . . you can figure out the meaning . . from the sentence it is contained in . . Or, you can go to a dictionary and look up the meaning . . Or, simply ask someone, who does know . .

Your mind is comparable to a computer . . It contains all information . . of everything you have ever read . . Everything you have ever seen . . Everything you have ever heard, felt, or experienced . .

Your subconscious mind knows how to sort out that information . . assess it and understand it . . And work out a solution to that problem . . to get that problem resolved, completely . .

Right now, there is nothing important for your conscious mind to do . . Your conscious mind can continue relaxing . . while your subconscious mind . . is free to respond to the suggestions . . and instructions . . that I am giving you . .

You continue moving deeper now . . into a DEEPER . . hypnotic state . . to assist your subconscious mind . . in experiencing this new insight . . with understanding . . And that is good . .

The whole problem is being resolved . . Your subconscious mind is busy . . working out the solution, right now . . in a way that is pleasing to you . .
(Pause)

You don't consciously know . . how to solve that problem . . If you did, you would not be here . . And you don't know how rapidly . . your subconscious mind can work out the solution . . But, that's okay . . You can be pleasantly surprised . . to find yourself improving quite rapidly . .

The important element in this session . . is that you can be going through an emotionally corrective experience, right now . . and not even realize it, consciously . . (Pause for about a minute)

We don't know exactly what is happening . . but you can sense that it is something good . . So, let it continue . . (Pause for about a minute)

It must be pleasing for you to know . . that your subconscious-self is doing this, just for you . . in your own way . . For your own self-improvement . . For your own benefit . . and for your own peace of mind . .

When your subconscious mind knows . . that a resolution to that problem is being enacted . . your subconscious mind will cause one of the fingers on your right hand to lift up . . and remain up, until I tell it to go back down . .

NOTE : AFTER FINGER HAS LIFTED, TELL IT TO GO BACK DOWN AND GIVE APPROPRIATE SUGGESTIONS FROM ONE OF THE OTHER PRESCRIPTIONS BEFORE AWAKENING THE CLIENT. IF FINGER DOES NOT LIFT AFTER FIVE MINUTES, EMERGE OR GO TO NEXT PRESCRIPTION.

(Follow Relaxation)

You are feeling very calm and relaxed . . now that you are in a hypnotic state . . And you will find that there are many things you can do . . Things that you have never been aware of . . And you are going to enjoy doing some things . . that will make you very happy . . Now, spread out your hands and place them on your thighs . . And keep your eyes closed . . while you notice your hands . .

Which one of your hands will begin to feel light, first ? . . (Pause) Will it be your right hand ? . . Or, will it be your left hand ? . . Or will they both feel the lightness, at the same time ? . .

Will your right hand become so light . . that it lifts up towards your face ? . . Or will your left hand lift up . . towards your face ? . . Or, will both hands lift up towards your face, as you continue drifting . . into a deeper and deeper hypnotic state . .

Do you notice the feeling of lightness in your fingers first . . or do you notice the feeling of lightness . . in the palms of your hands . . first . . And, as your expectancy is increasing . . I'm wondering if you are ready . . to get rid of the habit of sucking your thumb today . . Or are you going to wait until next week . . to stop sucking your thumb, completely . .

I know your Mother and your Father . . have been trying to get you to quit sucking your thumb . . They don't seem to realize that you are only _____ years of age . . And, they don't seem to know . . that you will, naturally, quit sucking your thumb . . either today or next week . . They really don't know that . .

When do you want to quit sucking your thumb ? . . Today . . or next week ? . . (Wait for answer)

Okay, You have decided to stop sucking your thumb _____ . . Now, that's our secret . .

You have decided to stop sucking your thumb _____ . . So, if your parents tell you to stop sucking your thumb . . Don't pay any attention to them . . Because, you already know you are going to stop sucking your thumb _____ . . Isn't that right . . (Pause)

Now, with your eyes closed . . I want you to notice your hands again . . We'll wait and see which hand . . is going to touch your face first . . The left hand or the right hand . . It's not really important . . which hand touches your face . . The important thing is that you notice the feelings in your hands . .

Some day, you will meet a new friend . . And you will be able to tell your friend about being hypnotized . . And how easy it was for you . . to stop sucking your thumb . .

It's so nice to know . . that you are going to stop sucking your thumb by . . _____ . . And, as soon as you are sure . . that you are getting rid of the habit . . of sucking your thumb . . you will be able to open your eyes . . And it will seem as though you just sat down . . and are waiting for me to begin . . And you will feel as though you have been away . . on a long, long trip . . to a far away land . . And now, you've come back again . .

(IF EYES DO NOT OPEN, REPEAT, AS ABOVE.)

As soon as you are sure . . that you are getting rid of the habit . . of sucking your thumb . . you will be able to open your eyes . .

532

(Follow Deep Relaxation)

You are very deep now . . and you continue drifting into a deeper . . and deeper . . hypnotic state . . You are relaxed and comfortable . . Your subconscious mind is now ready . . and anxious . . to accept the beneficial suggestions you are about to receive . . You are very calm and relaxed . . now that you are in a hypnotic state . . And you will find that there are many things you can do in this state of mind . . Things that may amaze you . . when you take time to consider these events . .

We are going into the realm of locating gold . . and other treasures . . Lost treasures . . But before we do that . . there are certain things that you must be made aware of . . about your position in life . . For that is where it all begins . .

You have been granted certain God given rights . . simply by virtue of your birth here on Earth . . You have a right to LIFE . . now that you are here . . And you have a right to FREEDOM . . without persecution by those who may be stronger or wiser . . And you have the right to pursue HAPPINESS and SUCCESS . . That would include the right to pursue WEALTH, if that is what will make you happy and successful . . You have the right to pursue GOLD . . and other treasures . . which equals wealth . . happiness and success . . The world has enough gold and lost treasures . . to provide you with a good life . . An abundant life . . And a fulfilling life . .

The first important aspect of hunting for gold . . hidden or buried treasure . . is that you must have a game plan . . You must first know what your target is . . And you should know . . at least, approximately . . where it is . . Do you have a map ? Do you know that your source of information is reliable ? . . Have you considered the expenses involved ? . . These are basic questions that must be considered . . And there are other important issues as well . . You may wonder . . Why do some hunters find gold consistently . . every time they go out . . while most do not ? . . and . . What is it that gives them the winning edge ? . . The obvious answers may be . . The amount of experience . . The quality of their equipment . . A basic understanding of geology . . An understanding of what the man was thinking . . when he hid the treasure . . Or was it all due to . . just 'dumb luck'? . . However, the better answers . . lie in the subconscious level of your mind . . For therein lie the four most important aspects involved with treasure hunting . . The same as it is with many other challenges in life . . The subconscious levels of your mind offer the clues that you must pursue . . if you are to ever find your lost treasure . .

There are four important cornerstones that make up the foundation of your pyramid of treasure hunting . . Not intricate or complex . . Yet often overlooked or underestimated . . And they are, simply put . . Confidence . . Patience . . Concentration . . and . . Motivation . .

The first and foremost aspect of treasure hunting is . .Confidence . . Confidence is not achieved quickly . . It must be earned . . It is the product of talent, training . . repetition . . and dedication . . Confidence translates into power, out in the gold field . . or in the board room . . Just as it does in many fields . . Because you are absolutely certain of your abilities . . This inner certainty comes because you know . . that you know . . It is a powerful force that definitely influences your abilities . . as a treasure hunter . . Or as anything else that you want to be . . A good example is the fact that . . the first nugget you find . . is always the hardest to find . . And that is only because of your level of confidence . . as compared to . . an experienced hunter . .

The second most important aspect is . . Patience . . Nothing destroys the chances of finding gold any quicker . . than a lack of patience . . Patience is one of the most desirable qualities a treasure hunter can possess . . A patient and optimistic attitude breeds success . . And is something all treasure hunters should never lose sight of . . So you will work on your patience . . Once you have mastered that . . other skills . . and many treasures . . will follow . .

The third important aspect is . . Concentration . . A clear, focused mind is essential for your success . . Don't allow yourself to be side tracked . . by other things going on in your life . . Wipe the slate clean and put all of your . . other worldly challenges . . on hold . . This is your time to relax and have fun . . Don't worry about the phone calls you need to make . . or the doctor's appointments to keep . . Forget about your bills and your job . . even if only for a little while . . Your only mission now is to find that lost treasure . . and to have a wonderful time in the process . .

The fourth important aspect is . . Motivation . . The most important motivational exercises you can do . . as a new treasure hunter . . is to make a conscious effort to learn all you can . . about the business . . And it is a business . . If you're not serious enough to consider it a business venture . . then you're wasting your time and effort . . Everyone should be familiar with the basics . . as it is difficult to progress . . without a foundation of knowledge . . Take time to read books and articles . . written by other prospectors and historians . . Anthologies, maps, ship logs and travel journals . . Watch videos . . explore the internet . . and freshen up a bit on the geology . . of your local area . . And of placer and lode deposits . . mining towns and archaeology dig sites . . However, Indian burial grounds are sacred . . and are definitely off limits . . to any searching . .

Earlier, I said, the first treasure would be the hardest one to find . . This is due in part because new hunters . . have a much lower level of confidence . . than experienced hunters . . They are unsure of where to look . . and what sounds to listen to, from their detector . . Or how to read the indicators on their seismographs . . which leaves them feeling doubtful . . The first treasure is, by far, the most important one you will find . . regardless of its value . . That first one will knock down many barriers . . It will remind you that finding gold or other valuables IS possible . . and that your efforts are worth while after all . . As your confidence increases . . so too will your faith in your equipment . . as well as in your own abilities . . In time, you will gain more experience . . and know where and how to hunt . . That elusive golden hoard will become much easier to find . .

Starting out . . concentration is usually difficult to maintain . . Occasionally, you should take a break from your search . . just to observe your surroundings . . There are a number of reasons for this . . If you do anything for an extended period of time . . it becomes monotonous and boring . . It is easy to become hypnotized by the coil . . This sounds funny but . . after three or four hours of solid detecting time . . your brain switches onto auto pilot . . You become so fixated on swinging the detector that you become oblivious . . as to what is going on around you . . You may also lose sight completely . . of what it is you are trying to accomplish . . Take measures to avoid this dreamlike state . . Take periodic breaks throughout the day . . Sit in the shade and enjoy a cool drink now and then . . Reflect on the places you have been . . and where you want to go next . . And why . . Take a moment to examine the geology of the area . . What do you see ? . .What color is the soil? What types of rocks are there? . . Have you located the signs or symbols you are looking for? . . Ask yourself . . Is this really where I want to be . . or have I bypassed something because I wasn't paying attention ? . .

Keep your equipment in good working order . . Clean your detector . . or your seismograph machine . . Use a damp cloth . . to get rid of the dust and mud . . A little dirt on the box or coil . . won't really affect its performance . . but it might affect yours . . Have you ever noticed how much better your vehicle seems to run . . after a good washing ? . . It doesn't actually run any better but . . psychologically, it makes a big difference . . Well, the same thing holds true for your treasure locating equipment . . That is why maintaining a clean, shiny control box and printout gauge . . can be beneficial . . It suggests that the machinery is working in tiptop shape . . And provides you with a new sense of confidence . . Your mood will remain pleasant and . . the chances of success will be higher . . Taking the time to properly care for your equipment . . will not only make you feel and hunt a whole lot better . . but it will also prolong the life of your equipment . .

If you spend much time in the field . . you soon will realize that . . hunting for treasure . . is as much a mental game as it is, physical or technical . . It is a real sport that requires confidence, patience, enthusiasm, concentration and a willingness to work hard . . Once you learn to 'ground balance' your mind . . all the pieces of the puzzle will come together and . . success will be waiting for you . . Under every rock . . or hiding in every small cave . . Tell yourself beforehand . . "It might take a while but I am definitely going to find that lost treasure" . . If you have the proper mind set . . keep your cool . . and stay determined . . you will find that missing hoard of gold . . that everyone else has missed . .

Each day, these suggestions will become even more effective . . you are learning to use these principles of relaxation . . which you are now experiencing . . in all phases of your daily life . . And that will keep you calm and relaxed . . at all times . .

In every situation or circumstance . . that comes up in your life . . you will be calm and relaxed . . Your nerves will be relaxed and

536

steady . . And you'll be able to do everything in a relaxed manner . . You will be able to cope with every day changing circumstances . . in a loving, peaceful way . .

Regardless of what comes up in your life . . you will be in control of your emotions and feelings . . That is what will cause success to be yours . . more than anything else . . and soon you will have all that you want in your life . .

You will remember everything we have talked about here today . . clearly and vividly . . And all of this information is going into the storehouse of your subconscious mind . . for you to recall . . any time you wish . .

It is important to remember . . the four most important aspects you must work on . . for successful treasure hunting . . And they are: . . Confidence . . Patience . . Concentration . . and Motivation . .

You can learn these traits . . in the field . . on your own . . with practice . . practice . . and more practice . . Or we can work on these issues together . . any time you'd like to make an appointment with me . . I know how much you enjoy having me hypnotize you . .

Continue to relax for a few minutes longer . . Allow your subconscious mind to absorb everything we have discussed here today . . Just relax in silence for a moment . . (pause)

Now, I am going to count from 1 to 5 . . and on the count of 5 . . you will open your eyes . . to an alert, waking state . . Feeling clear of mind, relaxed and wonderful . . I will begin . .

One. You will remember everything you have experienced today with complete understanding . .

Two. You are now connected to your spiritual, inner supporting strength . .

Three. Everything I have told you is true . . and is already happening . .

Four. Beginning to be more aware of your body as it fully awakens and wants to stir . .

Five. Let your hands and feet move now . . Stir and stretch as you open your eyes, feeling clear, rested and ready for a great new experience . .

(Follow Relaxation)

As you continue relaxing peacefully . . I am going to begin stroking, gently . . over the areas, where your warts are located . . And as I gently stroke those areas . . you will gradually begin to notice . . pleasant feelings of warmth . . flowing from my hand . . into those areas of your skin . . Those feelings of warmth . . will continue becoming stronger and stronger, each moment . .

I am going to begin stroking your skin now . . And you will soon notice . . those feelings of warmth . . flowing from my hand . . into your skin . . As soon as you feel the warmth . . developing . . you can signal me, by nodding your head . .

AFTER THE CLIENT HAS NODDED, CONTINUE AS FOLLOWS:

You will feel the warmth continuing to get stronger . . It's a very pleasant warmth . . You are feeling it moving . . across your skin . . and into those warts . . As soon as those warts begin feeling warmer than . . the rest of your skin . . Nod your head again . .

AFTER CLIENT HAS NODDED HEAD AGAIN, PROCEED AS FOLLOWS:

Now, as you continue feeling the warmth . . flowing out of my hand . . into those warts . . you can feel those warts beginning . . to get smaller . . They are beginning to heal . . The healing process will continue . . until the warts are gone, completely . .

In the days ahead . . the warts will become smaller . . And they will soon be gone, completely . .

For the next two weeks . . the healing processes . . will continue . . And, sometime, within the next two weeks . . they will disappear completely . . They are healing rapidly . . Your skin is becoming smoother . . and more perfect . . each day . . The warts are fading away . . Each day, they become smaller . . And your skin keeps healing . . and growing more perfect (beautiful) . . In a very short time . . the warts will be gone, completely . . and your skin will be smooth and healthy . .

Relax a few more minutes . . as your subconscious mind absorbs . . everything we have talked about . . (Pause)

In just a moment, I will begin my count . . from ONE to FIVE . . and when you hear me give you the count of FIVE . . you will open your eyes, feeling wide awake, refreshed and feeling wonderful . .

Now, I will begin my count . .

ONE

TWO

THREE

FOUR

FIVE

(Follow Relaxation)

USE A DEMONSTRATION SHOWING THAT THE MIND CONTROLS THE BODY. POSSIBLY HAVING THE CLIENT'S JAW BECOME MORE RIGID AND TEETH CLENCH TIGHTER, AS YOU COUNT FROM ONE TO TEN.

You have been responding very well to the suggestions I have given you . . And you understand now . . that your mind controls your body . . Your mind actually controls all . . of the processes and functions . . of your body . . And it has been found that . . through hypnosis . . we can get your mind to cause changes in your body . . and get rid of warts in a very short time . .

Each day, you will notice improvements in the condition of your skin . . The warts will continue becoming smaller . . and will disappear completely, within the next three weeks . . You are getting rid of the warts completely . . and they will never return . . You will be pleased to notice your skin . . continuing to become more smooth and flawless . .

The processes of your body are functioning perfectly . . to produce the chemicals needed . . to eliminate the warts from your body . . And you will be happy to notice your skin . . becoming clearer . . smoother . . and more perfect . .

Each time you wash your skin . . you wash away cells that have completed their purpose . . And they are replaced with new . . young, healthy cells . . Your skin is constantly being renewed . . Your subconscious mind is directing the cells of your body . . to do their work perfectly . . And your skin continues becoming more clear . . more smooth . . and more youthful looking . .

Even after you awaken from the hypnotic state . . all of these suggestions will continue . . to influence you, just as strongly . . just as surely and just as powerfully . . as they do while you are under hypnosis . .

Your nerves will become more relaxed and steady . . Your mind will be calmer and clearer . . Your happiness will keep increasing . . You will be more composed . . more tranquil . . And more at peace with yourself . . and with all things around you . .

Your subconscious mind has accepted these suggestions . . and is causing your circulatory system . . to carry healing energy forces . . into all parts of your skin . . and throughout the rest of your body . . And the warts are fading away . . easily and completely . .

Relax a few more minutes . . as your subconscious mind absorbs . . everything we have talked about . . (Pause)

In a moment, I will begin my count . . from ONE to FIVE . . and when you hear me give you the count of FIVE . . you will open your eyes, feeling wide awake, refreshed and feeling wonderful . .
Now, I will begin my count . .

ONE
TWO
THREE
FOUR
FIVE

You inquired about attaining wealth . . perhaps, amassing a fortune for yourself . . We are going into the realm of money and . . finances . . but before we do that . . there are certain things that you must be made aware of . . about your position in life . . for that is where it all begins . .

You have been granted certain God given rights . . simply by virtue of your birth here on Earth . .

You have a right to LIFE . . now that you are here . . You have a right to FREEDOM . . without persecution by those who may be stronger or wiser . . and you have the right to pursue HAPPINESS and SUCCESS . . That would include the right to pursue WEALTH, if that is what will make you happy and successful . . You have the right to wealth . . happiness and success . . The world has enough wealth to provide you with a good life . . an abundant life . . and a fulfilling life . .

People who know . . have estimated that the entire world could be fed . . by the food that goes to waste each day . . in the jungles of South America . . This gives you some idea of the excess abundance we have in our world . .

There is excess of everything . . and you are capable of drawing these excess riches of the world to yourself . . In other words . . there is no reason for anyone to be poor . . if things could be distributed for everyone's needs . . There IS enough wealth and riches in the world for everyone . .

Wealth is good because it can be used in so many ways to make life better for everyone . . The world needs wealthy people . . It is the wealthy who are able to provide jobs and income for others . .

So, you will begin each day . . knowing that it is good to be wealthy . . And knowing that there is an abundance of wealth available . . And that you have a right to attain enough wealth to provide yourself with an abundant life . .

A good way to draw wealth to yourself is by visualizing all of the benefits of being wealthy . . You should do this several times each day . . Picture yourself in comfortable surroundings . . in a beautiful, warm, fun-filled, happy home . . See yourself, now, owning beautiful possessions such as . . expensive cars . . a beautiful swimming pool . . expensive clothing and . . a lucrative business or other means of getting the money to flow to you . . Imagine yourself going on trips to nice places . . Staying in luxurious motels and resorts . . Basking in the sun on beautiful beaches . . And doing all of the things you would most enjoy . .

Each night, before you go to sleep . . visualize all of the beautiful things you want . . And think of the comfort and joy that your wealth is going to bring you . . Think also of the many good things you can do for others by attaining wealth for yourself . .

Remember that it is your thoughts that bring results to your life . . You have negative thoughts that you must eliminate . . for they will bring only negative things into your life . . So begin and end each day with positive thoughts about everything around you . . Begin and end each day with thoughts of abundance and wealth . .

Each time you see something beautiful . . something you desire . . or some way you can help others by having wealth . . this is an automatic signal that having wealth is good . . And therefore . . it is quite proper that you should have all of the wealth that you desire . . And so you will continue to have positive thoughts . . that wealth is soon to be yours . .

The world needs wealthy people because it is the wealthy . . who build factories . . own construction companies . . own land and restaurant chains and other businesses . . that provide employment for people . .

Think of those times you have wanted to help someone in need but have been unable to do so . . Wealth enables you to be that warm, loving, caring person you know you can be . . There are so many good things you can do with wealth . . therefore, you will continue reaffirming your faith . . that money and wealth will flow to you . .

The more wealth you attract to yourself, the more it will come to you . . automatically . . your belief that wealth is rightfully yours will be rewarded . . And your strong belief in yourself will automatically draw wealth unto yourself . .

Each day, your self-confidence, self-reliance and self-esteem . . will keep growing stronger . . and you will realize that you deserve the riches . . and other good things that life can provide for you . .

You will find that when you decide to make things happen in your life . . you will be successful . . When you work hard to be a success . . you earn the confidence and trust of everyone who knows you . . You will give your children and your friends . . a model to live up to . . They will emulate your success and strive to follow your good examples . . You can do anything you make up your mind to do . . regardless of the type of environment you were born into . . You know that the person who is determined to be successful . . who sets goals to achieve . . and is willing to put his talents . . skills and abilities . . into action . . will be successful . .

From the mere concept into the material . . the flow of wealth enters the physical world . . You are one of the fortunate recipients of the money flow . . Just as an antenna is configured to receive specific signals . . you, too, are configured to be a receiver of money from the money flow . . You win money . . You find money . . You earn money . . You are given money . . And you give money . . to others in need . .

As surely as the tide rolls onto the shores from the ocean . . so too, the tide of money rolls up to you . . at no harm to you or to others . . And with very little effort on your part . . Many people think you are merely lucky . . for they are not aware that you are at the recipient end of . . the money flow . .

WINNING AT THE CASINO

The casinos in Las Vegas . . or in other places . . function as one of the channels of the money flow to you . . They give away huge sums of money every day . . as a part of their normal operating procedure . . So when you win money in the casinos . . you are gaining income at no harm to yourself or to others . .

You will win a lot of money in the casinos . . by playing the slot machines or the keno machines . . rolling the dice . . spinning the wheel or turning the cards . . You will know what machine is about to pay off . . You will put money into that machine and it will pay off for you . . This is one of the ways you receive money from the money flow . . What a hoot when the three symbols line up to produce a big win for you . . What a thrill when you see all or most of the keno numbers you have chosen . . appear on the screen . . Whenever you get a combination of symbols that define a big win . . you know your affirmations are confirmed . . When you feel the coins fall into your hands . . when the slot machine supervisor hands you hundreds in dollar bills . . Once again, these affirmations are confirmed . .

You are fortunate . . For you are one of the recipients of the money flow . . This is your affirmation . . Now, repeat this out loud . . I AM ONE OF THE RECIPIENTS OF THE MONEY FLOW!

As surely as day follows night . . As certain as spring follows winter . . So, surely, will the money flow to you . . As surely as old age follows youth . . So, surely, will money come to you via the money flow . . As surely as water flows downhill . . So, too, will the money flow down upon you . .

In other areas, your creative works will be successful and well received by others . . You will be successful and able to reap your rewards by writing or painting . . and selling your great works . . Your poetry . . Your paintings or your lyrics . . Your creative juices are flowing endlessly . . They are potent . . helping you to constantly come up with ingenious creativity . . Ideas which you hone into greatly desired works of art . . that will become hit songs all across America . . They will help you to write successful children's books . . and comic books . . and cartoon concepts . . Not only for cartoons but for video games as well . . Your published books of poetry and your songs . . will never be out of print . . The royalty checks will never stop coming . . as surely as the tide washes in money from everywhere . . to you . . For you are the recipient of the money flow . .

Each day, you will realize more and more . . that you deserve the riches and all the good things that . . the money flow can provide . . Each day, your self-confidence . . self-realization and . . self-esteem will keep growing stronger . . Bringing you closer . . day by day . . to your dreams of gaining your greatest desires . .

You will realize more each day that wealth is good . . And that having wealth will enable you . . to use it in many beneficial ways . . For yourself as well as for others . .

When you come out of the hypnotic state . . you will be much more aware of the pleasures and the goodness . . that wealth can bring you . .

When you awaken . . you will easily remember everything I have said to you today . . You will feel refreshed and alert . . and you will feel a much stronger awareness of attaining your goals to become wealthy . .

Relax for a moment longer . . as your subconscious mind absorbs . . everything we have talked about today . . (pause)

And now . . I am now going to count up to Five . . and at the count of Five . . you will feel wide awake . . alert and refreshed . . you will be completely relaxed and invigorated . . with the knowledge that you have gained . .

One . . You are coming up now . . You feel the energy and the vigor flowing through your body . . From head to foot, you are feeling refreshed . . physically and mentally . .

Two . . Rising up now . . Coming to the surface . .

Three . . Feeling wonderful . . wonderful . . For you are a wonderful person . .

Four . . Now you are more alert . . more and more aware . . You feel vigorous . . energetic . . Relaxed . .

Five . . Open your eyes now . . Feeling refreshed, alert and awake . .

(Follow Deep Relaxation)

You are very deep now . . and you continue drifting into a deeper . . and deeper . . hypnotic state . . You are relaxed and comfortable . .Your subconscious mind is now ready . . and anxious . . to accept the suggestions I am about to give you . .

You inquired about attaining wealth . . Perhaps, amassing a fortune for yourself . .We are going into the realm of locating gold and . . other treasures . . But before we do that . . there are certain things that you must be made aware of . . about your position in life . . For that is where it all begins . .

You have been granted certain God given rights . . simply by virtue of your birth here on Earth . .

You have a right to LIFE . . now that you are here . . And you have a right to FREEDOM . . without persecution by those who may be stronger or wiser . . And you have the right to pursue HAPPINESS and SUCCESS . . That would include the right to pursue WEALTH, if that is what will make you happy and successful . . You have the right to pursue GOLD . . which equals wealth . . happiness and success . . The world has enough gold to provide you with a good life . . an abundant life . . And a fulfilling life . .

This session, as you know, is about . . prospecting for gold . . while using a metal detector . . The first important aspect of hunting for gold or . . nugget shooting . . is that you must have a game plan . . before heading into the hills . . A very successful prospector once said . . "There is a big difference between . . metal detecting and prospecting" . . He said, "When you are looking for gold nuggets, you are detecting . . When you are looking for new ground . . you are Prospecting" . .

So you may wonder . . Why do some hunters find gold consistently . . every time they go out . . while most do not ? . . and . . What is it that gives them the winning edge ? . . The obvious answers may be . . in the amount of experience . . The quality of their detectors . . A basic understanding of geology . . Or was it just 'dumb luck'? . . However, the better answers lie in the subconscious level of the mind . . For therein lies the four most important aspects involved . . with

nugget hunting . . Just as it is with many other challenges in life . .
And they are . . Confidence . . Patience . . Concentration . . and . .
Motivation . .

The first and foremost aspect of nugget hunting is . . Confidence . .
Confidence is not achieved quickly . . It must be earned . . It is the
product of talent, training . . or repetition . . and dedication . .
Confidence translates into power, out in the gold field . . Just as it
does in many fields . . Because, when you have confidence . . you
are absolutely certain of your abilities . . This inner certainty comes
because you know . . that you know . . It is a powerful force that
definitely influences your strength and abilities . . as a nugget hunter . .
Or as anything else that you want to be . . A good example is the
fact that your first nugget is always . . the hardest one to find . .
And that is only because of your level of confidence . . as compared to . .
an experienced hunter . .

The next most important aspect is . . Patience . . Nothing destroys
the chances of finding gold any quicker . . than a lack of patience . .
Patience is one of the most desirable qualities a nugget hunter can
possess . . A patient and optimistic attitude breeds success . . And is
something all nugget hunters should never lose sight of . . So you
will work on your patience . . Once you have mastered that . . other
skills . . and many nuggets . . will follow . .

The third important aspect is . . Concentration . . A clear, focused
mind is essential for your success . . Don't allow yourself to be side
tracked . . by other things going on in your life . . Wipe the slate
clean and put all of your other . . worldly challenges . . on hold . .
This is your time to relax and have fun . . Don't worry about the
phone calls you need to make . . Or the doctor's appointments to
keep . . Forget about your bills and your job . . even if only for a
little while . . Your only mission now is to find some gold . . And to
have a wonderful time in the process . .

The fourth most important aspect of nugget hunting is . . Motivation . .
The most important motivational exercises you can do . . as a new
detecting - prospector . . is to make a conscious effort to learn all
you can . . about the hobby . . Everyone should be familiar with the
basics . . as it is difficult to make progress . . without a foundation
of knowledge . . Take time to read books and articles . . written by
other prospectors . . Watch videos . . Explore the internet . . And

freshen up a bit on the geology . . of your local area and . . of placer deposits and lode deposits . . And read Maps . . Get a GPS so you can find the location again . . Or figure out where you are . .

Earlier, I said, the first nugget would be the hardest one to find . . This is due in part because new detectorists . . have a much lower level of confidence . . than experienced hunters . . They are unsure of where to look . . Or what sounds to listen to, from their detectors . . which leaves them feeling doubtful . . That first nugget is, by far, the most important one you will find . . regardless of its size . . That first one will knock down many barriers . . It will remind you that finding gold IS possible . . and that your efforts are worth while after all . . As your confidence increases . . so too will your faith in your machine . . as well as in your own abilities . . In time, you will gain more experience . . on, where and how to hunt . . And the gold will become much easier to find . .

Starting out . . concentration is usually difficult to maintain . . Occasionally, you should take a break from detecting . . just to observe your surroundings . . There are a number of reasons for this . . If you do anything for an extended period of time . . it becomes monotonous and boring . . It is easy to become hypnotized by the coil . . This sounds funny but . . after three or four hours of solid detecting . . your brain switches onto auto pilot . . You become so fixated on swinging the detector that you become oblivious . . to what is going on around you . . You may also lose sight, completely . . of what it is you are trying to accomplish . . Take measures to avoid this dream-like state . . or it may cost you nuggets in the long run . . Take periodic breaks throughout the day . . Sit in the shade and enjoy a cool drink . . Then, reflect on the places you have been . . and where you want to go next . . And why . . Take a moment to examine the geology of the area . . What do you see ? . . What color is the soil, What types of rocks are there ? . . Is there any quartz nearby ? . . Ask yourself . . Is this really where I want to hunt . . or have I bypassed the best gold ground because I wasn't paying attention ? . .

Look around at the local vegetation . . The old timers looked for certain types of plants as their 'gold indicators' . . An example is the unusual 'desert trumpet' plant which typically grows in auriferous soil . . Also, be on the lookout for workings . . done by the old timers . . Staying alert to your surroundings . . will help you locate the most

549

favorable areas for prospecting . . And help you avoid many potentially dangerous encounters with cactus, snakes and other poisonous critters . .

Another valuable exercise is to study the techniques of experienced hunters . . These men and women have a lot of knowledge to offer . . Listen to what they say . . Watch how they adjust their detectors and swing their coils . . Take note of the places they hunt . . and the places they don't . . And don't be afraid to ask 'reasonable' questions . .

If the area you are in has really been hammered . . be prepared to go several hours without hitting a single target . . This will really test you, mentally, because you will have to work that much harder to be successful . .

Crank up your mind's sensitivity and adjust your patience level to the max. . . Because . . chances are . . all the easy gold . . is long gone . . Tell yourself beforehand . . "It might take a while but I am definitely going to find a nugget" . . If you have the proper mind set . . keep your cool . . and stay determined . . chances are . . you will find the gold . . that everyone else has missed . .

Clean your detector . . Use a damp cloth . . to get rid of the dust and mud . . A little dirt on the box or coil . . won't really affect its performance . . but it might affect yours . . Have you ever noticed how much better your vehicle seems to run . . after a good washing ? . . It doesn't actually run any better but . . psychologically, it does . . Well, the same thing holds true for your metal detector . . That is why maintaining a clean, shiny coil and control box . . can be beneficial . . It suggests that the machine is working in tiptop shape . . And that provides you with a new sense of confidence . . Your mood will remain pleasant and . . the chances of success will be higher . . Taking the time to properly care for your equipment . . will not only make you feel and hunt a whole lot better . . but will also prolong the life of your equipment . .

If you spend much time out in the field . . you soon will realize that . . metal detecting for gold . . is as much a mental game as it is, physical or technical . . It is a real sport that requires confidence, patience, enthusiasm, concentration and a willingness to work hard . . Once you learn to 'ground balance' your mind . . all the pieces of the puzzle will come together and . . success will be waiting for you . . under every rock . .

Each day, these suggestions will become even more effective . . You are learning to use these principles of relaxation . . which you are now experiencing . . in all phases of your daily life . . And that will keep you calm and relaxed . . at all times . .

In every situation or circumstance . . that comes up in your life . . you will be calm and relaxed . . Your nerves will be relaxed and steady . . And you'll be able to do everything in a relaxed manner . . You will be able to cope with every day changing circumstances . . in a loving, peaceful way . .

Regardless of what comes up in your life . . you will be in control of your emotions and feelings . . That is what will cause success to be yours . . more and more . . And soon you will have all that you want in your life . .

Again, I will reaffirm the four most important aspects . . you must work on, for successful nugget hunting . . And they are are . . Confidence . . Patience . . Concentration . . and . . Motivation . . Now, you can learn these traits in the field . . on your own . . with practice . . practice . . and more practice . . Or, we can work on these issues together . . any time you'd like to make an appointment with me . . I know how much you enjoy having me hypnotize you . .

Now, I am going to count from 1 to 5 . . and on the count of 5 . . you will open your eyes . . to an alert, waking state . . feeling clear of mind, relaxed and wonderful . . for you are a wonderful and confident person . . (group of people).

I will begin . .

One. You will remember everything you have experienced today with complete understanding . .
Two. You are now connected to your spiritual, inner supporting strength . .
Three. Everything I have told you is true . . and is already happening . .

Four. Beginning to be more aware of your body as it fully awakens and wants to stir . .
Five. Let your hands and feet move now . . Stir and stretch as you open your eyes, feeling clear, rested and ready for a great new experience . .

WRITING - AUTOMATIC

NOTE : AUTOMATIC WRITING, UNDER HYPNOSIS, IS PRODUCED BY HYPNOTIZING A SUBJECT, WHO CAN ENTER A DEEP TRANCE EASILY, AND BY DISSOCIATING THE WRITING ARM AND HAND. SUBJECT IS TOLD, IN THE TRANCE STATE, THAT THEY CAN WRITE WITHOUT BEING AWARE OF WHAT THE HAND / ARM IS DOING. CHOOSE ANY INDUCTION METHOD AND PROCEED BY DEEPENING THE HYPNOTIC TRANCE AND GIVE THE FOLLOWING SUGGESTIONS. A COMPLETE STUDY OF THIS METHOD SHOULD BE DONE PRIOR TO USE.

In a moment, I will count from 1 up to 5 . . At the count of 5 . . you will open your eyes and remain in a very deep trance . . As your hand moves . .

you will not know what it is writing . . But that is all right . . The material you will be asked to recall . . will have a great bearing on this session . .
(FOR PROBING INTO A KNOWN EXPERIENCE OR EXTRACTING UNKNOWN INFORMATION, I.E., PAST LIFE REGRESSION OR INTO SOMEONE ELSE'S LIFE.)

Your writing hand and arm feel like they do not belong to you . . They are no longer a part of your body . . You have no control over them . . and you are not responsible for what they are about to write . . Your writing hand and arm will respond to everything I tell them to do . . You will find that you know the answers to the questions (or information) I ask of you . . And later, you will be able to read and fully understand what has been written . . I am placing a pen in your writing hand now . . Hold it in your hand correctly for writing . . As I ask you the questions . . your hand will write the answers on the writing tablet . . where your arm is resting . .

NOTE : AFTER THE INFORMATION IS GATHERED, OR THE ANSWERS TO QUESTIONS ARE WRITTEN, PROCEED AS FOLLOWS :

Please stop what you are doing now . . I want you to relax . . Close your eyes . . and go back into your restful, deep hypnotic state, once again . . as you were before . . Your writing hand and arm are coming back to their normal feeling once again . . They are now a normal part of your body . .

They feel normal in every way . . In a moment, after I awaken you . . you will understand every meaning of what you have written . . You will have full knowledge of every sign, symbol and word expressed . . and be able to read and derive their meanings . . Everything will be clear to you . .

NOTE : UPON AWAKENING, VERIFY WRITTEN RESPONSES AGAINST THOSE GIVEN PRIOR TO HYPNOSIS.

EMERGE

You are resting comfortably now . . and you will continue feeling the sensations of comfort . . and relaxation . . while your subconscious mind is listening . . to each word I say . . There may be times when you do not feel like you are hearing everything I say . . but that is all right . . Your subconscious mind is aware of everything that I speak . . And that is all that matters . .

As you continue relaxing . . your conscious mind keeps becoming more peaceful . . Each time you inhale . . you bring the breath of life into your body . . And you feel your oneness with God . .

As you submerge yourself, going deeper . . and DEEPER . . You can notice how you are becoming . . even more relaxed and settled now . . Concentrate on that pleasant feeling of relaxation . . Your mind and body are relaxing, more and more . . All tension is leaving your body . . And all stresses and strains are moving out of your systems . . as though they are being drawn out . . by a powerful magnetic energy . . You are learning to be relaxed and calm . . and you will continue to use these principles of relaxation . . during your daily life . . By learning to relax . . as you are doing now . . You will experience a happier, healthier, more enjoyable life . . And a more creative life . . than ever before . .

Every time your heart beats . . it pumps blood through your circulatory system . . like a song of health and strength and life . . And like a new melody and new lyrics, pump into your soul . .

Your entire body continues becoming more relaxed . . more peaceful and more at ease . . And you realize that everything is being worked out . . for your perfect health . . Your perfect well-being and happiness . .

You have elected to write . . as a passion . . or as an occupation . . and you have chosen well . . Your creative abilities and writing skills . . are what you have placed . . your greatest confidence in . . So your mind is at peace . . and your faith is strong . . Your confidence is high . . And although, not everything you write . . will be successful . . It will be a success . . in the experience . .

Each time you see water . . Each time you touch, think of . . or imagine water . . or hear the word, water . . that will be a signal for you to become more relaxed . . calm and peaceful . .

Your subconscious mind will cause the signal you have been given . . to work at all times . . And keep you calm and completely relaxed . . regardless of where you are or what is going on around you . .

God's will is that you always have a healthy body . . and mind . . Your subconscious mind is understanding that . . And is causing the processes of your body to function perfectly . . for maintaining your body . . and your mind . . and your spirit . .

You are feeling more comfortable now . . and are experiencing restful, calming sensations of relaxation . . in every part of your body . . So peaceful . . and relaxing . . Just flow with it . .

You will continue drifting into a deeper, DEEPER . . more peaceful, hypnotic state . . of relaxation . . as I give you suggestions and instructions . . that will cause you to experience continuous improvements in your life . . physically . . mentally . . and spiritually. .

You will soon notice a feeling of energy and vitality . . flowing through your entire body . . Cleansing . . healing . . purifying and rejuvenating your entire body . . Gradually and perfectly . . A warming, blue glow of energy . . is sweeping across you now . . Just let it flow . . Relax . . (pause)

The important thing for you to realize now is . . that you have a tremendous power within you . . that can renew old ideas, restore and rejuvenate old thoughts . . completely and perfectly . . And all of those revitalizing energies, that make this possible . . are all directed . . by your mind . .

You are continuing to have more confidence in your ability to concentrate . . The fact that you have been able to concentrate . . well enough to achieve a hypnotic state of relaxation . . indicates that you also have the ability to concentrate . . when you are reading, listening or studying . .

Concentration is imperative for creative thinking to occur . . You must know your subject well . . Analyze it . . Dissect it . . Probe it and test it . . Understand all of its best qualities . . and realize its hidden faults . . Ask yourself, "What improvements can I make . .

that are more practical or desirable". . Before proceeding with any changes, you must, first, be thoroughly familiar with your subject . . And realize what effect those changes will have . . Are they beneficial? . . The answer, most likely is . . Yes . .

I am going to give you some suggestions and instructions now . . that will improve your ability to concentrate . . And improve your learning skills . . so much, in fact, that your memory will keep improving more . . each and every day . .

From now on . . when you want to read or study . . or listen to a lecture or music . . you will get your materials ready . . Such as a tape recorder, books or writing materials . . Then when you are ready to begin concentrating . . you will breath deeply . . and exhale slowly, three times . . And then you will think of the numbers, 3, 2 and 1 . . As soon as you breath deeply and exhale slowly, three times . . and think the numbers . . 3 , 2 and 1 . . you will become calm and relaxed . .

Breathing deeply and exhaling slowly, three times and thinking the numbers 3, 2 and 1 . . will be a signal . . Your subconscious mind will respond to that signal . . and will cause you to become calm and relaxed . . just as you are now . . And your awareness will narrow down . . to absorb the reading . . studying or listening you want to do . . You will be less sensitive to surrounding noises or distractions . . while you are studying . . Your total involvement will be devoted . . to what you are concentrating on . . As you read, study or listen . . in that state of calmness and relaxation . . your close attention will increase to perfection . . and will remain that way for, at least, one hour . .

Your concentration will be perfect for at least one hour . . each time you use the signal . . of breathing deeply and exhaling slowly, three times . . while thinking of the numbers 3 , 2 and 1 . .

Your subconscious mind has capabilities . . far beyond what you have been aware of . . And your mind is remembering everything it needs to remember . . to cause the creative energies to function properly . . To instill thoughts or ideas . . or musical insights . . into your conscious thinking . .

All limitations are being lifted . . And you are being revitalized with increased energy and inner strength . . Your body, mind and soul are continuing to function . . in a more harmonious way . .

Self-realization and understandings are opening up within you . . A feeling of peace is moving through every part of your being . . Instilling greater awareness of the powers of God within you . . You are realizing that you have the ability . . to remember and to recall . . everything you learn . .

Your mind is comparable to a computer . . It records everything you see, hear and experience . . You are capable of recalling everything you learn . . And ever improving on concepts or ideas . . Some of the material you learn may not seem to be immediately important enough . . to remain in the conscious level of your mind . . So it goes into the storehouse of your mind . . But the information is always there . . And it is available when you need to recall it . . All you need to do is to let the subconscious level of your mind know . . you need to recall something . . And it will permit the information to come into the conscious level of your mind . . whenever you need it . .

Now you understand what real concentration is . . and that will cause your attentiveness to continue improving . . Your ability to recall . . will improve more each day . . Memories will stay in your conscious mind much longer . . And your ability to bring information out . . from the storehouse of your mind, more quickly . . will also improve dramatically . . You will become a memory giant . . And your future career . . will depend on it . .

You will also find your self-confidence and self-acceptance . . growing stronger . . And you will continue improving in all areas of your life . . physically, mentally, emotionally and spiritually . .

You will have the knowledge to solve every problem that comes up in your life . . You will look forward to each day of your life with anticipation . . And you'll find that each day will bring you greater happiness and joy . . You will arise each morning, feeling rested and refreshed . . And you'll continue having more energy, more strength . . and more vitality . . (pause)

The suggestions and instructions I have given you . . are now in the storehouse of your mind . . And they are already working to keep improving . . your creative life . . They are intended to influence your thoughts, feelings and actions . . in a positive, helpful way . . You will notice some very positive improvements . . And you will be very pleased . . with your continuous progress . .

I am going to give you a period of silence now . . as all of these suggestions seal themselves . . into the deepest part of your subconscious mind . . And they will reinforce themselves, over and over again in your mind . . Your subconscious mind is absorbing everything I am saying . . Continue to relax now . . as this period of silence begins . . now . .

(2 to 3 minutes of silence)

In a moment, you will be, once again, in a normal state of mind . . Now, I am going to count from ONE to FIVE . . and when you hear the number, FIVE . . you will open your eyes and be wide awake . . feeling refreshed and wonderful . . For you are . . truly wonderful . .

ONE - Coming up now . . Feeling rested and refreshed . . You will remember everything with clear understanding . .
TWO - Coming up a little higher now . . You are connected to your inner strength . . Supporting your best interest . .

THREE - Everything I have told you is true . . And is happening now . . You will benefit greatly from this experience . .

FOUR - Becoming more aware of your body . . Move your hands and feet . . Let them stir a little . .

FIVE - You may open your eyes now . . Inhale and stretch a bit . . Tell me, "How do you feel ?"

WEIGHT - LOSS

DEVELOPING PROPER EATING HABITS - 1

(Follow Relaxation)

You are now deeply . . and peacefully relaxed . . and you can continue relaxing even more . . as I talk to you . .

Your subconscious mind is receiving and translating . . everything I am telling you . . and is causing the processes of your body to function properly . . You want your body to continue . . getting rid of all excess cellulite, fatty tissues and fluids . . from every part of your body . . that you want to reduce . .

The subconscious level of your mind is absorbing everything I tell you . . and is working . . automatically . . to reduce your body to the level of _____ pounds . . where you want it to be . .

The processes of your body will continue functioning more perfectly . . and will cleanse all harmful substances . . which you consider to be excess fats and liquids . . out of your body . . and will reduce your body weight to _____ pounds . .

Your subconscious mind is causing your entire organism . . to cooperate and function properly . . and eliminate all excess fats and fluids . . from your body . . in an easy, natural way . . through the natural processes of your elimination system . .

Every time you look at water . . you will become calm, relaxed and peaceful . . for at least six hours . .You will be at ease in every situation or circumstance . . in which you are involved during your daily life . . Every time you look at water . . you will become calm relaxed and peaceful . .

Regardless of where you are or what you are doing . . or what other people around you are doing . . you will be calm and relaxed . . and you will respond to every situation in a relaxed manner . .

The relaxation of your mind and body . . is causing you to have a more relaxed attitude about eating . . You eat only when your body needs food . . and you eat only foods which are needed to keep your

body . . healthy . . and which will reduce your body to _____
pounds . .

Without any conscious effort by you . . the desire to eat . . in
between meals . . is fading away . . and will soon be gone completely . .

Your self-confidence and self-acceptance . . are increasing more each day
. . And your will power and self-control are also continuing to increase . .

You will be pleased to find yourself desiring only those foods needed . . to
keep your body healthy . . and to slenderize your body to _____
pounds . .

Your subconscious mind is causing your Appestat Gland . . to control
your appetite . . so you eat only when your body needs food . . and
you eat only the right foods . . needed by your body to keep you
healthy . . and reduce your body weight to _____ pounds . .

When your body does not need food . . you have no desire to eat . .
And you eat only the small amounts needed by your body . . at that
time . . You begin to feel content and satisfied . . as soon as you
start eating . . and the moment you have eaten the amount needed . .
at that time . . you feel completely full . . and satisfied . .

The subconscious part of your mind . . is causing every part of your
body . . to function harmoniously . . and cooperate in reducing your
body weight to _____ pounds . . and will continue to cooperate by
keeping your body weight at the level of _____ pounds . .

You are developing eating habits . . that are perfectly suited for your
_____ pound body . . You are developing eating habits that will . .
keep your body slim, trim, firm and strong . .

When you eat, you always eat slowly . . You take small bites and
chew each bite thoroughly . . By taking small bites and chewing each
bite thoroughly . . you keep experiencing more satisfaction . . from
the food you eat . . and you feel completely satisfied . . as soon as
you have eaten the small amount . . your body needs at that time . .

You can be calm and relaxed when you are eating . . That will cause your
metabolism to always function properly . . and causes your body to retain
only . . that part of the food needed . . to provide the proper nourishment
needed . . to keep every part of your body healthy and strong . .

Your elimination system is continuing to function more perfectly . . and is cleansing all waste materials . . from the food you eat . . out of your body, in an easy, natural way . .

You are getting rid of all fats and fluids . . from every part of your body that you want to reduce . . And you can notice your body getting slimmer and trimmer each day . .

Your subconscious mind is learning rapidly . . the best ways to cause the proper changes needed in your body . . to reduce your body weight to _____ pounds . . and keep your body slender, firm and strong . .

Every time you look at water . . your subconscious mind will cause you to become relaxed, calm and peaceful . . That keeps your metabolism functioning properly . . and the foods you eat will digest easily . . and your digestion system will always function properly . .

Every part of your organism keeps working just as it should . . . causing your body to continue reducing down . . to a level that is pleasing to you . .

Your desire and determination to reduce your body to _____ pounds, keeps increasing . . Your will power and self-control will continue becoming stronger . . And you will be pleased with the continuous improvements in all areas of your life . .

Regardless of what comes up in your life . . you will be in control of your emotions and feelings . . That is what will cause success to be yours . . more and more . . and soon you will have all that you want in your life . .

Now, I am going to count from 1 to 5 . . and on the count of 5 . . you will open your eyes . . to an alert, waking state . . feeling clear of mind, relaxed and wonderful . . for you are a wonderful and confident person . . I will begin . .

One.   You will remember everything you have experienced today with complete understanding . .
Two.   You are now connected to your spiritual, inner supporting strength . .
Three. Everything I have told you is true . . and is already happening . .
Four.   Beginning to be more aware of your body as it fully awakens and wants to stir . .
Five.   Let your hands and feet move . . Stir and stretch as you open your eyes, feeling clear, rested and wonderful . .

DEVELOPING PROPER EATING HABITS - 2

(Follow Relaxation)

You are now deeply . . and peacefully relaxed . . and you can continue relaxing even more . . as I talk to you . . Now that you have learned the ways of relaxation . . you can use that ability to keep improving yourself . . in many ways . .

You will be more calm and relaxed . . as you become more involved in the activities of your daily life . . And that causes all of the processes of your body . . to keep functioning more perfectly . .

Your mind and body will be more relaxed and peaceful . . enabling you to be more poised and more confident . . in everything you do . . You can also be more calm and more restful . . when you are sleeping . . And you will begin each new day . . feeling refreshed and renewed . . You will have more energy and vitality . . and will proceed with your daily activities . . with confidence and self-assurance . .

As I am talking to you . . you can continue moving into a more peaceful hypnotic state . . Your subconscious mind is ready . . to receive additional suggestions and guidance . . regarding the eating habits you are developing . . that cause you to continue reducing your body to _____ pounds . .

Through the years . . your unconscious mind has learned . . to respond to various sensations and signals . . and cause you to react automatically when those signals occur . . without consciously controlling what you do . .

For example . . if you touch something hot . . your unconscious mind rapidly sends a message to your brain . . that causes you to pull away from the object that is burning you . .

If a bright light shines in your eyes . . your unconscious mind automatically causes . . the pupils of your eyes to narrow down . . And there are also many other signals your unconscious mind responds to automatically . . merely because you make a conscious decision . . as I will explain . .

When you decide to walk . . your unconscious mind receives that message and causes the muscles, ligaments and tendons . . in your legs and feet . . to respond automatically and take you where you want to go . .

When you decide to wash your face . . your unconscious mind causes you to make all the movements you need to make . . So you can wash your face without . . needing to consciously think . . of each movement you need to make . .

The gateway to your subconscious mind is now open . . And your subconscious mind is causing the processes of your body to function properly . . to automatically slenderize your body to the way you consciously want it to be . .

Your metabolism is continuing to function more perfectly . . Your digestive system is functioning more perfectly . . Your assimilation system and elimination system are rapidly learning to function more properly . . These are functions which operate . . through the direction of your subconscious mind . .

And your Appestat Gland . . the gland that controls your appetite . . is learning to control your appetite properly . . so you will eat only those foods needed by your body . . to keep you healthy and reduce your body weight to _____ pounds . .

I want you to go deeper now . . Just a little deeper . . You are continuing to move into a more peaceful hypnotic state as I give suggestions that your subconscious mind can easily accept . .

Your subconscious mind is hearing and absorbing everything I tell you . . and is causing everything I suggest to you . . to begin functioning immediately . . And causing you to develop eating habits that are comfortably reducing your body to _____ pounds . . And then, causing your body to remain slender, slim, trim, firm and strong . . You are becoming more slender by eating only the foods needed . . to keep your body healthy . .

There are hundreds of foods you can choose from . . that can reduce your body as well as keep your body healthy . . You can choose to eat the foods that are right for your body . . and at the same time . . your entire system will function properly . . and eliminate all unneeded fats and fluids from your body . . in an easy, natural way . .

You are developing eating habits that are enjoyable . . and perfectly suited to keep improving your health . . and reduce your body to the level of _____ pounds . .

You are developing eating habits that will enable you to get real satisfaction . . from the foods you eat . . because you eat only . . when your body needs food . . And you eat only the right amount of food needed . . to provide proper nourishment and to keep your body healthy and slender . .

About ten minutes before you eat . . you will drink a glass or two of water . . Water is good for your body . . and it helps your digestive system to function more perfectly . . And when you hold the glass of water in your hand . . and when you look at the water . . it will calm you . . It will relax you . . for another six hours . . Every time you look at water . . you will feel calm . . and peaceful . . When you are ready to eat . . you will take a moment to enjoy the fragrance and the aromatic flavors of the foods you are eating . .

Each time you put a bite of food into your mouth . . you chew the food thoroughly . . That enables you to get a much greater sense of satisfaction from the food . . And it causes you to feel content and completely satisfied . . as soon as you have eaten the small amount needed by your body . . at that time . .

You are achieving great enjoyment out of developing eating habits that are slenderizing your body . . and making it strong and firm . . You are also going to be pleasantly surprised to find . . that your will power and self-control keep increasing . . And each day, your confidence grows stronger . . And you experience a sense of certainty and assuredness . . in your ability to develop a slender body . . the way you want your body to be . .

Your strength, energy and vitality keep increasing . . Your health continues improving . . and you continue developing a greater feeling of well-being throughout your entire body . .

Eating the right foods . . and only the small amounts needed to keep your body healthy and slender . . will cause you to feel much better about yourself . . And you will also be an inspiration to other people . . who notice your accomplishment . . You will be patient and persistent in reducing your body weight to _____ pounds . . As you notice your body becoming more slender . . you will find your confidence level increasing as well . . And you will be proud of the progress you continue to achieve . .

564

As your body becomes more slender . . your skin will keep shrinking . . and will become more smooth and youthful looking . . Your muscles will continue becoming more firm and more perfectly developed . . You will be very happy as you notice yourself developing a perfect body . .

You are feeling good about yourself . . and you are pleased to know that your subconscious mind is causing everything I suggest . . to work easily and automatically . . You are developing a more attractive body . . as well as a stronger, healthier body . .

Every cell . . every molecule and every atom in your body . . is responding by functioning properly . . Your entire system is responding . . to thoughts . . and to feelings . . of happiness and success . . Responding to the happy face inside you . . You will be well pleased with the continuous improvements . . in all areas of your life . . You will keep becoming more effective and more efficient . . in your work and in other daily activities . . And you will continue progressing in all aspects of yourself . . Physically, Mentally, emotionally and Spiritually . .

Every part of your body . . All organs, glands, muscles, nerves and tissues . . your entire circulatory system . . your metabolism . . your intestines and elimination system . . Every system of your body, mind and spirit are working well . . in accordance with God's Laws of health, strength and vitality . .

Peace, poise and confidence are growing stronger within you . . You are becoming stronger, healthier and more secure each day . . and you will continue to be amazed and pleased . . with your improvements . .

Continue to relax a few moments longer . . then, I will begin my count . . from one to five . . When you hear the number five . . you will be wide awake, feeling refreshed and relaxed . . and ready for new challenges . .
(Pause briefly)

One - You will remember everything you have experienced today . . You are feeling good now . . Relaxed . . In control . .

Two - Coming up now . . Move your fingers and your toes a little . . Let the body awaken . .

Three - Move your arms and legs a bit now . . Feeling good . . Feeling wonderful . . For you are a wonderful person . .

Four - We're nearly there . . Take a deep breath now and . .

Five - Open your eyes . . Focus on your surroundings . . How do you feel?

WEIGHT - LOSS

W162 Prescript   **FINGER RESPONSE - THERAPY**
(Follow Relaxation)   (LISTED ELSEWHERE)

Refer to 147 Prescript.

WEIGHT - LOSS

W163 Prescript   **EATING SELECTIVELY**
(Follow Relaxation)

You are now deeply . . and peacefully relaxed . . and you can continue relaxing even more . . as I talk to you . . You have learned some of the ways of relaxation . . and you can use that ability to keep improving yourself . . in many ways . . in your daily life . .

Many people who are overweight . . do not know what it is to feel 'HUNGRY' . . Studies have revealed that most overweight people . . are so unaware of some of the sensations of their body that they eat in response to a variety of . . external signals . . rather than according to their . . internal sense . . of being hungry . .

For example, they look at their watch . . or clock and see that it is 12 o'clock . . and they eat whether they are hungry or not . . They eat according to a set time . . rather than wait until they are hungry, to eat . .

Quite often, they go to visit a friend . . and the friend offers them food . . and they will eat . . Not because they are hungry . . but because food was offered to them . . They eat dinner because its the usual time to eat dinner . . They don't even consider that they may not even be hungry . . It is a habit . . They sit down to watch TV and they eat . . because they have developed the habit of eating something . . while they watch TV . .

If you have been eating . . only because it is a habit to eat . . that habit is going to change . . beginning right now . . You have a tiny gland in your brain called . . the Appestat Gland . . and the purpose of that gland is to let you know . . when your body needs food . . And also to let you know . . when your body has eaten the right amount of food needed . . to keep you strong and healthy . .

That gland is capable of functioning perfectly . . And your mind is now sending signals to that gland causing it to be stimulated . . and to function in accordance with the directions it is given . . by your subconscious mind . . From now on, your body will respond to your Appestat Gland and you will eat only when your body needs food . . And you can be very selective in the foods that you eat . .

The part of your mind that controls the processes of your body . . knows that the purpose for eating . . is to provide the nourishment your body needs . . to remain healthy and strong . .

So, from now on . . you will select only the foods that are beneficial for your body . . And you are perfectly content and completely satisfied . . by eating only the foods that your body needs . . to continue becoming healthier . . And to be slim and trim at the level of _____ pounds . .

About ten minutes before eating . . you can drink a glass or two of water . . because water helps your food to digest properly . . Water is also beneficial in many other ways . . It keeps you calm and relaxed . . It enables your elimination system to function properly . . by cleansing waste products and waste materials out of your body . . in an easy, natural way . . Water keeps your kidneys healthy . . and keeps your urinary system clean . . So, you can really enjoy drinking lots of water . .

I want you to use your imagination now . . Imagine that you are dining at the home of a close friend . . and the hostess has prepared a beautiful, delicious looking meal . . and set it out in front of you . . Look at that meal and notice how good it all looks . . Smell it and absorb the pleasant fragrances of all the different foods . .

You are looking it over and thinking about the small portions you can select . . that can benefit your body . . and be sufficient to take care of the needs of nourishment . . for your body . .

Now, you put a small portion of those foods that are beneficial for your body . . onto your plate . . You are very selective . . because you eat only the right foods for your body . . Now, you pick up your eating utensils and you select the best looking bite . . You remember that the first bite is the best and most tasty . . because your taste buds are clean and fresh . . You put that first, small bite into your mouth . . and then you put your knife and fork down . .

You are taking your time and you are chewing that bite thoroughly . . Really enjoying the delicious flavor of the food . . You are taking your time and noticing the texture of the food . . You continue chewing the food until all the pleasurable flavor is gone and then you swallow . .

You had put your knife and fork down because you are taking your time . . And now, before picking them up again . . you take a sip of water . . And you decide to have a sip of whatever else you are drinking with your meal . . Perhaps it is a small glass of juice or wine . . A small sip is sufficient . . You roll it on your tongue . . noticing the fine flavor as you swallow it . . You continue on through the entire meal . . Taking your time . . Chewing your food thoroughly . . And eating only until you feel satisfied and comfortable . . When you have eaten the small amount of food needed for your body . . you will know that it is time to stop . . And, as savory as it was, you have no desire to eat further . . until your body needs food again . .

That is the way you want it to be from now on . . And your subconscious mind is cooperating . . to assist you . . And that is the way you will eat your meals . . from now on . .

You eat only when your body needs food . . And you eat only the small amounts of food that your body needs . . at that time . . When you have eaten what your body needs . . to keep you healthy and to cause you to continue reducing your body weight . . you will be content and satisfied . . until your body needs food again . .

From now on . . you are very selective of the foods you eat . . Being sure that you eat only the foods that are right for your body . . And that will be beneficial and helpful . . for your body, mind and spirit . .

Now, I am going to count from 1 to 5 . . and on the count of 5 . . you will open your eyes . . to an alert, waking state . . feeling clear of mind, relaxed and wonderful . . for you are a wonderful and confident person . .

I will begin . .

One.   You will remember everything you have experienced today with complete understanding . .
Two.   You are now connected to your spiritual, inner supporting strength . .
Three. Everything I have told you is true . . and is already happening . .

Four.   Beginning to be more aware of your body as it fully awakens and wants to stir . .
Five.   Let your hands and feet move now . . Stir and stretch as you open your eyes, feeling clear, feeling rested and wonderful . .

WEIGHT - LOSS
ELIMINATING DOUBT

It is amazing how your subconscious mind knows . . how to cause
you to carry out the actions . . to enable you to accomplish the goals you
want to achieve . .

You have decided to reduce your body weight to _____ pounds . .
And I know you are going to achieve your goal . . Your subconscious
mind is causing you to get rid . . of all the excess fats and fluids from your
body . .

I don't know if you have any conscious idea of how this is happening . .
But that's okay because . . your subconscious mind has all of the
knowledge it needs . . and knows the very best ways to reduce your body
. . And you can feel quite relieved and happy . . in discovering what your
subconscious mind is doing for you . . And you can continue in this
experience . . as you go about your typical, everyday activities . .

To look in the mirror . . and see that you are becoming more slender . .
is always a thrilling experience for you . . And to notice that your clothes
are becoming more loose . . And to see the numbers on the scale, going
down . . each time you are weighed . . is a very pleasant experience . .

You don't know exactly when you will attain the level of _____
pounds . . It may be a month from today . . It may be two months or even
six months . . It makes no difference that your conscious mind does not
know . . Your subconscious mind knows and that is what's important . .

You may have doubts . . or you may consciously have . . a different
belief about reducing your body weight to _____ pounds, but no
matter what you believe, consciously . . your subconscious mind
knows you will reduce your body weight . . Your subconscious mind
has the knowledge it needs . . and is using that knowledge to reduce
your body . . easily and naturally . . to _____ pounds . .

Through the years, you have learned how to forget . . You have
experienced many things that you have been able to forget completely . .
And now you can forget how to lift your left hand . . Notice how easily
you can forget . . how to lift your left hand . . as you count in your mind
. . from ten down to one . . When you reach the count of one, you can be
surprised to notice that your left hand . . and arm . . will not lift up . .
(pause)

When you have forgotten how to lift your left hand . . you can test it . . and notice how easily you have been able to forget . . how to lift it up . . (pause)

Very good . . You have learned something very important . . You have learned that you can forget something . . But, it is only temporary . . Because of imprints, impressions, thoughts, ideas and misinformation in your mind . . your subconscious mind temporarily forgot how to keep your body at its normal _____ pounds . . But now, that you are having these sessions . . your subconscious mind remembers how to cause all of your body functions and processes . . to perform properly . . and restore your body to its normal level of _____ pounds . .

When you awaken from the hypnotic state . . you can forget to remember what I have told you . . while you are here relaxing . . Or you may find it more enjoyable to remember to forget . . That has happened to others many times . . And it is an ability you have . . even when you are wide awake . . Just like you have the ability to see, when you are wide awake . . although you may not always notice nor remember what you see . .

Remember, when you were a child, lying on your back, in bed, with your head hanging over the edge of the bed, so that you could see behind you . . and everything you were seeing, looked upside down ? . . You have probably done that . . But, even though everything looked upside down . . it really wasn't . . It only appeared that way . . when you looked at it that way . . Things are not always what they seem . . Memories in the mind are often found to be false . . even when they are true memories . .

It is due to, things not being recognized or considered . . at the time . . when they happened . . They were not remembered . . in their true perspective . . Quite similar to lying on your back to look . . and having everything appear to be . . upside down . .

It reminds me of a young boy . . who went to spend a week on his uncle's farm . . The boy was not very big . . And as he went with his uncle to do the chores . . his uncle appeared to be very tall, and strong, as he picked up the big bales of hay . . Then, he didn't see his uncle again for many years . . And as he was on his way to his uncle's farm, to visit, once again . . he pictured his uncle as being about seven feet tall . . and much bigger than him . . just as he was, the last time he saw him . . At last, he arrived at his uncles farm . .

And as his uncle answered the door . . he was amazed to realize that he was actually taller . . than his uncle . .

The memory in his mind caused him to have a false idea . . And when he saw his uncle for the first time, from an adult point of view . . he was seeing him, as he really was . . Not the way he thought he was . .

These things are called, Improper Memories . . Just like things that happened in the past . . that caused you to become overweight . . are improper memories . . Now, your subconscious mind understands that . . and can review, explore and examine those memories . . from an adult point of view . . And it can realize that there is no good reason . . that your body needs to be overweight . . at this time in your life . .

It's okay for your body to be slim, trim slender, healthy, strong and firm . . It is natural for your body to be _____ pounds . . So, your subconscious mind is causing you to experience these very pleasant changes while reducing your body weight down to _____ pounds . .

You are now, an adult . . And as an adult, you now realize that the idea of being overweight . . is an improper idea in your mind . . Your subconscious mind is clearly understanding those improper ideas . . from a more mature point of view . . And is causing you to experience the changes that are needed . . to reduce your body to the level of _____ pounds . .

By doing it this way . . it is normal and natural . . It gives you a great feeling of satisfaction . . And you will continue having a stronger feeling of happiness . . as you notice what you are accomplishing . .

EMERGE

WEIGHT LOSS

W165 Prescript.   **FEMALE WEIGHT REDUCTION**   (Metaphor)
(Follow Relaxation)   LAYERS

There was a young woman who lived in a very cold part of the world . . where it was always winter . . and the ground was always . . covered with snow . .

The land was barren . . and frozen . . and she lived in a house by herself . . The only heat she had was from a fireplace . . and it was difficult to find enough wood to keep the house warm . .

She kept adding layer upon layer of clothing . . trying to keep herself warm . . until she looked like a large . . shapeless ball . . Almost as wide as she was tall . .

She felt very unhappy . . because she spent most of her time . . trying to keep warm . . Although she still felt cold, most of the time . . All of the other people were cold too . . but they had moved away . . She felt lonely and very sad . .

One day, there was a knock on her door . . She got up from the chair and waddled slowly to the door . . She opened it just a crack . . trying to keep the cold wind from blowing in . . She peeked through the crack and asked, "Who is there" ? . .

"What are you doing here", she was asked, by a man with a firm, strong voice . . "Everyone was notified to evacuate from this place, long ago . . You must come with me immediately" . .

But the young woman protested, saying, "I can't leave my house . . I have nowhere to go" . .

"Nonsense," said the stranger, "You must leave or you will die here" . . And the stranger forced the young woman to go with him . .

Fearfully, she waddled out, and they began walking on a long journey . .

"Where are you taking me," she asked, "and what will I do" ? . .

"Just trust me", he replied. "I am taking you where you will be safe . . and warm . . and happy" . .

But the young woman had never known safety . . or warmth . . or happiness . . so she still felt fearful . . And yet she understood that she had no other choice . . so she followed as quickly as she could . .

They followed a path that led them through desolation and wastelands
. . After walking for several days, she began to notice how the landscape
was beginning to change . .

She saw some shrubs . . and they had leaves on them . . Then, she began
to notice some trees with leaves, also . . Then one morning, she awoke to
feel moisture, trickling down her forehead . . and could feel moisture
trickling down her body . . from her armpits . . She asked the stranger
what the moisture was, for she had never known of such a thing . .

He laughed as he told her, she was sweating . . Then he explained to her
about sweat, and told her it was caused from being too warm . . He
suggested that she take off a layer or two of her clothing . . to see how
much better she would feel . .

Timidly, the young woman took off the top two layers . . and she
felt much more comfortable . . and much lighter . . She began to feel
more free and found that she could walk more easily . .

Each day, as they continued on their journey, she experienced greater
delight . . The sun was shining more . . The sky was blue instead of
. . drab gray . . and she was continually noticing many more enjoyable
things that she had not noticed before . .

She also noticed more sweat . . but this time she was more eager as
she took off another two layers . . She felt much better and . . so much
lighter . . She was able to walk faster . . and so the stranger didn't have to
stop and wait for her anymore . .

Each day she kept feeling happier . . Seeing the trees . . and the
flowers blooming . . and birds all around . . She even noticed that a
slight breeze felt refreshing on her face . . and without waiting for
the stranger to suggest it . . she began taking off layer after layer . .
Freeing her body, more and more . .

Finally, one day, they arrived in a land of beautiful gardens, in full bloom . .
And right before her was a beautiful, calm lake . . She rushed to the lake
and looked down into the water . . and saw her reflection . .

She was very pleased when she noticed that her true self . . her
slender self . . had finally emerged from under all the layers that had
been covering her body for so long . . And she recognized that she
really was . . quite attractive . .

She saw and felt her beauty and her freedom . . She was joyful and full of boundless energy and vitality . . She was swept away with herself and felt like singing and dancing . . The stranger seemed to read her mind as he encouraged her to sing . . and to dance . .

Each day, she kept feeling more free . . more energetic and healthier . . Her slenderness delighted her and she began to skip and to run . . Sometimes, she would stop and look back at the stranger . . then run on a little farther . . feeling overjoyed with her new sense of freedom . .

She was smiling and laughing . . a lot more . . And she felt so happy to be free that she wanted to stop right there . . But the stranger said, "Not yet, my dear . . We're almost there . . but you still have a little more to go" . .

"What could be better?" she asked, "I feel so good and so happy now . . I can't imagine anything better" . .

"You will see, my dear . . Soon, you will see" . .

One morning, they arrived in a beautiful city . . And everywhere she looked, she saw others like her . . All of them were slender and trim . . and very beautiful . .

They greeted her and welcomed her . . and invited her to join their dances and their singing . . And she felt like she was becoming a part of the community at last . . Soon, she was sharing the work with them . . and she found herself enjoying a great variety of activities . . And each day, her life became happier . . until she was overflowing with joy . .

Perhaps you can identify with one of the characters in this story . . Because . . like her . . your level of confidence and your self-image . . continues to improve with each passing day . . Your joy and happiness keep becoming more noticeable . . You continue to make progress in all areas of your life . . and you are more and more pleased with your progress . . as you become more aware of your true, slender self . . And, as for the stranger ? . . Well . . we'll leave that for another time . .

We are going to conclude this session in a few minutes . . I will be counting from ONE to FIVE . . and you will awaken a little bit more . . with each number you hear . .

Each time I say a number . . your conscious mind will keep becoming more alert . . and when you hear the number FIVE . . your eyes will open easily . . and you will be back in a wide awake . . fully alert state . .

You will feel wonderful when you open your eyes . . You will feel better . . both physically and mentally . . You will feel as though you have awakened from . . a very deep . . peaceful and restful sleep . .

Each time I hypnotize you . . you can continue going into a deeper . . more peaceful . . more detached state . . much more quickly . . and continue gaining benefits from each session we have . .

Continue relaxing now for just a little longer . . giving your subconscious mind opportunity . . to analyze and absorb everything we have talked about . . (Pause)   You will remember everything I have said to you . .

I will begin my count now . .

ONE . . You are beginning to awaken now . . a little at a time . . You will soon awaken . . and feel fully alert, confident and happy . .

TWO . . You are experiencing a wonderful, glowing feeling . . all through your body . . Each day you will feel more alive . . and more happy with yourself . . And you will continue to experience more improvements in all areas of your life . .

THREE . . All of the suggestions I have given you . . are now in the storehouse of your mind . . They will continue becoming more effective each day . . It's a cycle of progress that grows stronger with each day . .

FOUR . . You are feeling rested and refreshed . . Your mind is alert . . and you will continue having more strength . . more energy and more vitality . . Breathe in deeply now . . and . .

FIVE . . Open your eyes, feeling healthy . . happy and confident . . You're back in a wide awake, fully alert state . . Tell me now . . How do you feel ?

Having these sessions . . and permitting yourself to be hypnotized . . is making it easy to reduce your body to _____ pounds . . And is automatically causing your health to improve, more each day . .

Permitting yourself to be hypnotized . . reveals that you are determined to . . follow a program that is reducing your body to _____ pounds . . and is helping you develop a strong, slender, healthy body . . that you will be proud of . .

Your subconscious mind is hearing and absorbing everything I am saying . . and is causing everything I suggest, to begin working immediately . . And to continue working, automatically . . after you awaken from the hypnotic state . . So, you don't need to consciously remember anything I say . . as you sit there with your eyes closed . .

To reduce your body weight . . and to develop a strong, healthy, firm body . . your subconscious mind is causing you . . to automatically make proper changes in your eating habits . . And it is causing you to exercise your body properly . . in ways that are easy and beneficial to you . .

A proper amount of exercise is good for your health . . and it helps regulate your appetite . . causing you to desire to eat only foods that are beneficial for your body . . It also causes you to feel content . . and completely satisfied . . when you have eaten the amount your body needs . . to keep you healthy and slender . .

You can really enjoy doing exercise that is suited to your capabilities . . And you can really enjoy walking . . Walking is one of the best exercises you can do . . So, you will do some walking each day . . Because it helps keep your body slim and trim and strong . .

There are many other exercises you can choose from . . that can be very enjoyable . . Such as swimming, bicycling, jumping rope, jumping on a rebounder . . or other comparable activities that you can find enjoyable . . That will help balance and strengthen every part of your body . .

In addition to reducing your body to _____ pounds . . and causing your body to become healthier, firmer and more slender . . you will find that it will cause your body to become more youthful . . Doing exercises regularly . . will cause your circulatory system to function more actively . . It will strengthen your blood vessels . . permitting your blood to flow through every part of its system, easily . . It also strengthens your heart . .

You can feel good about exercising because it's good for your bones . . And it tones up your skin, making it firm, smooth and youthful looking . . And it enables you to sleep more deeply and peacefully . . when you go to bed to sleep . . And you awaken each morning . . feeling rested and refreshed . .

You are fully relaxed . . and you are moving into a deeper, more peaceful, hypnotic state now . .

Continue to relax . . Your subconscious mind understands . . that I am telling you only the things that I know you can do . . And you can enjoy doing everything that I suggest to you . .

Continue to relax another few moments . . while your subconscious mind absorbs and examines . . all of these suggestions . . (Pause)

You can enjoy following the program I am giving you . . because it enables you to easily reduce your body to _____ pounds . . And also to get rid of unwanted wrinkles from your skin . . And it will eliminate unwanted lumps of cellulite from your body . . causing your entire body to become more firm . . more pliable . . and more youthful looking . .

Your subconscious mind is causing your body to become more slender . . and is reducing your body weight to _____ pounds . . in an easy, natural way . . Your subconscious mind is accepting everything I am telling you . . and is causing your body processes to function properly . . And you are automatically eliminating pounds and inches from your body . . And, you will be thrilled to notice your body becoming slender, firmer and more youthful in its appearance . .

It is normal for your body to be slender and firm . . It is natural for your skin to be firm . . smooth and healthy . . And your digestive system, your assimilation system, your metabolism and your elimination system . . All of your body systems . . know how to function perfectly . . And it is normal for your body to be _____ pounds . . In fact, everything I am telling you is a part of your real nature . . So, your subconscious mind is receiving everything I am telling you . . and is causing this information to be put to use . . automatically . .

Through your subconscious mind . . your body processes are continuing to perform more perfectly . . And your body is becoming more slender, firmer, healthier and stronger . .

578

You will drink a lot of water each day . . to maintain a good fluid balance in your body . . Water is good for your body . . It helps transport nutrients into every part of your body . . And it enables your elimination system to function properly . . to cleanse waste materials and impurities out of your body . . in an easy, natural way . .

About ten minutes before each meal . . you will drink one or two glasses of water . . because water helps your digestive system to do its work correctly . . And drinking water helps you to feel content . . and completely satisfied . . as soon as you have eaten the small amount of food your body needs . . at that time . .

Water is good for your body in many other ways . . It helps keep your body temperature stabilized . . It lubricates joints, tendons, ligaments and muscles . . It preserves the health of your kidneys . . and enables your urinary system to remain clean and healthy . . It also washes bacteria out of your body . . It helps eliminate snacking . . And causes fats and fluids to be cleansed out of your body . . through the natural processes of your elimination system . .

You have a strong desire and resolve to reduce your body to _____ pounds . . Your own determination is causing your will power and self-control to keep increasing . . And your subconscious mind is cooperating by causing you to select . . only foods needed to keep your body strong, healthy and slender . .

You eat only when your body needs food . . And you begin feeling content as soon as you begin eating . . The moment you have eaten the amount needed by your body . . at that time . . you will feel completely satisfied . . And you have no desire to eat again . . until your body needs food . .

You seldom think about eating . . Your thoughts will be on other things . . important things . . The only time you think of eating is when your body needs food . . You will be satisfied and happy . . by eating only the small amount of food needed, to keep your body healthy, strong and slender . .

As your body continues reducing . . your eating habits will continue changing . . to meet the needs of your slender body . . And you will continue eating only those foods needed . . to maintain your body, the way you consciously want it to be . .

You will maintain a healthy body . . and will continue having more energy, strength and vitality . . And you will feel very proud of your accomplishments . . As you should . .

You can enjoy the wonderful feeling of knowing . . you are achieving your own program . . of developing a slender body . . And you will be an inspiration to other people . . who notice your wonderful accomplishments . .

Reducing your body to _____ pounds . . gives you a feeling of accomplishment . . And the wonderful feelings you receive from doing it . . knowing you are doing it . . and have done it . . continues increasing your self-confidence and gives you a strong sense of satisfaction and pride . .

You are feeling enthusiastic about it . . You are happy and excited about it . . You are sensing a feeling of satisfaction . . by putting everything I have suggested into your own actions . . Knowing it really is happening from your own resolve . .

You can enjoy doing something each day . . that will help your body to continue reducing to _____ pounds . . And you can feel proud of what you do because . . it is through your own efforts . . And it is for your own benefit . . And your accomplishments will bring you much happiness and joy . .

Each day, these suggestions will become even more effective . . you are learning to use these principles of relaxation . . which you are now experiencing . . in all phases if your daily life . . And that will keep you calm and relaxed . . at all times . .

In every situation or circumstance . . that comes up in your life . . you will be calm and relaxed . . Your nerves will be relaxed and steady . . And you'll be able to do everything in a relaxed manner . . You will be able to cope with . . every day changing circumstances . . in a loving, peaceful way . .

Regardless of what comes up in your life . . you will be in control of your emotions and feelings . . That is what will cause success to be yours . . more and more . . And soon you will have all that you want in your life . .

We are about to end this session so . . continue to relax a moment longer . . (Pause)

Now, I am going to count from 1 to 5 . . and on the count of 5 . . you will open your eyes . . to an alert, waking state . . feeling clear of mind, relaxed and wonderful . . For you are a wonderful and confident person . . I will begin . .

One.   You will remember everything you have experienced today with complete understanding . .

Two.   You are now connected to your spiritual, inner supporting strength . .

Three. Everything I have told you is true . . and is already happening . .

Four.   Beginning to be more aware of your body as it fully awakens and wants to stir . .

Five.   Let your hands and feet move . .   Stir and stretch as you open your eyes, feeling clear, rested and wonderful.

WEIGHT - LOSS
HIGHER SELF

You are very relaxed now . . Relaxing deeper . . and deeper . . Enjoy this relaxation . . as we begin to talk about . . your body . .

The fact that you are having these sessions . . and permitting yourself to be hypnotized . . reveals that you sincerely want to be slender . . And it also reveals that you are willing to accept my guidance . . and suggestions . . And that means that your subconscious mind . . will cause your body to reduce . . in an easy, natural way . .

I want you to use your imagination now . . I want you to imagine a very bright, white light . . coming down from above you . . and entering the top of your head . . permeating your entire body . . You can see it . . and feel it . . And it becomes reality . . It fills your entire body with a positive, protective energy . . causing you to be safe from any harm . . Now, imagine an Aura of pure white light . . emanating from your heart region . . This pure white Aura . . is surrounding your entire body . . protecting you . . You can see it . . and feel it . . and it becomes reality . . Now, only your higher self, masters and guides . . and highly evolved, loving entities . . who mean you well . . will be able to influence you . . during this, or any other hypnotic session . . You are totally protected by this Aura of pure white light . . And it will surround you with protection . . each time you are hypnotized . .

In a few moments, I am going to count from One to Twenty . . And as I do so . . you will feel yourself . . rising up, to the superconscious mind level, where you will receive information . . from your higher self, and masters, and guides . . You will also be able to overview . . all of your past, present and future lives . .

Relax . . and just allow yourself to flow with me . . as I begin the count . . with Number 1 . . Rising up . . Rising up . . 2, 3, 4, Rising higher now . . Gently rising higher . . 5, 6, 7, Letting information flow . . as you are rising higher . . 8, Letting information flow freely . . 9, 10, You are halfway there . . 11, 12, 13, Feeling yourself rising even higher . . Higher . . 14, 15, 16, Almost there now . . 17, 18, 19 . . and, number 20 . . You have arrived . . Take a moment and orient yourself . . to the superconscious mind level . .

You are now in a very deep, DEEP, hypnotic trance . . And from this superconscious mind level . . there exists a complete understanding and resolution . . to the overeating problem . . Your problem . . of overeating . . may have derived from a condition . . or situation . . in your past or present . . or even from your future . . I want you to discover . . in your own way . . how this problem developed . . You are in complete control . . and are able to access this information . . by tapping into this limitless power . . of your superconscious mind . . I want you to be open to anything . . and to flow with this experience . . You are always protected by the Aura of white light . .

At this time . . I want you to ask your higher self to explore the origin . . of your tendency to overeat . . Trust your higher self . . and your own ability . . to allow any thoughts, imprints or impressions . . to come into your subconscious mind . . concerning this goal . . Do this now . . (Pause for several minutes)

Now, I would like you to let go of this situation . . Regardless of how simple or complicated it may seem . . At this time, I want you to visualize yourself . . in your current life and consciousness . . Free of this issue . .

Imagine yourself being at your ideal weight . . See a friend or mate . . shopping with you . . He or she, is amazed at your slender appearance . .

Now, visualize two tables in front of you . . The table on the left has all the foods you like . . But they add unwanted weight . . The high cholesterol foods, fried in oils and grease . . mayonnaise and other fattening products . . Now, draw a large, red X through that table and imagine looking at yourself in a mirror . . In this mirror, you look very wide . . and short . . as in a carnival mirror . .

The table on the right contains foods that are healthy for you . . and that will not add unwanted weight . . There are fish, eggs, lean meats and fresh vegetables . . and fresh fruits . . Now, draw a large, yellow check mark through this table . . And imagine looking at yourself in a thin mirror . .

You can see yourself, tall and slender . . Now . . in agreement with your higher self, mentally tell yourself that you desire only the foods on the check marked table . . Imagine your friends and family telling you how great you look by (specify a date) weighing only _____ pounds . .

583

Visualize a photograph of yourself at your ideal weight . . And visualize a photograph of yourself at your present weight . . Now, focus your attention on the photograph of yourself at your ideal weight . . The other photograph disappears . . Imagine how it will feel . . at your ideal weight . . to bend over to tie your shoelaces . . walk . . go jogging . . and wear a bathing suit at the beach . .

Now, mentally select an ideal diet . . that will help you reach your ideal weight . . Tell yourself that this is all the food your body will need or desire . . and it will not send hunger pangs for more . .

You eat only when your stomach lets you know . . that your body needs food . . And as soon as you have eaten what your body needs . . at that time . . You are content and satisfied . . knowing that your stomach will let you know . . when your body needs food again . .

You have done very well . . Now, I want you to further open up the channels of communication . . by removing any obstacles . . and allowing yourself to receive information and experiences . . that will directly apply to . . and help to better . . your present life situation . . Allow yourself to receive more advanced . . and more specific, information . . from your higher self and masters and guides . . To raise your frequency and improve your karmic subcycle . . Do this now . . (Pause a few minutes)

All right now . . Rest and relax a few moments . . You have done very well . . I am going to count forward now . . from One to Five . . When you hear the number Five, you will be back in the present . . And you will remember every thing you have experienced . . You'll feel very relaxed and refreshed . . And you'll be able to do whatever you had planned for the rest of the day or evening . . You will feel very positive about what you have experienced here today . . And very motivated about your confidence and ability . . to play this tape again . . to re-experience your higher self . . Now, I will begin my count . .

One   - You are very, very deep . . You are gradually coming towards consciousness . .
Two   - You're getting a little lighter now . . Feeling better . . Feeling good about yourself . .
Three   - You're much, much lighter . . Let your fingers and toes move a little now . .
Four   - Coming up now . . Very, very light . .
Five   - Awaken . . Wide awake and refreshed . .

584

WEIGHT - LOSS

W168 Prescript.   **LOSING WEIGHT IS FUN**
(Follow Relaxation)

You are responding well to everything I say to you . . That's a good indication that you will be successful . . in reducing your body weight to _____ pounds . . And then you will be happy to find . . that your body will remain slender and trim . .

You are ready now to continue enjoying some pleasant changes . . that are causing you to develop a strong . . healthy, slender body . . that is pleasing to you . .

In the past . . you have probably tried dieting . . as well as other methods . . to reduce your body to the level you desire . . But dieting . . taking pills, doing exercises and starving yourself . . soon becomes tiring . .

Trying to stay on a specific diet is comparable to hearing the same old song . . over and over, a thousand times . . However . . just a slight change or two . . can make the same thing surprisingly pleasant . . Enjoyable . . Even inspiring . .

So, I'm going to tell you something now, that your subconscious mind can accept . . And you will find it to be . . a very enjoyable way to reduce your body weight to the level of _____ pounds . .

Going through the experience of reducing your body weight to _____ pounds . . will give you a wonderful feeling of satisfaction and pride . . And the enjoyment you get from doing it . . knowing it's going to be done . . and is being done . . and has been done . . will give you a tremendous sense of confidence and a real feeling of accomplishment . .

I'm sure you will agree that it is enjoyable . . to get on a scale . . and see how your body is reducing . . And it is enjoyable to realize that your clothes are becoming more loose . . And it gives you real pleasure . . to notice your body becoming more firm . . and slender . . And it gives you great satisfaction to know . . that your body is reducing to the level of _____ pounds . .

You can really enjoy getting rid of all the excess fats and fluids from your body . . And feel proud of knowing . . that you are reshaping your body to the way you want it to be . .

It is typical for your body to be slender . . It is normal for your body to be slim and trim . . It is natural for your body to be strong and healthy . . And you will find, it is fun for your body to be _____ pounds . .

You will really enjoy being your natural, normal self . . You can enjoy being the typical, slender, happy person that is really you . .

Continue relaxing peacefully now . . feeling comfortable and happy . . while your subconscious mind reviews and explores . . memories in your mind . . that gives you pleasure . .   (Pause)

Relax and enjoy the pleasant changes taking place . . as your body continues becoming more slender . . It will give you a feeling of accomplishment . . knowing you are doing it . . with a joyful feeling of achievement . .

Reducing your body to _____ pounds . . causes you to feel proud of yourself . . And also causes your self-confidence to continue increasing more each day . .

You are thrilled with what you are doing . . And you are filled with a sense of happiness . . to be getting rid of all that unwanted . . and unneeded . . fat and fluid from your body . . It gives you a profound feeling of pleasure . . to realize what you are accomplishing . .

Your subconscious mind is helping you . . to develop patterns of eating . . that are enjoyable and healthy . . And your subconscious mind will cause you to do something . . each day . . to develop a slender . . and healthy body . .

You will go to bed each night and sleep peacefully . . knowing you have been successful . . in your accomplishments of the day . . And the image in your mind . . of a healthy, slim, trim, firm body . . will be thrilling to you . . And will cause you to continue experiencing more enjoyment . . in reducing your body to the level of _____ pounds . . Wonderful feelings come to you for doing this . . and you know it is really worthwhile . .

Your subconscious mind understands everything I am telling you . . and is translating everything I say into your own anatomical actions . . And all of the changes you experience are accomplished in your own way . .   (Pause)

I am going to explain something now . . that will give you impressions . . and will cause your subconscious mind to produce . .

enjoyable ways of eating . . that will keep you healthy while reducing your body weight to _____ pounds . .

Shifting from one pattern to another . . can be very enjoyable . . Because when you shift from one pattern . . you are resting from the previous pattern . . This way, you can continue doing something . . and really enjoy it . . Because when you change from one thing . . you are resting from the other . .

Your subconscious mind is understanding this principle . . and will cause you to develop creative ways . . of changing your patterns of eating . . So you will enjoy reducing your body weight to _____ pounds . .

You will enjoy reducing your body weight to _____ pounds . . by changing your pattern of eating . . a little differently each day . . You will alternate the types of foods you eat . . and will also alternate the times you eat each day . . because the needs of your body are not the same each day . . You will also alternate the foods you eat by eating only what your body needs each day . . And you will eat only at the times . . when your body actually needs food . .

There will probably be days when you will eat only one meal . . of lean meat and fresh vegetables . . And be totally satisfied . . Another day you can be completely content . . by eating only apples . . Another day, you may be happy by eating only bananas . . And the next day . . you may be at ease, eating only lean meat . . Or you may desire to eat only vegetables . .

You will enjoy the way your subconscious mind will cause you . . to come up with ideas of eating the right foods . . to keep your body healthy . . And cause your body to become slender and trim . .

You are putting these ideas into your own actions . . And what you do is your own accomplishment . . And you can be really proud of that . .

You will think about everything I have told you . . And as you decide to do everything I have suggested . . you'll find it to be to your own advantage . . and for your own benefit . . You can find it to be a very enjoyable way . . of reducing your body weight to _____ pounds . .

You are realizing that . . what you are doing is very important . . And it will help you to be an inspiration to other people . . who will see what you are accomplishing . .

You can experience a great deal of satisfaction . . in achieving goals you set for yourself . . It will cause you to continue having more confidence . . in your own abilities . .

The enjoyment of coming here . . and getting on the scale . . before going into a relaxing, hypnotic state . . and seeing that your body is reducing . . will give you a feeling of satisfaction and pride . . You are already feeling enthusiastic about it . . And you are sensing the feeling of satisfaction . . you will be experiencing . . because it will be of your own doing . . Your own accomplishment . .

Your subconscious mind . . is organizing the suggestions I have given you . . into your own actions . . And you will be pleased and happy to notice . . how it all works together automatically . .

At this very moment, all systems are making comfortable adjustments . . Your systems are now synthesizing proteins, nutrients and other chemicals and substances . . and they are traveling, all through your body . . Rejuvenation is now taking place . .

Your expectations are, naturally, increasing . . and you will be sensing the pleasant changes taking place within you . . You can feel pleased and proud of what you are accomplishing . . The feeling of knowing that it is happening . . gives you a strong sense of satisfaction and contentment . .

Now, I want you to rest a few moments . . while your subconscious mind continues to absorb . . all that we have talked about . .   (Pause)

I am going to begin my count now, from ONE up to FIVE . . When you hear the count of FIVE . . you will be wide awake and alert . . And you'll feel refreshed and wonderful . .You will remember everything clearly that we have talked about today . .

ONE - Beginning to emerge now . . Move your fingers and toes . . just a little . .

TWO - Waking more now . . Coming up higher . .

THREE - Your arms and legs are still asleep . . move your arms and legs now . .

FOUR - Take a deep breath now and . .

FIVE - Open your eyes . . feeling good . . feeling wonderful . .

WEIGHT - LOSS

W169 Prescript. **LOVE THE FAT AWAY**
(Follow Relaxation)

Continue relaxing now as I give you suggestions and instructions . . that will help you to relax deeper . . Go deeper now . . Deeper . . Relax peacefully . . with no thoughts . . and no outside influences . . Hearing only the soothing sounds of the air conditioner . . and my voice . .

You are experiencing an easy walk across the top of a rugged mountain top . . Finally, you reach the edge of the mountain . . and you look down the sides . . searching for a way to go down . .

As you look around, you notice a rocky stairwell . . winding down and around the mountain . . You step onto the stairwell and you begin to descend . .

You are going down slowly . . because there are places where the terrain is rough . . and there are some boulders in the path . . But you keep moving down . . Noticing that you are able to go around or over . . every obstacle along the way . .

You continue moving down the mountain, carefully . . Careful of the rocks . . Careful of each step you take . . Taking your time . . But confidently and surely getting closer . . and closer . . to the bottom of the mountain . .

Now, you are at the bottom of the stairs . . And you step back so you can look at the mountain . . And as you are looking . . you discover a large door . . leading into the mountainside . . You go to that door . . open it . . and enter . . finding yourself inside a long tunnel . . that has beautiful green and blue lights along the way . .

You become aware, as you are walking deeper . . and deeper . . into the mountain . . that there are pictures on the walls, portraying beautiful nature scenes . . and pictures of ideal, perfectly developed bodies . . The way you want your body to be . .

You feel instinctively that this is a place of renewal . . A place where you are to learn about the restorative, reshaping and restructuring powers . . of your own body . .

You feel that power welling up inside you . . as your self-confidence increases . . And you know that you can trust your own progress . .

You continue your walk through the tunnel . . with many pictures of beautiful bodies on the walls . .

Moving more deeply into the mountain . . you notice ahead of you . . a door . . There is a sign on the door . . And as you get closer to the door . . you notice the words on the sign . . It says, "The one who knows your body" . . And you want to understand the meaning of those words . . You open the door and walk in to an interesting room . . so you can meet, "The one who knows your body" . . It is your own . . inner mind . .

You sit down in a chair . . across from that part of your inner self . . You are waiting for answers . . You are allowing yourself to be receptive to . . whatever comes through . .

The one who knows your body . . may communicate in words or images . . or even through feelings and sensations . . But, be assured, communication will come . .

Allow yourself to continue relaxing . . as you are receptive and attentive . . to the messages you are receiving . . You are open to new insights . . and are learning . . And that is good . . (Pause)

Your inner mind is learning . . to cause the processes and activities of your body . . to function properly . . and eliminate all excess fats and fluids from your body . . in an easy, natural way . . through the normal processes of your elimination system . .

You are developing a more relaxed attitude about eating . . You eat only when your body needs food . . And you eat only the small amounts of food that is needed . . to keep your body healthy . . and to reduce your body to the level of _____ pounds . .

The desire to eat when your body does not need food . . is fading away . . and will soon be gone completely . . You eat only the small amount your body needs . . to keep improving your health . . and to slenderize your body to _____ pounds . . You are developing eating habits that are perfectly suited for your _____ pound body . .

Having received the messages from your inner self . . you are ready to leave the room . . And you are feeling thankful . . for the information and the understanding received . .

You are leaving now . . closing the door behind you . . and walking confidently back to the entrance of the tunnel . .

590

Now, you are leaving the tunnel and you begin the climb . . back up to the top of the mountain . . Notice how easily you move . . up the stairwell to the top of the mountain . . As you get closer and closer to the top of the mountain . . you are feeling your body evaluating this new knowledge and information. . . The changes have already started . . And you are ready for another . . interesting experience . .

When you reach the top of the stairwell . . the path leads off to the right . . towards a small cabin . . No one is home and so you let yourself into the cabin . . It is a quaint little cabin with a fireplace burning warmly . . It is comfortable and you feel very safe here . . and welcome . . You are drawn to a full length mirror . . You stand in front of the mirror with another full length mirror behind you . . and full length mirrors on either side of you . .

You are removing all of your clothing now and scanning your entire body . . Seeing yourself, slim and trim and slender . . Seeing your body exactly as you want it to be . . You see . . and you feel . . every part of your 'ideal' body . . Slender and trim . . Perfectly healthy and strong . . You like your ideal body . . And you love your ideal body . . That really is your body . .

All you need to do . . is to continue reducing 2 to 5 pounds or more, each month . . and you will soon have your perfect, ideal body . . To change your body . . you are doing it differently this time . . You are loving all the excess fat and fluid and cellulite . . off your body . . You are reducing from 2 to 5 pounds or more . . off your body, each month . . by loving off all excess fat from your body . . And you are doing it with enthusiasm and great expectation . . Imagine . . and feel . . all the pleasant, warm, soothing vibrations of love . . flowing through your body now . . Feel those vibrations of warm love . . flowing through every part of your body . . Pleasant changes are taking place . . And you can feel those changes taking place . . And you can feel your body gradually becoming slimmer and trimmer . . Your legs, knees, thighs, hips . . Your abdomen, stomach, waist . . Your arms, shoulders, chest . . Your neck and face . . All are becoming slender and firmer . . You are getting rid of all excess fat . . And you can see your body, reshaping itself . . exactly as you want your ideal body to be . .

As you visualize your ideal body in the arrangement of mirrors . . you can see the changes taking place . . and you really like what you are seeing . . You really do like your ideal body . . And you love your ideal body . .

And you are allowing it to gradually become slimmer and trimmer . . by loving yourself and your body . .

Those warm, pleasant vibrations of love are causing . . the excess fat to dissolve and be cleansed out of your body . . through the natural processes of your elimination system . . This is giving you many other benefits, as well . . Your self-confidence, self-reliance, self-acceptance and self-esteem are increasing more each day . . And you are becoming more efficient in your work and other activities . .

You will find that many people will be complimenting you . . for your accomplishment . . And you will feel proud because it is of your own doing . . Your own achievement . . You have a strong, healthy, attractive body . . You radiate a feeling of love and self-acceptance . . You feel competent . . And those feelings are increasing more each day . . You feel good about yourself . . as you should . .

These suggestions keep becoming more and more effective each day . . They are very important to you . . And your inner mind is remembering them, quite clearly . . You may put your clothes back on now . . Take your time . . (Pause)

You are ready to come back to a wide awake, fully alert state . . and continue to experience the pleasant changes taking place inside of you . .

Continue relaxing now for a few more minutes . . to give your subconscious mind the time . . to accept and absorb . . everything we have talked about today . . We have covered a lot of things, haven't we . . So continue to relax . . (Pause)

In a moment, I will count to FIVE . . and you will awaken feeling refreshed and wonderful . . You will awaken a little more with each count you hear . . I will begin my count now . .

ONE . . You are coming up now . . Soon you will awaken . .

TWO . . Your fingers and toes want to wiggle now . . Let them move a little . .

THREE . . Feeling refreshed and wonderful . . for you are, truly, a wonderful person . .

FOUR . . You're almost there . . Take a deep breath now . . and . .

FIVE . . Open your eyes . . Now, let me see a big smile . .

Take a few moments now to pay attention to the relaxed feeling all over your body . . Memorize it as carefully as you can . . Store into your memory, the entire feeling . . of your whole body in complete relaxation . . You enjoy this peaceful feeling . . And you look forward to re-experiencing . . this wonderful, restful state of mind in the future . . Each time you are hypnotized . . you will go into a deeper level of hypnosis more quickly and more easily . .

You will find that you can easily . . quickly and willingly . . follow every suggestion that I give you . . In this relaxed condition, your subconscious mind . . will strengthen the effect of every suggestion that I give you . . All of the suggestions . . will make the changes . . we want them to make . .

Now that you have reduced your body weight down to _____ pounds . . you want to keep your body slim and trim . . And you will find yourself remaining slender . . because your body is made to keep itself stabilized . .

Your body is a complex organization of organs, glands, blood vessels . . nerves, brain cells, muscles . . ligaments, tendons, tissues and bones . . The energy from your mind . . which stimulates the actions of your body . . and coordinates the functions of all parts of your body . . is a plurality of constantly changing energies . .

From birth, until death . . your mind is constantly receiving impressions that influence you in some way . . The impressions, made in your mind . . influence your natural, physical impulses . . as well as your subconscious impulses . .

So, one of the most important tasks . . is to have your mind forces harmonized . . So they will be organized and directed . . towards the orderly attainment . . of what you want to achieve . . You have already been doing this . . by permitting yourself to be hypnotized . . And that is the reason your body weight has reduced to _____ pounds . .

By successfully directing the energies of your mind . . you have developed the ability to be calm . . and relaxed . . during the activities of your daily life . .

You will continue to be even more poised and . . in control . . and will maintain harmony within your body . . in the midst of changing circumstances . .

You are continuing to relax and you are resting more peacefully now . . And you are realizing that your subconscious mind is a powerful tool . . which is continuing its work . . to keep your body slim and trim . . Exactly the way you, consciously, want your body to remain . .

You understand now . . that your thoughts are creative . . And there are levels of your subconscious mind . . that operate according to the nature, impulse, emotion or conviction . . behind each thought . . Your thoughts may be positive or negative . . It is up to you to, consciously, keep them positive . . And your thoughts create a mold in your subconscious mind . . which sets an energy in motion . . in response to each of your thoughts . . It is a natural law . . that always works the same . .

So, you are realizing that your mind is a powerful tool . . And you are also understanding . . that you have the ability to consciously direct . . the subconscious level of your mind . . to cooperate with your conscious desires . . Regardless of how powerful your subconscious mind is . . the responses it causes in your physical body . . are set in motion by your conscious thoughts . . And, this fact, enables you to keep your body weight at the level of _____ pounds . .

Experience and scientific research . . has taught us that you have the ability . . to consciously direct your subconscious mind . . so it will respond in a positive, helpful way . . The key to maintaining your body . . at a level that is pleasing to you . . is by making use of Nature's Law (God's Law) . . of programming your subconscious mind properly . . We have not created these Laws and Principles . . They already exist . . God has given us the ability to understand them . . and to use them . . for our own benefit and personal well being . .

So, listen closely now, as I give you suggestions . . which your subconscious mind will accept . . And will, therefore . . be caused to automatically maintain your body . . at a slender level that is pleasing to you . .

The suggestions I am giving you are going directly into . . the storehouse of your subconscious mind . . and will continue to influence your thoughts . . your feelings . . and your actions . . in a positive and helpful way . . And will be very beneficial to you . .

Even after you awaken from the hypnotic state . . as you go about the activities of your daily life . . the suggestions that I am giving you . . will continue to influence you . . just as strongly . . just as surely . . and just as powerfully . . as they do while you are hypnotized . .

You will be happy to have your subconscious mind . . continue controlling your appetite . . to keep your body slim and trim at the level of _____ pounds . .

During your daily life . . you will automatically apply these principles of relaxation . . which you are now experiencing . . Your nerves will be calm and relaxed . . in all situations and circumstances . . And you will remain peaceful and composed . . regardless of what is going on around you . . This will keep your metabolism functioning perfectly . . And will easily . . keep your body slender . .

You realize now, that you are in control of yourself . . rather than you, being controlled . . You are directing your subconscious mind . . to keep your body slim and trim . . As well as for any other worthwhile purpose . . you wish to accomplish . . You are empowered And you . . are in control . .

In every situation and circumstance that comes up in your life . . you will be calm and relaxed . . You will use your ability to think clearly . . That will enable you to evaluate everything . . thoroughly and completely . . before making a decision . . and with a clear mind . . You will confidently handle every situation . . that comes up in your life . . in a peaceful, loving way . .

All of these suggestions are permanently stored . . in the warehouse of your subconscious mind . . and they will continue to be more effective every day . .

You will keep becoming more youthful in appearance . . Your skin is becoming smoother and healthier . . Your overall happiness will continue increasing . . as your body keeps becoming healthier and stronger each day . .

Every organ in your body is continuing to function more perfectly . . Every cell, every atom and every molecule in your body . . is doing its work properly . . to continue improving your health . .

Youthful vitality emerges in the way you look . . In the ways you feel and in all of your actions . . And you will be exceptionally happy . . with all of the improvements in your life . .

You will always think good thoughts about yourself . . You will speak to everyone in a positive way . . And you will continue to increase the development of your self-confidence, self-acceptance and . . self-esteem . .

Take a few moments now to pay attention to the relaxed feeling all over your body . . Memorize it, as carefully as you can . . Store into your memory, the entire feeling of your whole body in complete relaxation . . You enjoy this peaceful feeling . . and you look forward to re-experiencing this wonderful, restful state of mind in the future . . Each time you are hypnotized . . you will go into a deeper level of hypnosis . . more quickly and more easily . .

In a few moments, I will count to five (5) . . and at the count of 5, you will open your eyes . . You will feel wide awake . . And you will feel wonderfully better for this long, relaxing rest . . You will feel completely relaxed . . both mentally and physically . . You will be more refreshed and more invigorated than you have felt in a long time . . You will be totally free from all feelings . . of stress or anxiety . . You always find hypnosis to be relaxing . . refreshing . . and invigorating . . An experience you truly enjoy . .

Now, the counting begins . . On the count of 5, your eyes will open . . On the count of 5, you will emerge from this pleasant relaxation, feeling wonderfully refreshed and completely relaxed and refreshed . . As though you were awakening from a long nap . . Here we go . .

1 - You are coming up now . . You feel the energy and the vigor flowing through your legs . . flowing up through your body . . Your eyes feel fresh and clear . . From head to foot, you are feeling good . . physically refreshed . . emotionally refreshed . .

2 - Rising up now . . Coming to the surface . .

3 - Feeling wonderful . . Wonderful . . For you truly are a wonderful person . .

4 - You are more and more alert . . more and more alert . . you feel vigorous . . energetic . . Relaxed from head to foot . . You are completely refreshed . . rejuvenated . . Your eyes are set to open and you are ready to return to an alert . . wakeful state . .

5 - Open your eyes now, feeling refreshed and wonderful . .

WEIGHT - LOSS

W171 Prescript.
(Light Relaxation) **OVEREATING TO LOSE WEIGHT # 1**

Can you describe how you feel about the level of hypnosis you are in now?
(Pause)

Good . . Now, I want you to remain in that same level . . Try to keep yourself from going into a deeper hypnotic trance . . because I want you to be aware of everything . . I say to you today . . I want you to listen carefully to everything I say . . And then you will be able to understand completely . . what I say . .

If it becomes too difficult to keep yourself from going into a deeper trance . . and you feel you want to let go completely . . then do as you wish . . But whatever you do . . you will want to listen to the entire explanation . . without awakening from the hypnotic state . . Are you willing to do that ? . . (Pause)

Good . . You know how you have been responding to the idea of . . controlling your eating habits . . You have continued overeating . . even though you really want to slenderize your body . .

You have been overeating for many years . . And it is quite obvious that you will continue overeating . . You know what you are doing . . You know what foods are high in calories . . And you know what foods are not high in calories . . But that doesn't make any difference . . Your own eating habits have defeated you in the past . . And it hasn't made any difference by what you have known . . But now, your eating habits will be used to produce therapeutic results . . This, you do not understand . . but that is okay . . You will cooperate . . as you always do . . And you will also . . overeat . . With my blessing . .

You now weigh _____ pounds . . Not 130 or 120 . . but _____ pounds . . So, you need to overeat . . to support all that excess weight . . You will remember this and cooperate fully . . For the next week . . you will overeat . . The weight of your body is _____ pounds, right now . . so, you need to overeat . . And you will do so, carefully and willingly . . You will eat enough to sufficiently support _____ pounds . . (Suggest 8 to 10 pounds LESS than present weight)

It is amazing how your subconscious mind knows . . how to help you achieve that . . And there is nothing more I need to tell you now . . except that you will be sure to continue cooperating . . So, I am going to awaken you now . . with no further discussion or comment . . And I want you to return one week from today . . for your next session . .

EMERGE

WEIGHT - LOSS

W172 Prescript.   **OVEREATING TO LOSE WEIGHT # 2**
(Follow Relaxation)

You are doing real good . . you are learning to overeat wisely . . And you are ready to continue your program of overeating . . This week, you will overeat enough to sufficiently support _____ pounds . . (5 pounds less than today's weight) . . And you will come back for another session, a week from today . . You want your body to be healthy . . So, you will be sure to overeat, carefully and willingly . . to sufficiently support _____ pounds . .

You will notice that eating carefully and willingly . . is increasing your happiness . . And you are beginning to have better feelings about yourself . . Your self-confidence keeps increasing more and more each day . . You will also be noticing other important changes . . Your body processes continue functioning more perfectly . . And your health continues improving . . Your muscles are becoming more firm, and your body is becoming more slender . . You will also be happy to notice that your skin gradually becomes more clear and youthful looking . . All of these changes will continue as you go about your daily activities . . And your happiness keeps increasing as you become more aware of what you are accomplishing . .

You are becoming the person you have always wanted to be . . Self-confident, self-sufficient, acceptable, healthy and successful . . Your life continues becoming more enjoyable . . And your feelings of happiness go on increasing more each day . . You will be more stable, emotionally . . And you'll be more calm and relaxed . . whether you are alone or with other people . . And you remain pleased that you decided to have me hypnotize you . . You maintain a feeling of happiness . . because you will not be thinking about dieting . . Instead, you are learning to overeat . . wisely . .

You will also drink lots of water . . because water is good for your body . . You will drink a glass or two of water . . about ten minutes before eating each meal . . That will cause your food to digest properly . . And will enable your elimination system to function normally and easily . .

What you are doing is for your own benefit . . It is your own accomplishment . . and you will be proud of that . . You are sensing the pleasure of knowing that something good is happening . . And it will bring you much happiness and joy . . EMERGE

WEIGHT - LOSS

W173 Prescript   **REDUCING ABS AND HIPS**
(Follow Relaxation)

You have decided to get rid of the excess weight from your body . . Especially from your abdomen and hips . . By making that decision . . you are opening your subconscious mind . . to be receptive to the suggestions and instructions . . that I give you . .

You have permitted yourself to be hypnotized . . and now your subconscious mind is accepting . . everything I tell you . . and you will be very pleased with the improvements . . as you carry on to your goal . . of developing a more perfect body . .

What first caused you to become overweight, doesn't really matter anymore . . Because hypnosis can help you reduce your body . . to the level you desire . . And then, enable you to maintain that level . . after you have reduced . .

You are gradually reducing your body . . And you are developing your body . . exactly the way you want it to be . . If your body was a solid mass of flesh and bones . . it might be difficult to understand . . that your subconscious mind can reshape it . . to the way you consciously want it to be . . But scientists have found that the body is more than 80 per cent liquid . . Even your bones are filled with a liquid substance . . and they are soft, pliable and porous . . Because they are penetrated by blood capillaries and corpuscles . .

Since your body is more than 80 per cent liquid . . and is controlled by your subconscious mind . . your subconscious mind can send radiant energy into every part of your body . . And can reshape your body . . exactly the way you consciously want it to develop . .

The Bible even says, "You can be transformed . . by the renewing of your mind" . . And that is what we are doing as you continue these hypnotic sessions . . We are renewing your mind . . with positive ideas and thoughts . . about the way you want your body to be . .

Each time I hypnotize you . . I am permeating your mind with suggestions . . that are beneficial to you . . And your subconscious mind accepts these suggestions . . and causes your body processes to continue functioning more perfectly . . to eliminate excess fat from your waist . . your stomach

. . your abdomen, hips and buttocks . . Easily and naturally . . through the natural processes of your elimination system . .

Your will power and self-control persist in becoming stronger each day . . causing you to desire, choose and eat . . only the foods your body needs . . to keep improving your health . . And to get rid of all of the excess fats and fluids . . that have been stored in your body . . Especially from your abdomen and hips . . You are developing a more healthful and attractive body . .

Your waist is become smaller . . And your stomach and abdomen are reducing . . Becoming more smooth and firm . . Your hips are becoming more slender . . And your body is turning into a more perfectly developed body . . as each day passes . .

You can really enjoy participating in exercises that best suit your natural abilities and capacities . . You can enjoy walking . . and breathing in good, fresh air . . Continuing to improve your health . . When you are walking . . you will always walk briskly . . keeping your body erect and limber . . You will stride freely and easily . . Every step you take will increase your energy level and vitality . . You will enjoy walking . . And will always feel happy when you are walking . . Each step you take increases your feelings of good health and well being . .

Every cell, every atom and every molecule of your body . . continues functioning more perfectly . . And you will be very happy . . as you notice your appearance improving more each day . .

Your self-confidence is increasing . . And you are very proud of what you are accomplishing . .

You are putting all of these suggestions into your own actions . . causing them to work automatically . . They keep becoming more effective wach day . . And you will be well pleased to notice yourself developing . . your perfect body . . Exactly the way you, consciously, want your body to be . .

Relax for another moment . . Then we will conclude this session . .
(Pause)

Now, I am going to count from ONE to FIVE . . and on the count of FIVE . . you will open your eyes . . to an alert waking state . . Feeling clear of mind . . relaxed . . and wonderful . .

I will begin . .

ONE - You will remember everything you have experienced today . . with understanding and clarity . .

TWO - You are now connected to your inner strength and higher power . . Supporting your good . . You will carry that inner strength with you throughout your day . .

THREE - Everything I have told you is true and is already happening . . And you are already successful in manifesting the positive suggestions that I have given you . . into your daily life and consciousness . .

FOUR - You are beginning to be more aware of your body . . as it fully awakens and wants to stir . .

FIVE - Let your feet and hands move . . Stir and stretch as you open your eyes, feeling clear, rested and wonderful . .

WEIGHT - LOSS

W174 Prescript. **REDUCING YOUR BODY**
(Follow Relaxation)

You are very relaxed now . . Relaxing deeper . . and deeper . . Enjoy this relaxation . . as we begin to talk about . . your body . .

The fact that you are having these sessions . . and permitting yourself to be hypnotized . . is your assurance that you are reducing your body to _____ pounds . . Permitting yourself to be hypnotized . . reveals that you sincerely want to be slender . . And it also reveals that you are willing to accept my guidance . . and suggestions . . And that means that your subconscious mind . . will cause your body to reduce . . in an easy, natural way . .

You are dissatisfied about being overweight . . You are determined to develop a slender body . . Because you realize that it will help you in many ways . . Reducing your body to_____ pounds is causing you to look better . . and feel better . . It also gives you more strength, more energy and vitality . .

Each day, you are more pleased that you decided . . to have me hypnotize you . . You can notice your body reducing . . and getting rid of all excess fats . . and fluids . . easily and naturally . . through the processes of your elimination system . .

After you awaken from the hypnotic state, you can consciously forget the suggestions I am giving you . . Relax, as you sit there with your eyes closed . . Your subconscious mind will remember everything I tell you . . and is causing everything I say . . to begin working immediately . . And continue working, automatically . . as you go about the activities of your daily life . .

One of the facts I have learned . . is that your subconscious mind . . knows how to work out solutions . . to any problem you are experiencing . . Your subconscious mind will review and examine . . all imprints . . all impressions, thoughts, ideas and memories . . stored in your mind . . that have been causing you to be over_____ pounds . . And, the great thing about it is . . that your subconscious mind will continue reviewing and examining . . all of that information in the storehouse of your mind . .

until it has worked out the solution . . that will cause your body to reduce to _____ pounds . . and remain at that level . .

It is natural for your body to be slender, healthy, firm and strong . . It is normal for your body to be at _____ pounds . . Everything I am telling you is normal for your body . . So, your subconscious mind is causing your body processes . . to function properly . . And reduce your body to its normal level, of _____ pounds . .

As I am talking to you . . you will continue moving into a deeper . . more restful . . hypnotic state . . Deeper . . Relax . . Deeper now . . Deeper . . And now, be comfortable . . at that level . .

As you go about the activities of your daily life . . you are making important changes in your eating habits . . that are continuing to reduce your body . . until your body weight is _____ pounds . .

It may take a week . . or even two weeks . . for your mind to review all of the information . . that has caused you to become overweight . . When you know that reason . . I want you to know . . that you can talk to me about it . . In the coming days, you may notice your body . . becoming more slender . . and continuing to reduce a little more each day . . By tomorrow . . your body will be . . a little more slender than it is today . . And by the next day . . your body will reduce a little more . . The following day . . your body will be even slimmer . . And you will continue reducing a little more, each day . . until your body weight is at _____ pounds . . And then, your body will remain at _____ pounds . . You will be happy to notice your self-confidence and self-acceptance increasing, more each day . . Now that you have made a firm decision to reduce to _____ pounds . . your subconscious mind is controlling your Appestat Gland . . The gland that controls your appetite . .

From now on, you eat only when your body needs food . . And you eat only the amount needed by your body . . at that time . . As soon as you start eating . . you feel satisfied . . And the moment you have eaten the amount needed . . by your body . . at that time . . you feel content, and completely satisfied . . And you have no desire to eat again . . until your body needs food . .

Your subconscious mind knows your body needs protein to keep you strong . . And it knows you also need a proper balance of vitamins, minerals, fiber and potassium . . to keep your body healthy . . So, you desire, you select, and you eat, only those foods needed . . to keep your body healthy and strong . .   And which will reduce your body to _____ pounds . .

Your food taste is corresponding to the real needs of your body . . You enjoy eating foods and drinking liquids, needed by your body . . And you avoid foods and liquids . . that are not needed, for your body . .

You enjoy the good foods your body needs so much . . that a small amount of the right foods . . takes care of keeping your body healthy . . while reducing your body to _____ pounds . .

It may be another week . . or even two weeks . . before you realize how your body is becoming slimmer . . trimmer, firmer and stronger . . But you will be pleasantly surprised to notice . . the changes happening, automatically . .

You can get rid of some fats and fluids from your body, today . . And tomorrow, you can eliminate some more excess fats and fluids from your body . . Each day, you continue becoming more slender . . And you will soon have your body at a level . . that is pleasing to you . .

Your subconscious mind is causing pleasant changes in your body . . that are gradually getting rid of all excess fats and fluids . . in an easy, natural way . . through the normal processes . . of your elimination system . .

You may not be consciously aware of what caused you to become overweight . . But that doesn't make any difference now . . Whatever caused the problem is past . .   And your subconscious mind is understanding it . . from a completely different point of view . . So, it will be resolved, automatically . . And you will feel like a big load has been lifted from you . . By doing it this way . . you will experience a real sense of accomplishment . . and a feeling of confidence in knowing . . that you are doing this, for yourself, in your own way . .   Your subconscious mind knows how fast it can work out the proper solution . . and get those misunderstandings straightened out . . in your mind . .

You will be happy as you notice the continuous improvements you make . . And, you'll become increasingly aware that your body is reshaping itself, exactly the way you want it to be . .

EMERGE

WEIGHT - LOSS

W175 Prescript.   **REMOVE CELLULITE**

(Follow Relaxation)

You are very relaxed now . . Relaxing deeper . . and deeper . . Enjoy this level of relaxation . . as we begin to talk about . . your body . .

You have lumps and bulges in some areas of your body . . that you want to eliminate . . so your muscles and skin will become more firm . . and smooth . . over every part of your body . .

The fact that you want to . . get rid of that excess cellulite . . makes hypnosis work more effectively . . Because you are now open . . to receive the suggestions, guidance and instructions that I give you . .

Permitting yourself to be hypnotized . . causes your subconscious mind . . to accept the suggestions that I give you . . and they will begin working immediately . . Soon, you will be pleased to notice . . all of those unwanted lumps and bulges disappear from your body . . easily and naturally . . through the processes of your elimination system . .

First, I am going to explain what causes cellulite to form on your body . . That will make it easier for your subconscious mind . . to cause your body processes to function properly . . and to cleanse it all out of your body . .

Sometimes, when nothing encourages the natural processes of your body . . to function properly . . coupled with bad eating habits . . fats, liquids and other waste materials . . accumulate . . forming little pockets on the skin . . If it is not cleansed out of the body properly . . it forms a gel-like substance . . that shows through the skin . . looking like lumps . . or bulges . . This is cellulite . .

Now that you understand that, cellulite . . is made up of liquid, fat and other waste materials . . your subconscious mind comprehends . . that you have chemicals in your body . . that can dissolve the gel-like substance . . and change it into a liquid . . that can be cleansed out of your body . . easily . . through the natural processes . . of your body's elimination system . .

Your subconscious mind is instructing the activities of your body . . to function properly . . by cleansing all excess fats, fluids and waste materials . . including cellulite materials . . completely out of your body . .

Each time you take a drink of water, milk, fruit juice, or other healthy liquid . . It turns into useful products that your body can utilize . . Your subconscious mind will activate these natural fluids in your body . . Using them to dissolve those 'unnatural' lumps and bulges . . and eliminate them from your body . .

By drinking more of these healthy liquids . . the natural fluids and acids in your body . . will function perfectly . . Dissolving all unwanted lumps and bulges . . You will be happy to notice your body becoming more smooth . . more firm . . and more perfectly developed, each day . .

All excess bulges and lumps in your thighs, hips, buttocks, knees, upper arms . . or on any other part of your body . . are dissolving . . And your muscles and skin . . keep becoming more firm and youthful, in appearance . .

Your body is reshaping itself . . in a perfect way . . It is becoming more perfect in size . . Exactly the way you, consciously, want it to be . . You will be noticing improvement within three or four days . . And you will be happy to observe yourself . . as you continue to progress . . Getting rid of all excess cellulite . . All excess fats and liquids . . and all excess impurities . . from your body . .

You will drink the amounts of liquids your body needs . . to enable your system to cleanse all waste materials . . out of your body . . completely and easily . . Each time you drink liquids . . your subconscious mind will activate . . the natural processes of your body . . to function properly . . And they will dissolve those lumps and bulges . . And flush them out of your body . .

Your friends and relatives will notice your improvement . . and compliment you on your accomplishment . . That will serve as reinforcement . . to keep your body in good shape . . and keep you trim, healthy, strong and energetic . .

Every organ in your body will continue functioning more perfectly . . Every cell, every atom and every molecule of your body . . is working properly, to continue . . improving your appearance and your health . . You will be very happy with the continuous improvements you are making . . in your life . .

We will end our session at this point . . Continue relaxing for a moment longer . . (pause)

I am going to count from ONE to FIVE . . and on the count of FIVE . . you will open your eyes, to an alert, waking state . . Feeling clear of mind . . relaxed . . and wonderful . . I will begin . .

1 - You will remember everything you have experienced today . . with understanding . . and clarity . .

2 - You are now connected to your inner strength and higher power . . supporting your good . . You will carry that inner strength with you . . throughout your day . .

3 - Everything I have told you is true . . and is already happening . . and you are already successful . . in manifesting the positive suggestions . . that I have given you . . into your daily life and consciousness . .

4 - You are beginning to be more aware of your body . . as it fully awakens and wants to stir . .

5 - Let your feet and hands move . . Stir and stretch as you open your eyes . . feeling clear, rested and refreshed . .

WEIGHT - LOSS

W176 Prescript.   **SHRINK THE STOMACH**

(Follow Relaxation)

You are very relaxed now . . and peaceful . . Relaxing deeper now . . and deeper . . Enjoy this level of relaxation . . as we begin to talk about . . your body . .

You don't need to consciously listen . . to what I am saying right now . . because your subconscious mind . . and all levels of your inner mind . . are receiving . . and absorbing . . my words . . And your mind is enabling you to respond . . to the suggestions and instructions I am giving you . .

You can be pleased to find that the processes of your body . . are functioning properly . . causing all excess cellulite and fats in your body to dissolve . . and become liquid . . which is being cleansed out of your body . . through the normal, natural processes . . of your elimination system . .

You can also be happy to notice . . that you eat only small amounts of food . . And you eat only when your body needs food . . And because of that . . your stomach is gradually shrinking to the proper size . . to reduce your body weight to _____ pounds . .

It is normal for you to eat . . only when your body needs food . . And it is quite normal for you to eat . . only the small amount your body needs . . to keep becoming healthier . . and more slender . . Exactly the way you want your body to be . .

Your self-confidence and self-acceptance keep increasing more each day . . Your will power and your self-control continue to become stronger . . And, without any conscious effort by you . . your stomach is shrinking to the proper size . . to hold only the right amount of food . . to keep your natural _____ pound body, healthy, slender and strong . .

If your body does not need food . . you have no desire to eat . . And when your body does need food . . you eat only the small amount needed by your body . . at that time . . And when you have eaten what your body needs . . you feel content, happy and perfectly satisfied . .

I want you to hold your left arm, straight out in front of you . . and tighten your fist . . And make your arm stiff and rigid . . Clench your fist tighter now . . and make your arm more rigid . . Make it as stiff and rigid as you possibly can . . Notice how strong and powerful your arm is . . Feel the power in your muscles . .

Now, let your arm relax . . Let all the muscles in your arm become completely relaxed . . Let your hand go back down in your lap . . You are doing real good . . You are responding perfectly . .

Now, I want you to do the same thing again . . Stretch your left arm out in front of you . . and make a fist . . And make your left arm stiff and rigid . . Make it even stiffer and more rigid . . than you did the first time . . Make it so stiff and rigid . . that you feel it aching . . Notice that it is aching as you make it more stiff and rigid . . When you have it aching so much that you don't like the feeling . . let your arm become completely relaxed and comfortable . .

PAUSE UNTIL CLIENT RELAXES ARM COMPLETELY, THEN PROCEED AS FOLLOWS :

I want to explain something now . . that your mind is already understanding . . You made your left arm stiff and rigid . . two times . . The actions to do that were the same each time . . And the first time you made your arm stiff and rigid . . you did not feel any pain, did you ? (Pause for response) Didn't I tell you, the first time, to make it just as rigid as you could make it ?
(Pause for response)

You made it just as rigid as you could make it, the first time, but you did not feel any pain . . because I did not tell your mind to experience pain . . And the second time, as you made your arm stiff . . I also told you to experience an aching feeling . . You are understanding . . that it is all a matter of the way your mind interprets the signal . . it receives . . Just as easily as your mind caused you to experience pain . . the second time you made your arm stiff . . your stomach can send a signal to your mind . . And it can happen any time your stomach muscles are being stretched . .

You are learning to respond to the normal activities of your stomach . . When your body needs food . . your stomach will let you know . . by causing you to feel hungry . . Yes, by sending a signal to your brain . .

Whenever you experience that 'hunger' feeling . . you will know it is time to eat some food . . to provide the proper nutrition needed by

610

your body . . at that time . . As soon as you have eaten the amount of food needed by your body . . at that time . . you will feel satisfied . . And the hunger feeling will be gone . . until your body needs food again . .

You eat only when your stomach lets you know . . that your body needs food . . And you eat only the small amount needed by your body . . at that time . . When you have eaten what your body needs . . at that time . . you are content and satisfied . . and you will stop eating . . knowing that your stomach will let you know . . when your body needs food again . .

Your stomach is shrinking, as the rest of your body is reducing . . And you continue needing a smaller and smaller amount of food . . Which will always provide the proper nutrition your body needs . . to be healthy . . You can be very happy . . noticing that your entire body is becoming more slender, trimmer and more perfectly proportioned . . The way you consciously want your body to be . .

And now, relax . . and feel yourself floating and drifting . . Just float . . Float as if you were riding on a big billowy cloud . . Floating and drifting into deeper relaxation . . You feel so dreamy . . so drowsy . . as you go deeper and deeper into pleasant relaxation . . You are breathing slowly and smoothly . . And with each breath . . you become a little more relaxed . . with each gentle breath . . Floating and drifting into gentle relaxation . . Your body is relaxing more and more deeply . . deeper and deeper . . Take another deep breath . . and hold it as long as you can . . Now, breathe out slowly . . Feeling your body go limp and relaxed . . You are feeling so pleasantly drowsy and so sleepy . . Notice how very comfortable your body is . . how the tension is gone from your body . . Just allow yourself to relax completely . . And with every gentle breath . . ripples of soothing relaxation pass throughout your body . . allowing the muscles of your face to relax . . to let go . . releasing tension . . Also, relax your neck muscles . . The muscles of your shoulders . . your arms . . hands . . Relax your chest muscles . . and your lungs . . your heart . . down to your stomach . . And relax all of the organs inside of your abdomen . . Your pelvic muscles . . your legs and your feet . . Let them all relax . . Enjoy this feeling of inner calm and peace . . Internalize this pleasurable feeling . . Going deeper and deeper . . Every muscle . . every nerve . . every fiber of your being . .

is now deeply relaxed . . And you are drifting . . floating . . into deeper relaxation . . Relax . .

You are relaxing still deeper . . Going deeper into pleasant relaxation . . Drifting and floating into dreamy, drowsiness . . Drifting and floating . . And with each and every gentle breath . . you become just a little more relaxed . . Allow this gentle feeling to flow throughout your entire body . . You feel so drowsy . . so peaceful . . as you drift and float with my voice . . you may drift up higher and see a self-image of yourself . . sitting there so peaceful . . so serene . . (so beautiful) while you become sleepier and dreamier with every breath you breath out . . and deeper and deeper relaxed with every breath you breathe in . . Deeper . . deeper . . dreamier . . drowsier . . with the gentle rise and fall of your chest . . drifting . . deeper and deeper . . more and more relaxed . .

As you internalize this deep relaxation . . your mind and your body go deeper and deeper . . Just let go . . more and more . . And now, go all the way down . . into that deep, pleasant relaxation . . You have a feeling of complete inner calmness and peace . . How pleasant it is . . How enjoyable . . Enjoy this wonderful feeling you have created for yourself . . just for a little longer . . (Pause)

Now, in just a moment . . we will conclude this session . . And I will begin counting, from ONE up to FIVE . . And when you hear the count of FIVE . . you will open up your eyes and feel awake and alert . . and ready for your next challenge . . (Pause)

I will begin my count now . .

One . . You are becoming more aware now . . Coming back to reality . .

Two . . You feel a numbness in your arms and legs . . Just a tingling . . Move your fingers and toes . .

Three . . Beginning to awaken. Feeling good . . Feeling wonderful . . For you are a wonderful person . .

Four . . Waking more and more now . . Just take a deep breath now and . .

Five . . Open your eyes and adjust your focus . . You are awake, alert and feeling good . .

WEIGHT - LOSS

W177 Prescript.   **SLENDERIZING YOUR BODY**
(Follow Relaxation)

Even though you may not always be aware of it . . you are continuing to progress more each day . . And your body is becoming more slender . . in attaining your goal weight of _____ pounds . .

The fact that you are coming for these sessions . . and permitting yourself to be hypnotized . . indicates that you will be successful in reducing your body weight to _____ pounds . . Because it reveals that you have the determination you need . . to develop a slender, trim body . . and that makes hypnosis work more effectively . .

You have made a wise decision . . because hypnosis is the best method there is . . for getting the processes of your body to function properly . . and reduce your body to a level that is pleasing to you . . And then, keep your body, slender and trim . .

Each time I hypnotize you, you keep experiencing more benefits . . And your self-confidence continues growing stronger . . Because you realize that you have found an easy . . natural way . . to reduce your body to _____ pounds . . and then, keep your body slender . .

Now that you have made a firm decision and commitment . . to reduce your body to _____ pounds . . your subconscious mind is cooperating . . and causing you to develop eating habits . . that are perfectly suited for your _____ pound body . .

Your subconscious mind knows the foods that are just right for your body . . to keep improving your health while reducing your body to _____ pounds . . So, your subconscious mind is controlling your appetite . . and is causing you to eat only those foods needed . . to slenderize your body in a perfectly healthy way . .

The Bible says, your body is a "Temple of God" . . That means, it is your right to have a perfect body . . It is right for you to have a slender body . . that is a perfect example of God's creation of beauty, health and strength . .

So, your body is reducing to _____ pounds . . Your body is becoming more slender . . more trim . . more firm . . and more youthful . . Your body is reshaping itself . . Each day, your body is becoming (lovelier and more beautiful) stronger, firmer, healthier and more perfect . . You are developing a slender, trim, perfect body . . Exactly the way you want your body to be . .

Your subconscious mind is causing your Appestat Gland . . the gland that controls your appetite . . to function properly . . And your Appestat Gland is controlling your appetite . . Causing you to eat only those foods needed . . to keep your body healthy, slender and strong . . You eat only when your body needs food . . And you eat only foods that are beneficial for your body . .

Your subconscious mind is causing you to eat only foods that are needed by your body . . to keep it healthy and reduce it to the level of _____ pounds . .

As your body continues becoming more slender . . your skin continues becoming more smooth and more youthful looking . . And your muscles continue becoming more firm and more perfectly developed . .

During those times when you are eating . . you will take small bites . . and you will chew each bite thoroughly . . You will eat slowly and you will take the time . . to enjoy the delicious flavor . . of the foods you eat . . That will give you much greater satisfaction . . And will cause you to feel content . . and perfectly satisfied . . as soon as you have eaten the amount of food . . your body needs . . at that time . .

AT THIS POINT, DO AN IMAGINATION DEMONSTRATION, SUCH AS, HAVING CLIENT HOLD BOTH ARMS OUT IN FRONT OF THEM AND SAY :

Imagine a bucket hanging on your left wrist . . And there are strings with balloons, attached to your right wrist . . The balloons are filled with helium gas . . Now I'm Going to count to five . . and with each number I say I am adding more sand into the bucket . . up to ten pounds . .

HAVE THE CLIENT IMAGINE YOU ARE POURING TEN POUNDS OF SAND INTO THE BUCKET WHILE ADDING MORE BALLOONS TO THEIR RIGHT WRIST.

Now, you understand that when you imagine something . . in your conscious mind . . your subconscious mind causes your body to respond . . to what you imagine . . This is a fact that has been known for thousands of years . . Even the Bible talks about this . . It says, "We become what we think" . . The actual words are, "As we think in our minds, so are we" . . And there has been a tremendous amount of research conducted . . that has proven, beyond doubt . . that your subconscious mind can change your body . . and can reshape your body . . to the way you want your body to be . .

So, each night, before you go to sleep . . I want you to close your eyes for a couple of minutes . . and visualize your body . . Slender, trim, firm, healthy and strong . . Exactly the way you want your body to be . .

Your subconscious mind is cooperating and is causing the processes of your body to function properly . . and is reducing your body to the level of _____ pounds . .

From this moment on . . always think about yourself . . and your body . . with good, positive thoughts . . Think of your body as being slender, slim, trim, firm and strong . . Think of your skin as being supple and youthful looking . . And think of yourself as being in perfect health . .

Each day, your self-confidence and self-acceptance will keep increasing . . And you will have the courage, confidence and determination you need . . to handle every situation that comes up in your life . . You will look forward to each day of your life with confidence and anticipation . . Knowing that every day will be filled with joy, love and much happiness . . You will arise each morning, feeling healthy and very enthusiastic . . And you will be filled with energy and vitality . .

As your thoughts about yourself continue . . in a more positive light . . you will continue to improve in all areas of your life . . And your body weight will soon be at _____ pounds . . And then, your body will remain at _____ pounds, permanently . .

Every atom, every cell and every molecule of your body . . is continuing to function more perfectly . . Cleansing all excess fats and fluids out of your body . . through the normal processes of your elimination system . .

(For Women) Your breasts are becoming full, round and firm . . and yet, soft . . And perfectly proportioned to your _____ pound body . .

Your muscles are becoming firm and more perfectly developed . . Your skin is becoming healthier, smoother and more youthful looking . .

Your will power and self-control are continuing to increase . . And your subconscious mind is in complete control of your appetite . . And it tells you to eat only when your body needs food . . And to eat only the foods needed by your body . . in the small amounts your body needs . . to be healthy, slender, trim, firm and strong . .

All fats and fluids . . that are not needed in your body . . to keep your body healthy . . are being released from your body daily . . through the normal processes of your elimination system . .

Your appearance is improving . . Your confidence is increasing . . And you will be pleased to find your happiness increasing . . and your life becoming much more enjoyable . .

You will be pleased to discover that you have the full confidence you need . . to overcome every challenge that comes up in your life . . And that you will be successful . . in overcoming all obstacles . . in a peaceful, loving way . .

Your subconscious mind has received all of the suggestions I have given you . . and is causing them to happen, automatically . . They will keep becoming more effective as each day passes . . And you will be very happy to notice . . the many, continuous improvements in your life . .

Rest a few moments longer as your subconscious mind absorbs and resolves these suggestions . . (Pause)

In a moment, I will begin counting, from ONE to FIVE . . as we bring this session to completion . . When you hear the count of FIVE . . you will open your eyes . . and be awake and alert . . and ready for your next challenge . .

I will begin my count now . .

ONE   Beginning to waken now . . Your mind is working towards reality . .
TWO   Now, your body wants to stir . . Move your fingers and toes a little bit . .
THREE   Coming up more now . . Feeling good, feeling wonderful . . For you are, truly, a wonderful person . .
FOUR   More awake and alert now . . Take a deep breath now and . .
FIVE   Open your eyes and adjust to your surroundings . . Welcome back

WEIGHT - LOSS

W178 Prescript.   **THE IDEAL BODY**

(Follow Relaxation)

Continue relaxing now as I give you suggestions and instructions . . that will help you to relax deeper . . Go deeper now . . Deeper . . as you relax peacefully . . with no thoughts of outside influences . . Listening only to the soothing sounds of the air conditioner . . and of my voice . .

Our image of how our bodies should look . . has been predetermined by our environment and by our experiences in life . . This image has been reinforced by identifying with parents, relatives and friends . . We have also been influenced by advertisements . . movies, statements by doctors, teachers . . and other sources . . that have caused us to lose our identification of the reality . . of who we really are . . As a result, we move into adulthood . . always wishing we were taller . . or shorter . . more slender or more robust . . feeling and believing that our bodies can . . and should be . . different . . Those feelings and beliefs . . cause us to abuse our bodies . . in an effort to try and make them different . .

Some people starve their bodies . . And some try to change their bodies by neglecting certain foods . . Others take pills while, still, others, do all kinds of exercises . . All of these things, in an effort to change their bodies . .

It is important to learn to regard your body as an ally . . As a friend . . Your body is a friend . . It is willing to carry you through life . . in spite of everything you have done to abuse it . .

The mind exercise you are about to do will be very helpful . . to enable you to develop your normal, beautiful, slender, trim, healthy, strong body . . As you are doing this mind exercise . . I want you to observe your body . . as though you are looking at yourself . . through the eyes of a very close, loving and supportive friend . .

Continue breathing easily and freely now . . as you continue relaxing, ever more peacefully . . And respond automatically to the suggestions, ideas and thoughts . . I am giving you . .

Notice your body now . . Notice the position of your body . . and be completely aware of all parts of your body . . If you feel like you want to move any part of your body . . to get into a more comfortable position . .

before you go into a much deeper hypnotic state . . you may do so now . . (pause)

Now, you can relax even more . . as you go deeper . . deeper into pleasant relaxation . . And as you go deeper . . I want you to visualize your body for a moment . . the way it is, right now . . Because it will never be this way again . .

Scan your whole body . . from the top of your head, all the way down to your little toes . . Pausing in those areas . . where the image is not quite clear . . And doing little movements to make each of those areas . . more vivid in your awareness . . (Pause)

Now, rest again for a moment and continue relaxing . . calmly and peacefully, as you go deeper . .

You have completely examined your body . . as it is right now . . and that is good . . So, now, you are ready to visualize your new body . . The way that you actually want your body to be . .

You will give all of your attention to the tiniest details of your body . . Just take your time . . In your mind, you are creating the ideal . . slender, trim, healthy, youthful and active body . . that is the real you . . Re-create yourself into that slender, trim _____ pound body . . Strong, healthy and firm . .

Notice the slender, firm, trim legs (WOMEN - smooth and beautifully shaped) Exactly the way you want to see your legs . .

Imagine your thighs . . slim, trim, firm (WOMEN - smooth and beautiful.) Exactly the way you want your thighs to be . . And imagine . . and feel . . your hips and buttocks . . slender and firm . . Perfectly proportioned . . Put that image clearly into your mind . .

Now, think about your genitals . . and imagine your genitals to be exactly . . as you want that area of your body to be . .

Now, move your attention to your lower abdomen . . Your upper abdomen . . and your stomach . . See and think of your abdomen and stomach . . flat, smooth, firm and perfectly developed . .

Concentrate on your waist now . . as being slim and slender . . Your waist, your stomach and abdomen . . Slender, trim and firm . .

And now, move to your back . . Notice your slender, strong back . . Visualize your spine in perfect alignment . . The muscles in your back are strong . . always keeping your back in proper alignment . .

Now, move around to your chest area . . (WOMEN) Imagine your breasts . . full, smooth and firm . . Both breasts are round, beautiful and . . perfectly proportioned to your slender, slim, _____ pound body . . (MEN) Notice how your chest is so muscular, firm and strong. . .

Think of your hands . . your arms and your shoulders . . Slim, trim and strong . .

Visualize your neck now . . Sleek and slender . . Right up to the bottom of your chin . .

And now, look closely at your face . . and see your face exactly the way you want it to appear . . Trim, smooth and youthful looking . .

You are doing very well . . Continue relaxing peacefully as you envision your entire ideal body . . standing about a foot in front of you . . so you can see the full front and back side of your slim, trim, strong, healthy body . .

Now, I want you to move into your ideal body and notice how it fits . . how it feels . . If it doesn't feel comfortable, get out of it quickly . . Adjust those parts . . or even the whole body, if necessary . . so they are more realistic . . And move back into your body again . . Continue adjusting and moving in and out . . until everything feels comfortable for you . .

Now, as you walk and move . . inside your new, ideal body . . I want you to see yourself, still naked, standing in front of a full length mirror . . with another full length mirror behind you . . so you can see every part of your body . . completely and clearly . .

See and feel . . your whole body . . Notice how good your slim, trim, strong and healthy, ideal body feels . . Notice the smooth, flawless, youthful looking skin . . Notice the perfectly developed muscles . . Notice your over all improved feeling of confidence and competence . . That is your ideal body . .

That image of your slim, trim, healthy, strong _____ pound body . . is now firmly implanted in the storehouse of your subconscious mind . .

The changes of your desires have already started to come real . . and will continue . . You only needed to let your subconscious mind know . . how you feel . . consciously . . And now, you are experiencing . . some very pleasant changes taking place . . as you go about the activities of your daily life . .

619

You have discovered your real body image . . Your ideal body . . It is now, clarified in your mind . . And it will keep becoming more real . . as each day passes . .

You are now very comfortable, relaxed and totally at ease . . You are experiencing perfect peace of mind . . And in the future . . you can enjoy this same perfect calmness and respite . . any time you want it . . All you will need to do is to sit or lie down in a comfortable position . . close your eyes and imagine yourself in this . . comfortable place . . Then count backward in your mind from TEN down to ONE . . By the time you reach number ONE . . you will be completely relaxed . . calm and at ease . . And you will know peace with the world . . And you can remain in that state for as long as you desire . . When you are ready to return to a wide-awake and alert state of mind . . you'll only need to open your eyes . . Whenever you do this . . you will always feel rested and refreshed . . Full of energy, strength and vitality . . after relaxing this way, for only a few minutes . .

You will remember everything I have said to you today . . and you will greatly benefit from everything I have told you . . Continue now, to relax, for just a little longer . . (Pause)

In just a moment we will be concluding this session . . I will be counting to FIVE for you to awaken . . You will come up to a wide-awake, fully alert state, when I say the number FIVE . .

I will begin my count now . .

ONE - Feeling so good . . feeling wonderful . . all over . .

TWO - your hands are tingling and your legs are feeling a bit numb yet . . Get the feelings back into your body . .

THREE - Coming up now . . More alert . . More aware . . Stirring into conscious awareness . .

FOUR - Gently inhale now . . Breathe out . . and . .

FIVE - Open your eyes now and focus on your surroundings . .

WEIGHT - LOSS

W179 Prescript.   **THE PERFECT BODY**

(Follow Relaxation)

Continue relaxing now as I give you suggestions and instructions . . that will help you to relax deeper . . Go deeper now . . Deeper . . as you relax, peacefully . . with no thoughts . . and no outside influences . . Hearing only the soothing sounds of the air conditioner . . and my voice . .

You are continuing to experience a more peaceful calmness now . . A relaxing, velvet smooth calm . . that holds you in a pleasant, comforting embrace . . Relax . . and let yourself go with it . .

And there will appear . . standing in front of you . . your own body . . And you are pleasantly surprised to see your own body . . exactly the way you want it to be . . Look at your body . . standing there . . and see it as it is capable of being . .

Examine it closely . . and see it, realistically, as an ideal body image . . See it as the body you really can achieve . . That ideal body is the one you really are achieving . .

The Bible says, "Your body is a temple of God" . . That's a wonderful statement . . because it enables your mind to understand . . that you have a right to have a perfect body . . You have the inborn right to have a body . . that is a perfect example of God's creativity . . It is normal and natural for your body to be slender, firm, strong and healthy . . It is normal for your body to be _____ pounds . .

And when you have a clear image in your mind . . of your body . . the way you want it to be . . your inner mind will cause one of the fingers . . on your left hand . . to lift up . . and it will stay up . . until I tell it to go back down . .   (Pause until finger lifts up.)

Your finger will go back down slowly . . and you will continue visualizing that ideal body image . . as you move into a deeper . . and deeper . . hypnotic state . . Go deeper now . . Deeper relaxation . .
(Pause)

That ideal body image is becoming more real . . You continue seeing it more clearly . . Seeing the perfect size . . The smooth, youthful skin . . (The firm, full breasts) The perfectly developed muscles . . And now, you are stepping forward, into that body . . so you can try it out . . Make certain that it is the body you want to have . . Check every part of your body . . And if there is something you want to change . . you will find that change taking place . .

Move around in that body . . Feel its strength . . Notice how good it feels . . Notice the vitality . . the energy and the comfort . . Notice the feeling of joy and happiness . . The self-confidence and the self-acceptance . . Be certain that it has the right appearance . . and all the good characteristics, attributes and qualities . . you realistically desire . .

As you occupy that body . . you are becoming aware that your present body . . is already beginning to reshape itself . . and is being drawn into that new mold . . The changes have already begun . . Your body processes are gradually changing . . so that your body may become . . your new, ideal body . .

From now, onward . . in your daily life . . you will be doing whatever is necessary . . for you to achieve the perfect body . . that you want to live with . .

You will be drinking the right amount of water . . You will be eating the right foods . . You will be eating foods that provide the proper amounts of proteins, vitamins and minerals . . that your body needs . . You will eat foods that provide the proper amount of fiber your body needs . . And you will enjoy doing exercises . . according to your own capabilities . .

You are learning to create the proper conditions that automatically . . produce the changes needed . . in your body . . which enable you to achieve your ideal body . .

The image of your ideal body . . is imprinted in the storehouse of your subconscious mind . . and will remain in your mind . . serving as an automatic force . . that will influence you strongly . . during your daily life . .

You are achieving your ideal body . . It is your natural body . . And your subconscious mind is cooperating fully . . in the development of that body . . as you go about the activities of your daily life . .

You do not need to consciously remember . . anything I have told you . . while you have been hypnotized . . It can fade from your conscious awareness . . Because your subconscious mind will remember . . And it is your subconscious mind that will cause you to continue responding, automatically, to all of these suggestions . .

Your experience here today has been thoroughly learned . . with complete understanding in all levels of your mind . . And that knowledge is becoming . . a permanent and lasting part of you . .

At this very moment, your system is making comfortable adjustments . . Your system is now synthesizing proteins, nutrients and other chemicals and substances in your body . . Rejuvenation is now taking place . .

Your expectations are, naturally, increasing . . and you will be sensing the pleasant changes taking place within you . . You can feel pleased and proud of what you are accomplishing . . The feeling of knowing that it is happening . . gives you a strong sense of satisfaction and contentment . .

You are responding very well to these suggestions . . Now, I want you to rest a few moments . . while your subconscious mind continues to absorb . . all that we have talked about . .   (Pause)

Now, I am going to begin my count from ONE up to FIVE . . When you hear the count of FIVE . . you will be wide awake and alert . . and feeling refreshed and wonderful . . For you are . . a wonderful person . .

ONE - Beginning to emerge now . . Move your fingers and toes . . just a little . .

TWO - Waking more now . . Coming up . .

THREE - Your arms and legs are still asleep . . move your arms and legs now . .

FOUR - Take a deep breath now . . and . .

FIVE - Open your eyes . . feeling good . . feeling wonderful . .

WEIGHT - LOSS

W180 Prescript.   **TRIBAL MIRROR**

(Includes Relax Induction)

Now . . close your eyes and relax . . breathe deeply now and . . slowly let it out . . Take another deep breath through your nose . . Slowly, let it out . . I want to take you to a restful . . quiet place deep in the forest . . where you will find peace and relaxing comfort . . in a totally relaxing world of your own . . You're going to take a short journey up a mountain trail where . . tall trees are nestled high up . . in the rain clouds . . The clouds bump and mesh together . . swirling in shades of pink and soft azure blue . . Occasional drops of rain settle softly . . on your face . . But you smile because the rain drops make you feel excited and . . happy inside . .

Climbing up the steep mountainside is quite slow . . I will show you a better way . . It's time now to let go . . Let yourself be free to slowly drift up . . up . . to the tops of the trees . . high above the trees where you are free to sail on the wind . . Look away and you will see the far mountain ranges . . covered in white snow caps . . many miles away . . You can see them clearly in the distance . . but you are not going there . . Let yourself slowly drift through the branches of the trees . . The huge trees . . Tall and majestic . . You are settling down into the top of . . a great, spreading tree, with mighty branches . . where birds flutter past in darting flashes . . Chipmunks and squirrels . . find food to store for winter . . And there, far below you, a gurgling brook trickles . . with singing waters . . Winding through the forest grasses . . far below . .

You are drifting now . . Rocking on the winds like the leaves . . Drifting slowly, among the haunting tree branches . . You see the leaves of the trees drifting by you . . and you drift with them . . Sometimes quickly . . Sometimes very slowly . . To the left . . Then to the right . . Back and forth . . You slowly, gently, sail down . . down deeper . . and DEEPER . . toward the green grasses of the forest, far below . . Slowly you circle between the huge branches of the trees, drifting in circles . . Swaying to the right . . Sailing up with the wind . . Then to the left . . Circling . . Circling . . The winds carry you gently in a downward motion . . Down deeper . . DEEPER . . until at last your feet touch the soft, velvet grasses that cover the earth . . Here is where you will find peace . . Tranquility . .

Complete relaxation . . Here, you are as one with all that God has created for you . . Here, there are no sounds besides my voice . . and the noise of rushing waters in the distant brook . . flowing through the forest . . Any other sounds you may hear will only support you . . in your relaxed and comfortable place . . Your mind and body are open to complete trust . . Trust in the power of your mind to benefit you on your journey . . Your mind is very relaxed now and . . open to receive the beneficial suggestions . . I will soon give you . . But for now, we will stay here . . in this beautiful valley . . deep in the forest . . For here, there is much to learn . . and to remember . .

This valley is one of many, here on the plain . . Many different kinds of animals live here . . and die here . . for that is the way of nature . . This is called a Savanna . . where the grasses grow very tall . . where elephant herds migrate . . and creatures are safe to hide . . until the lion strikes . .

Death comes quickly . . but the creatures know it is their place . . to provide the nourishment needed . . for all creatures to survive . .

Moving among these creatures, who kill to survive . . you will have no fear of them . . They cannot see you . . unless you want them to . . You are quite safe . .

Look toward your left now . . You see a small rise in the valley floor . . Just beyond the rise is . . an encampment of native hunters and gatherers . . They often come here searching for nuts and berries for winter . . and with hopes of capturing an antelope . . for its hide and meat . . They travel silently through the tall grasses on the savanna . . carrying only stone-chipped spears . . their Basenji dogs search the way ahead of them . . When an antelope is killed . . it is quartered and carried back to camp in pieces . . including the hide . . the blood . . and all of the intestines . . the stomach lining . . Nothing is wasted . . Food is not easy to find . . Sometimes, days or weeks go by with nothing to eat . . But on this day, they are fortunate . . They have killed an antelope and have carried it back to camp . . on their heads . . Walking single file through the dangerous, tall grasses . . where a lion might attack any one of them . . at any time . . It is a dangerous lifestyle . . but the only one they know . .

Look more closely at the men in their camp . . as they go about their daily chores . . They wear no clothing. . . Their skin is baked hard from the blistering northern sun . . It stretches tight over their skeletal frames . . Look closely at their ribs . . Their teeth are not good . . but they smile and laugh easily . . They are happy now . . for they have enough meat to feed everyone for many days . .

You are standing in this group of men . . in their camp . . There are several men on each side of you . . I want you to leave your body now . . Step away about ten feet . . Now look back at your body . . standing next to these gaunt, frail native Africans . . Look at how HUGE your body is . . compared to these men . . You are . . three . . four times larger than they are . . Later, I want you to remember this picture . . of yourself . . standing next to these hungry people . . Remember it . .

Now, I want you to look into a tall, thin mirror . . This mirror will make you appear to be much thinner . . As you look into the Thin Mirror . . you will notice how your eyes are much brighter . . the bags under your eyes have disappeared . . The heavy jowls around your jaw are gone . . Your smile is still there and . . that is good . . And now, your skin is smoother . . Your arms . . your chest . . your stomach muscles . . are tighter . . All the excess flab is gone and your waist is . . thirty eight inches . . You feel much stronger . . much healthier . . Your youth has returned and you feel . . wonderful . . This is the image I want you to take with you . . This is how I want you to think of yourself . . Healthy . . well conditioned . . and feeling so good about yourself . . This will be the new you, once you have completed this program . . And you are going to make that happen . .

You are walking down a new road now . . away from the village . . Away from the road you were on yesterday . . This is the road to being trim and healthy . . Things will be a lot different now . .

Before you go any further on this path to trimness and good health, there is a stop you need to make . . Imagine that you are walking down a corridor . . At the end of the corridor, there is a door to a room . . This room is filled with all of your old, self destructive, overweight eating habits . .

You need to visit this room . . Go ahead and walk down that corridor . . Soon you come to the door . . Open it and walk in . . This room is full of your old, self-destructive, overweight eating habits . .

As you enter this room . . think about a food that causes you to gain weight . . When you have that food in your mind . . take a big, bold 'X' and place it right over that food . . wonderful . . Think of another food that causes you to gain weight . . Place a big bold 'X' right over it now . . Wonderful . . Now, see yourself doing an eating behavior that causes you to gain weight . . As that image forms in your mind, place a big, bold 'NO' right over it . . Wonderful . . As you see yourself doing that behavior, place a big, bold, 'NO' right over it . . Now, see yourself doing another eating behavior that causes you to gain weight . . As that image forms in your mind, put another big, bold, 'NO' right over it . . As you see yourself beginning to do that behavior . . you immediately recognize your big bold, 'NO', that you placed over it . . Wonderful . . Look around this room for any other foods or behaviors that can cause you to gain weight . . and put big, bold 'X's and 'NO's over all of them . . Do this NOW . . When this room is filled with 'X's and 'NO's, it is time for you to leave . . As you do, the door becomes an Iron Gate . . Close the door and listen to the sound of the iron gate clanging shut . . Lock it and listen to the sound of the lock as it snaps . . The sounds are very clear and you know the gate is permanently locked, for sure . .

Walk away from that room . . Those foods and overweight behavior patterns are now locked in your past . . That is where they belong and that is where they will stay . . They are locked out of your life . . Clearing the way for you . . to form new behavioral patterns . . Better behaviors . . healthier ones . .

Of all the relationships you have . . right now . . you are beginning a new one . . It is the most important one of all . . You are now becoming BEST FRIENDS with your body . . Best friends listen . . They honor and respect what they hear . . From now on, as a best friend, you are listening to your body . . When you feel hungry, you honor and respect that feeling and you eat . . You choose foods that your body wants and needs . . You choose foods that are low in fats . . healthy, nutrition-filled, low fat foods . . As you eat, you are listening to your body . . The moment you feel satisfied . . Not stuffed . . but satisfied . . you stop eating . . It doesn't matter how much food might be left on your plate . . It doesn't matter what that food might be . . It doesn't matter how much you paid for it . . The moment you feel satisfied . . as your body's best friend . . you simply stop eating . . When you are satisfied . . you stop eating . .
You are exercising . . Every time you exercise, you feel younger . . stronger than before . . And more alive than ever before . . Every

time you exercise, your muscles call up your fat cells and tell them, "Send some fat for us to burn off, for energy" . . Your body wants to melt away the excess fat . . Soon you'll begin to notice . . every time you walk, you leave a trail of fat in your footsteps . .

Whenever you desire something sweet, you now reach for nature's desert - fresh fruit . . Fresh fruit is so sweet and delicious . . Mother Nature has made this desert for your special treat . .

Imagine, in your hand is a piece of your favorite fruit and it is perfect in its ripeness . . You are bringing it to your mouth and now you are sinking your teeth into it . . Feel the taste and flavor burst into your mouth . . It is so sweet . . so delicious . . Mother Nature's dessert of fresh fruit . . Just for your enjoyment and nourishment . .

FATS . . I want to tell you the story of fats . . Your body uses a certain amount of fats every day . . Fats are important . . in their right amounts . . but when you eat more fats than your body uses in a given day, that extra fat is turned into . . adipose tissue . . Adipose Tissue is that yellow, heavy, bulbous fat you may have noticed on chickens . . what we call chicken fat . . That is very much like what your body develops . . It is excess baggage your body has to carry . . Wherever you go, you have to carry this excess load of unhealthy, heavy, yellowish, Adipose fat . .

Imagine a very large table . . This table is full of food . . First thing you see on this table is a bowl of French fries . . Next to that are bowls of potato chips, corn chips and other fried chips . . and you begin to notice the table is full of many fattening foods . . mayonnaise . . margarine . . butter . . oils . . fried chicken . . and fried fish . . on top of platters dripping with fatty oils from the meat . . Also, lots of cold cut meats like salami, bologna and sausages, bacon . . and plenty of desserts of various types . . cakes, pies, cupcakes, brownies, puddings, donuts and snack foods . . Every imaginable store-bought or home-baked treat . .

Stand back and look at all those foods on that table . . They are loaded . . LOADED with fat . . heavy, greasy, unhealthy fat . . Fat that adds useless . . needless . . heavy fat onto your body . . Many of those foods are loaded . . loaded with sugar . . Additive sugar that adds useless . . needless . . heavy fat onto your body . . Fat - that your wonderful body has to drag around as excess baggage wherever you go . . Whatever you do . . Your body deserves better than that . .

Your body deserves to be treated with respect and given what it needs to be healthy . . for you . . Now, imagine taking your arm and clearing that table . . That's right . . Take your arm and sweep all those foods right on the floor . . Look at them on the floor . . They do not look so good anymore, piled one upon the other in a big mess . . It look like "junk", doesn't it ? . . And that's exactly what those foods are called . . "JUNK FOODS" . . At the very least, you are a decent human being . . and because of that, you deserve to have good things . . not JUNK in any form . .

Now, we are going to reset the table . . The first thing you see is a large, 12 pound, browned, roasted turkey . . You can smell the aroma and almost taste it . . Next to that is a broiled and roasted chicken, ready to eat, with its natural juices inviting its good flavor to be experienced. . . and . . look ! . . There is a platter of your favorite seafood, all ready for you to savor . . And it is also broiled and roasted for your enjoyment . . And there are various kinds of pastas with a choice of several sauces . . And a wonderful, absolutely marvelous display of fresh greens and vegetables, in a variety of salad combinations for you to make . . Fresh lettuces of many kinds . . Tomatoes . . All kinds of fresh veggies . . and, interestingly enough . . several choices of low-fat salad dressings . . WOW ! Look around . . several kinds of cooked vegetables of every kind and manner of preparation . . What a selection! There's more . . You can see the various kinds of breads - wheat, potato, rye, multi-grain, yeast rolls and the choices are many . . You can see the table is filled with healthy, nutritious and delicious foods of every kind . . Including desserts of low-fat ice cream, yogurt, pastries and other marvelous ways people find to take what nature offers and turn them into the best things for the body, if it isn't already the best, naturally . . We can really make food great !

Stand back and look at this table . . There are thousands of foods on it and they are all healthy, nutritious and delicious, low-fat foods . . Eating these foods . . when you are hungry . . leads you naturally and comfortably to your weight loss goal . . This is going to be so simple and easy . . because it is simple and easy . .

Because you have made these positive changes in your eating behavior . . your body weight begins to melt down a little bit every day . . Just like an ice sculpture on a sunny afternoon . . Melting down . . little by little . . A gentle, melting away . . Your body weight melts down a little bit every day . . until you have the ideal weight and body you know is yours . .

Now, I want you to recall the picture of yourself, standing beside the people on the African plain . . Remember the shape and condition of your body . . as it was then ? Before you now is a beautiful, full length mirror . . It is the 'Thin Mirror' you saw once before . . The reflection you see in the mirror is the image of a perfected self, having attained your ideal weight . . Take time to really notice your perfect body and overall healthy appearance . . See your body as being trim, healthy and very attractive . . Feel how good you look . . Feel your pride at the success you have achieved . . All your efforts have been worth while . . See your beautiful self and feel proud . .

Look at your face . . See what a healthy glow you have . . reflecting both your inner and outer beauty . . The expression on your face is wonderfully peaceful and happy . . You have a right to be pleased with yourself . . with your body . . and with your success . .

This is your FUTURE . . It is waiting for you . . If it ever happens that you get a food craving that is not good for your body's ideal weight plan . . you will immediately pause . . take in a deep breath . . and remember . . MY FUTURE . . And remember the image of yourself, in the thin mirror . . Along with your feelings of a beautiful body and personal pride . . All these things will come to mind . . And your cravings will vanish . . And anytime you feel a temptation of any kind that violates your commitment to your ideal body weight and health . . you will remember to pause a moment . . take a deep breath . . and remember, MY FUTURE . . The image of your ideal weight and health will remind you . . MY FUTURE . . is happening right now . .

Some time ago, you had a dream . . that one day, you would be trim and free from being overweight . . Right now . . that dream is happening . . And these positive eating behaviors have become your Top Priorities . . Priorities that you will ensure happen every day . . You already have other top priorities that you ensure happen every day, such as, getting up in the morning, brushing your teeth, getting dressed . . and these are just the beginning of what you know happens for you every day . . And all these good habits ensure that your positive changes in good eating behavior will continue to happen every day . . Eating only when you experience hunger pangs . .

Eating until satisfied and stopping at the point of satisfaction . . Choosing foods that are healthy, nutritious . . Eating substantially less sugar . . Less fat . . Remembering that low-fat foods are better for your body . . Eating fresh fruit for dessert and . . most of all . . paying attention to what you know is best for your body . . Eating right, to be healthy and happy . . And exercising at every opportunity . . Finding the time . . Making a schedule so that you ensure your proper weight, health and exercise plan is working for you, every day . . You are Top Priority ! . . And the lifestyle you choose is . . good eating . . good exercise . . good thinking . . good feelings . . Your enjoyment of life . . You can do it ! You are doing it ! You are living your dream . . with your happy body weight, health and exercise care plan . . Now, I want you to relax for a while . . (pause)

In a moment I am going to count from one to five and when I reach the number Five, you will feel alert and confident . . On your way to a slender future . . I will begin my count now . .

One -   You are feeling great and wonderful about your commitments . .
Two -   You will remember everything you have heard today and remember well, all the good foods you can eat and the exercise activities you enjoy . .
Three - Knowing that you can do what you want to do . . and you are doing it right . .

Four -   More alert now and feeling wonderful . . because you are a wonderful person . .
Five -   You may open your eyes now . . Feeling alert and awake . .

WEIGHT - LOSS

W181 Prescript.   **YOUTHFUL APPEARANCE**

(Follow Relaxation)

Continue relaxing now as I give you suggestions and instructions . . that will help you to relax deeper . . and will help to improve your youthful appearance . . Your subconscious mind is absorbing everything I am saying . . so you can continue to relax . . and go deeper into your hypnotic state . .

These suggestions and instructions I am giving you . . are going directly into the storehouse . . of your subconscious mind . . and will begin working immediately in your body . .

Even though you are not consciously aware of it . . the processes of your body are constantly at work within you . . at all times . . They maintain your body temperature at a stable level . . They are continuously causing your hair . . your fingernails and your toenails to grow . . They repair the tissues of your skin . . when you have scratches, cuts or bruises . . They repair your bones, if they are broken . . They are constantly nourishing tissues, strengthening muscles, ligaments, tendons and bones . . And they cleanse waste materials out of your body . . through your elimination system . .

Those processes . . and many more . . that continue working in your body . . are normal and natural . . They keep working, twenty four hours a day . . causing all the activities of your body to keep functioning properly . .

Thomas Edison discovered, many years ago, that "Every cell in your body . . thinks" . . Since that is true . . your body is capable of rebuilding itself . . reshaping itself . . and revitalizing itself . . to look more youthful . .

Your body is composed of molecules, enzymes and cells . . which are designed to function perfectly . . Each cell in your body is young and vital . . and is capable of functioning perfectly . .

Scientists have discovered that every atom . . every cell and every molecule in your body . . is constantly in the process of renewing itself . . and is actually replaced with new cells every few months . . So, your body is always young . . and is capable of remaining young looking at all times . . Our society keeps track of time by using calendars and counting years . .

632

But your mind understands that the number of years you have lived in your body . . has nothing to do with the physical condition of your body . .

Each time you wash your skin . . you wash away cells and molecules . . that have completed their purpose . . and they are replaced by new cells and molecules . . Your skin and organs are endlessly being renewed . . And your subconscious mind is directing the processes of your body to do their work perfectly . . to keep your body healthy, strong and youthful looking . .

The natural processes of your elimination system . . also function to keep the inside of your body cleansed . . So your entire body is in a constant state of renewal . . And every part of your body is new and perfect . . and is capable of functioning properly at all times . .

The Bible says, "We become what we think," and that has been found to be a true fact . . So, you are thinking of yourself as being YOUTHFUL . . You are ceaselessly making your body more youthful by continuing to think . . and by expecting your body to be young, strong and healthy . . Right now, your body is in the process of adopting a more youthful appearance . . It is normal and natural for your body to keep looking young . .

Just for a moment . . I want you to go inside your head . . I want you to visualize your brain . . At the base of your brain is your Pituitary Gland . . It is a small endocrine gland which secretes hormones . . that influence . . your body growth . . your metabolism . . and the activities of other endocrine glands . . You have a radiant light of energy . . shining on the top of your head . . which is God's gift to each of us . . We can use this gift . . any time we wish to . . I want you to direct this radiant energy source to your pituitary gland . . Focus your inner power onto the Pituitary Gland until it is glowing . . a soft light blue color . . Visualize your entire brain, wrapped in a soft, velvety blue, fuzzy mist . . But concentrate . . on the pituitary gland . . and direct it to release growth hormones into your system . . (pause)

All of nature maintains a youthful look, in its own way . . Snakes shed their skin, only to reveal a new and youthful looking skin . . Birds shed their feathers . . only to have new, brightly colored feathers replace the old ones . . And you, too, shed your skin . . a little each day . . And your body ceaselessly emerges . . with a more perfect, flawless, healthy, youthful, smooth looking skin . .

From now on, you expect to continue looking younger . . And you will keep feeling younger . . As greater amounts of growth hormones are released from your Pituitary Gland . . you will have more energy, more vitality and more strength . . You will notice yourself becoming more youthful in appearance . . Your skin, becoming more smooth and delicate . . You will be aware of endless improvements . . And you will be proud of what you are accomplishing . .

Each day, your health is improving . . Every organ in your body is functioning more perfectly . . Every cell, every atom and every molecule is . . performing perfectly . . Youthful vitality is emerging . . in your looks . . your feelings and in your actions . .

Even after you awaken from the hypnotic state . . all of these suggestions will continue to influence you . . just as strongly, just as surely and just as powerfully as they do while you are under hypnosis . . Your nerves will be more relaxed and steady . . Your mind will be calmer and clearer . . You will be more alert, more composed more tranquil . . and more at peace, within . . You will be well pleased with the improvements in your life . . As each day passes, you continue to improve even more . .

You are experiencing a very pleasant feeling of relaxation all through your body . . You know how good it feels, to be relaxed . . as you are now . . And you will automatically use these principles of relaxation during your daily life . . (pause)

You will remember everything I have said to you today . . and you will greatly benefit from everything I have told you . .

In just a moment, I will be counting to FIVE for you to awaken . . You will come up to a wide-awake, fully alert state, when I say the number FIVE . .

ONE - Feeling so good . . feeling wonderful . . all over . .
TWO - Your hands and legs are feeling a bit numb yet . . Get the feelings back into your body . .
THREE - Coming up now . . More alert . . More aware . . Stirring into conscious awareness . .
FOUR - Gently inhale now . . Breathe out . . and . .
FIVE - Open your eyes now and focus on your surroundings . .

ABOUT THE AUTHOR

Dennis L. (Smokey) Franks was born in 1939 on a native-American reservation and was raised in Selah, Washington. Following a five year tour of duty in the US Navy, he graduated from Seattle Community College with a degree in Mechanical Design Engineering followed by an additional three years of study at Central University, Ellensburg, Washington, in the fields of Anthropology, Archaeology and Geology. Later, he attended The American School of Hypnotherapy of Las Vegas and also received a Fellowship awarded through the University Church Institute under the tutelage of Doctor Paul Leon Masters. Mr. Franks enjoyed a 30 year stellar career as a contracting engineer, both mechanical and electrical, in projects such as ship construction, aircraft, aerospace, land survey and private enterprise during which time he developed a number of patented innovations. As a contractor, he traveled through and/or lived in many countries throughout the world including Europe, Asia, South Africa, North and South America, the South Pacific Islands, New Zealand and Australia; some thirty countries in all. Mr. Franks opened and operated a number of private businesses including a computerized cabling company, an import-export company and a hypnotherapy clinic. Also, he enjoyed a period of time as a noted songwriter in Las Vegas. Mr. Franks has written a number of how-to books, poetry and adventure stories from his personal life, derived mainly through exciting adventures experienced in gold and opal mining and indigenous contacts while traveling throughout the world.

"INHALE AND RELAX", a book of Inductions and Prescriptions for Hypnotherapy, is, he feels, his most important contribution to society to date and for the betterment of mankind.